AF352559

HEALTH-HARMING LEGAL NEEDS

A Guide for Canadian Primary Health Care Clinicians

Edited by Rami Shoucri and Jennifer Stone

Health-Harming Legal Needs equips primary health care professionals with the tools to recognize and respond to legal issues that are injurious to health, particularly among low-income patients. Co-developed by medical and legal experts, this book advances health equity through the integration of legal support into clinical care.

Utilizing a practical, case-based approach, the book helps clinicians identify when legal issues such as eviction, denial of social benefits, immigration status, family breakdown, discrimination at work, or involvement with the criminal-legal system may be undermining their patients' health. It also focuses on several patient populations with unique legal needs, including pediatric patients, people living with HIV, Indigenous peoples, and people living with intellectual or developmental disabilities. It demystifies the legal systems with which patients interact and builds clinician confidence in navigating and leveraging community legal support. Central to the book is the introduction of health and justice partnerships, a flexible, collaborative model that brings legal and health professionals together to address the root causes of poor health. By fostering shared understanding and joint dialogue across sectors, the text shows how meaningful legal-health collaboration can enhance patient care, reduce provider burnout, and promote equity and access to justice.

Through real-world examples and actionable guidance, the book underscores that legal support can make a decisive difference in moments that feel hopeless – for both patients and care teams. It ultimately encourages clinicians to see legal advocacy as part of a holistic approach to care and offers a road map for integrating this perspective into their practice.

RAMI SHOUCRI has been a family physician in the St. Michael's Hospital Academic Family Health Team since 2016 and is an assistant professor in the Department of Family and Community Medicine at the University of Toronto.

JENNIFER STONE is an adjunct professor in the Faculty of Law at the University of Toronto and executive director of Neighbourhood Legal Services.

Health-Harming Legal Needs

A Guide for Canadian Primary Health Care Clinicians

EDITED BY RAMI SHOUCRI
AND JENNIFER STONE

UNIVERSITY OF TORONTO PRESS
Toronto Buffalo London

© University of Toronto Press 2025
Toronto Buffalo London
utppublishing.com
Printed in Canada

ISBN 978-1-4875-4973-2 (cloth)   ISBN 978-1-4875-5692-1 (EPUB)
ISBN 978-1-4875-4976-3 (paper)   ISBN 978-1-4875-5061-5 (PDF)

Library and Archives Canada Cataloguing in Publication

Title: Health-harming legal needs : a guide for Canadian primary health care
   clinicians / edited by Rami Shoucri and Jennifer Stone.
Names: Shoucri, Rami, editor. | Stone, Jennifer (Executive director of
   Neighbourhood Legal Services), editor.
Description: Includes bibliographical references and index.
Identifiers: Canadiana (print) 20250181622 | Canadiana (ebook) 2025018169X |
   ISBN 9781487549732 (cloth) | ISBN 9781487549763 (paper) |
   ISBN 9781487556921 (EPUB) | ISBN 9781487550615 (PDF)
Subjects: LCSH: Medical care – Law and legislation – Canada. |
   LCSH: Social medicine – Canada. | LCSH: Indigenous peoples –
   Legal status, laws, etc. – Canada. | LCSH: Indigenous peoples –
   Health and hygiene – Canada.
Classification: LCC KE3646 .H3933 2025 | LCC KF3821 .H3933 2025 kfmod |
   DDC 344.7104/1 – dc23

Cover design: Kristjan Buckingham
Cover image: iStock.com/Amorn Suriyan

We wish to acknowledge the land on which the University of Toronto Press
operates. This land is the traditional territory of the Wendat, the Anishnaabeg,
the Haudenosaunee, the Métis, and the Mississaugas of the Credit First Nation.

University of Toronto Press acknowledges the financial support of the
Government of Canada, the Canada Council for the Arts, and the Ontario Arts
Council, an agency of the Government of Ontario, for its publishing activities.

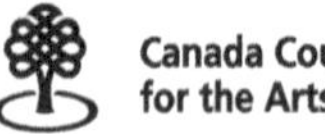

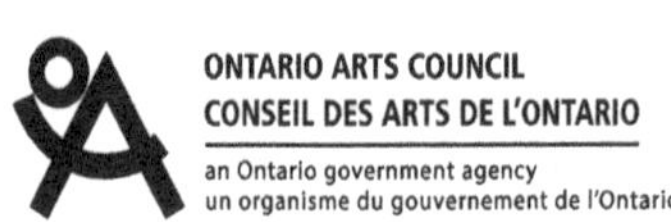

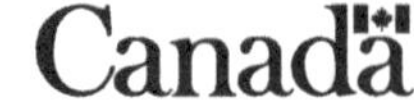

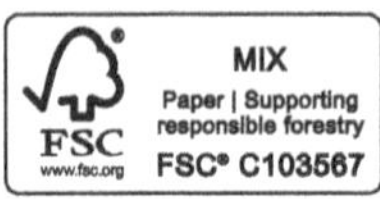

Contents

List of Illustrations   ix

Acknowledgments   xi

Introduction   3
RAMI SHOUCRI AND JENNIFER STONE

1 Forming Partnerships and Effectively Collaborating with
   Legal Professionals in the Care of Patients   13
   RAMI SHOUCRI AND JENNIFER STONE

2 Law 101: An Introduction to the Canadian Legal and
   Constitutional Framework for Health Care Providers   30
   BETH BILSON

3 Health, Law, and Indigenous People   56
   CHRISTA BIG CANOE AND SUZANNE SHOUSH

4 Health and Justice Partnerships for Health and Home   78
   ANDREW BOND AND BENJAMIN RIES

5 Work and Health   104
   NABILA F. QURESHI AND ANDREW PINTO

   Indigenous Legal Expert Reflection on Chapter 5   136
   SARA MAINVILLE

6 Income, Social Benefits, and Health   138
   GARY BLOCH, ANU BAKSHI, AND LOUISE SIMBANDUMWE

   Indigenous Legal Expert Reflection on Chapter 6   182
   DOUGLAS VARRETTE

7 Immigration Status and Health 186

MICHAELA BEDER, DILAN BRAR, RITIKA GOEL,
VANESSA REDDITT, JENNIFER STONE, DIANA GALLEGO
(ADVISOR), AND LUIS ALBERTO MATA (ADVISOR)

8 Family Law and Health 238

ANITA VOLIKIS, JAMIE AHN, AND KATHLEEN DOUKAS

Indigenous Legal Expert Reflection on Chapter 8 278

CAITLYN E. KASPER

9 Health, Social, and Structural Determinants of Health in the
Context of Traumatic Brain Injury and the Criminal-Legal
System in Canada 283

FLORA I. MATHESON, PROMISE HOLMES SKINNER,
AND CHRISTINE CARTHEW

10 Common Legal Issues Affecting People Living with
HIV/AIDS 310

ROBIN NOBLEMAN, DEBBIE RACHLIS, RYAN PECK,
DEVAN NAMBIAR, AND GORDON ARBESS

11 Health Justice in Paediatric Practice: Children's Rights
and Social Justice for Patients and Their Families 372

SARAH GANDER, LEE ANN CHAPMAN,
AND MELANIE LAKING

12 Estate, Financial, and Personal Care Planning for
Marginalized and Isolated Populations 406

NAHEED DOSANI, EDGAR-ANDRE MONTIGNY,
AND MERCEDES PEREZ

Indigenous Legal Expert Reflection on Chapter 12 450

KATE FORGET

13 Health Care Decision-Making Involving People with
Intellectual and Developmental Disabilities in Primary
Health Care: Solidarity to Promote Capabilities While
Mitigating Vulnerabilities 454

WILLIAM F. SULLIVAN, MERCEDES PEREZ,
JOHN HENG, AND PAULA HUTCHINSON

Conclusion   479
JENNIFER STONE AND RAMI SHOUCRI

Appendix 1: Legal Aid and Other Legal Resources in Canada   488

Appendix 2: HELPS Brain Injury Screening Tool   499

Appendix 3: Sample Advocacy Letter for Supported Decision-Making   501

Glossary   503

Contributors   507

Index   519

Illustrations

Figures

0.1 Basis for Understanding Access to Justice as a Social
Determinant of Health   5
3.1 A Basic Medicine Circle Diagram (Anishinaabe Wheel)   60
4.1 The Housing Continuum   83
4.2 Selected Interconnected Aspects of Modern Housing Law
and Practice   84
4.3 Potential Intervention Points to Prevent Homelessness
for Individuals   93
6.1 Quick Guide to Navigating Income Supports   148
6.2 Letter-Writing Tips for Practitioners   168
6.3 Five Pillars of Financial Empowerment   173
7.1 Visual of Pathways (and Pitfalls) to Citizenship   189
7.2 Refugee Claim Process in Canada   192
7.3 Canada Immigration Levels (2017–21)   193
7.4 Permanent and Temporary Economic Newcomers in
Canada (2000–20)   194

Tables

1.1 Legal Information versus Legal Advice   21
2.1 Distinguishing Features Regarding Undue Hardship in
Accommodations   46
3.1 Examples of Health Access and Outcome Discrepancies for
Indigenous People in Canada   66
4.1 Overview of 2018 World Health Organization *Housing and
Health Guidelines*   81
4.2 Canadian Tenant Protection Laws by Province and Territory
(as of 2023)   85

4.3 Housing Law Issues by Collective versus Individual
Orientation   87
5.1 Forum and Limitation Periods for Employment Standards
Complaints by Jurisdiction   110
5.2 Forum and Limitation Periods for Human Rights Claims in
Employment by Jurisdiction   114
5.3 Forum and Limitation Periods for OHS Complaints by
Jurisdiction   116
6.1 Highest and Lowest Adequacy of Welfare Incomes among
Provinces (2023)   149
6.2 Identification in Canada: Jurisdictions and Services   151
6.3 Poverty Rates among Persons with Disabilities with
Marginalized Identities (2019)   157
6.4 Legal Resources for Major Disability Income Support
Programs   163
6.5 Legal Definitions of Disability   165
6.6 Words to Use to Communicate the Standard of Proof   167
7.1 Length of Financial Responsibility Undertaking for Sponsored
Individuals   197
7.2 Immigration Status and Access to Health Care and Health
Insurance   201
7.3 Immigration Status and Its Impacts on Safety   204
7.4 Immigration Status and Access to Primary and Secondary
Public Schooling   206
7.5 Immigration Status and Access to Post-Secondary
Schooling   207
7.6 Access to Income and Employment Supports Based on
Immigration Status   210
7.7 Criminal Justice Based on Immigration Status   212
8.1 Time Limits for Initiating Spousal Support Claims by Province
or Territory   249
8.2 Child and Spousal Support Resources   267
8.3 Parenting Resources   267
8.4 Family Violence and Intimate Partner Violence Resources   268
10.1 Privacy Legislation That Applies to Health Care Providers in
Canadian Jurisdictions   319
10.2 Publicly Funded Drug Plans in Canada That Cover
Antiretroviral Medication   339
12.1 Some Unique Aspects of Powers of Attorney across Canada   412
13.1 Screening for Decision-Making Vulnerabilities of People with
IDD Using a Supported Decision-Making Approach   471
A.1 Legal Aid and Other Free or Low-Cost Legal Resources in
Canada, by Province (as of December 2020)   488

Acknowledgments

The editors are immensely grateful for all of the contributors to this project over the years:

- the chapter authors, who took time out of their busy clinical, legal, and academic practices to collaborate and share their expertise;
- the University of Toronto's Department of Family and Community Medicine, who supported earlier versions of this work through a Louise Naismith Grant;
- the research team at the St. Michael's Hospital Department of Family and Community Medicine, Ann Burchell and Andrée Schuler, for their guidance and support;
- the visionary partners of the Health Justice Program and their leaders who have supported this project from the beginning: Neighbourhood Legal Services (Melodie Mayson, Jack DeKlerk, and Jennie Stone), Aboriginal Legal Services (Christa Big Canoe and Emily Hill), ARCH Disability Law (Ivana Petricone, Robert Lattanzio), HIV and AIDS Legal Clinic of Ontario (Ryan Peck), and the St. Michael's Academic Family Health Team (Karen Weyman, Linda Jackson, and Jacqueline Chen);
- the original and current Clinical Champions for the program, Nav Persaud and Katie Dorman, respectively, and the original and current social work leads, Celia Schwartz and Christine Barta, respectively;
- the first on-site lawyer for the program, Johanna McDonald, and administrative assistants Sheleca Henry and Marcello Ferraro;
- the various members of our Education subcommittee who have guided our education work over the years, including Gary Bloch, Christa Big Canoe, Judith Peranson, Helen Anderson, and Emily Hill;

- Legal Aid Ontario for their ongoing financial support of the Health Justice Program;
- our contacts and supports at University of Toronto Press, including Jodi Litvin, Lohit Jagwani, Kathie Porta Baker, and Janice Evans for their support, attention to detail, and guidance; and
- our student researchers acknowledged in the chapters, as well as Maryam Hassan and Xin Meng, for their additional research.

We would also like to thank our inspirational and collaborative colleagues at the Health and Justice Community of Practice in Ontario – in particular, the leadership of Amy Slotek, Lisa Turik, Michele Leering, and Aidan Johnson, who have built a foundation and a vision for growth and sustainability. We hope that this guide will support these efforts across Ontario and Canada. In addition, we thank the Law Foundation of Ontario for its ongoing financial support of the Community of Practice to sustain and scale up these partnerships.

Our patients and clients have been our greatest teachers, challenging us to collaborate more deeply, improve the way we serve, and transform the systems that stand in their way.

Finally, we would like to thank our families for their patience and support as we worked through the various drafts, edits, and deadlines for this project: Ilene and Adrian for Rami, and Jeff, Oscar, Edie, and Iris for Jennie. Thank you!

A Note to the Reader

This guide is meant to inform and provoke a case-finding approach. It is full of legal information, which cannot be taken as legal advice.

HEALTH-HARMING LEGAL NEEDS

A Guide for Canadian Primary Health Care Clinicians

Introduction

RAMI SHOUCRI AND JENNIFER STONE

Malalai, a 37-year-old woman, and her husband Ali (also your patient) are both new to the country and parents to two young children, also in your practice. Malalai begins to tell you of conflict in her relationship.

Jim, a 64-year-old man on social assistance for a chronic mental health condition, is coming in for his routine check-up. He is unaware of the upcoming potentially drastic changes to his financial situation.

Jessica comes to see you in tears, not sure whether she will be fired from her job as she deals with an illness.

Kim asks you about cheaper versions of their chronic medications because they just lost their job. They also wonder whether it was just a coincidence that their boss recently found out they are transgender.

Successive patients are telling you that they might be getting evicted – Angela because she fell behind on rent when her partner had a relapse of their addiction, Erica because she was too sick to maintain her apartment.

Jamal's father wonders if something in their social housing explains his recurrent asthma exacerbations.

Billy, who is Indigenous but without "status," comes in for a review of his diabetes, which does not seem to be responding to the medications you are prescribing.

The goal of this book is to empower primary health care professionals to identify and effectively address these and other important and common health-affecting social needs that may have legal solutions; we call these "health-harming legal needs."

Legal support can be invaluable in many situations that seem hopeless for primary care patients and their providers: fighting eviction, securing disability benefits, accessing full citizenship status, navigating family courts in times of crisis, and stabilizing family decision-making for vulnerable adults, to name a few. We revisit and elaborate on the (fictional) patients described here and others over the course of the book to highlight the common and important health-harming legal needs that arise in primary care.

The objectives for this text are to allow primary health care professionals to

- identify when a health-harming social need might have a legal solution, including for common and important social determinants of health (SDOHs), such as income, housing, and personal and family security;
- identify situations that are at high risk of deteriorating into intractable legal problems and how to access preventive services;
- empower you to connect with available community legal resources for patients in your area; and
- identify community- or system-level issues and how to participate in advocacy efforts to address them.

In the following chapters, we elaborate on several of the well-known SDOHs to help you identify those that commonly have the most significant impact on the health of your patients and have potential legal solutions. We also focus on several patient populations that often face unique or additional social and potentially legal challenges, including those living with HIV, Indigenous people of Canada, and the paediatric population. In future editions, we hope to dedicate chapters to the care of other populations who often face health-harming legal needs, including sexual and gender minorities.

This book is meant to provide a framework, tools, and an approach to these issues for primary care practitioners. In practice, partnering with local legal professionals is the key to supporting individual patients, continuing education about these issues, and effectively advocating for organizational and systemic change.

Health-Harming Legal Needs in the Context of the Social Determinants of Health

SDOHs have been defined as "the conditions in which people are born, grow, live, work, and age."[1(p. 3)] A growing literature is establishing an evidence base for what health providers have long understood to be a critical part of what makes people healthy and what makes them sick: "income, wealth, employment status, educational attainment, race or ethnicity, and other individual-level characteristics strongly predict who acquires a range of diseases, who dies of these diseases, and who dies prematurely from all causes."[2(p. e478)]

Figure 0.1. Basis for Understanding Access to Justice as a Social Determinant of Health

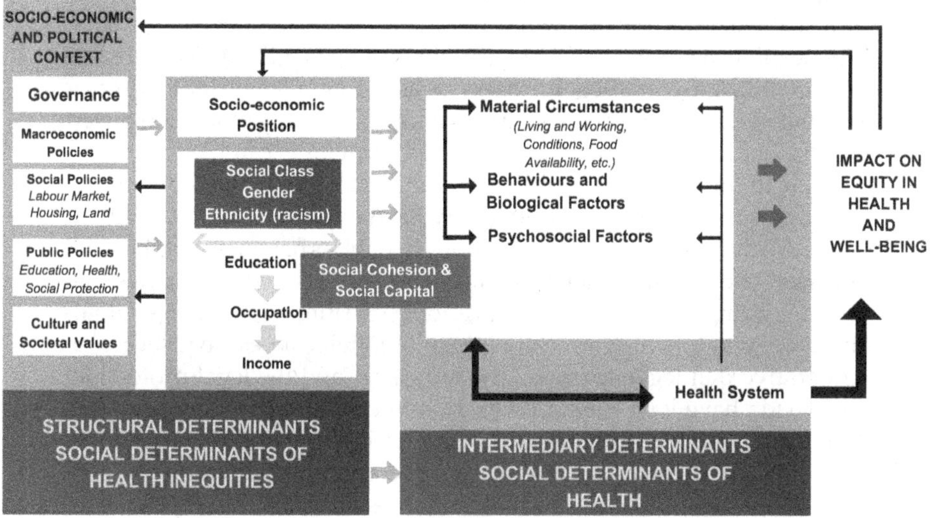

As a primary care clinician, these issues can feel overwhelming. However, with some tools and knowledge, you can assist your individual patients, especially low-income or otherwise marginalized ones, as they navigate the world in which their health is determined. If you can assist them with modifiable social conditions that significantly affect their health, not only will their well-being improve, but your job will be easier.[3]

Helping individual patients in your practice with these issues is critical but only a start because the underlying structures that created the disadvantage or marginalization go unchallenged in this patient-to-patient approach. The conceptual framework for action on the SDOHs of the World Health Organization's Commission on the Social Determinants of Health recognized this and emphasized that it is important to "distinguish between the social causes of health and the social factors determining the distribution of these causes between more and less advantaged groups."[4(p. 5)] As illustrated in Figure 0.1, it is not just housing, income, education, and so forth but the structures that define the (inequitable) distribution of these resources that really merit attention.

Throughout this text we attempt to highlight the upstream structures or policy choices that determine the degree of (in)equity in the distribution of SDOH-related resources in Canada. Indeed, one of the primary potential benefits of partnering with legal professionals is the potential collaboration in advocacy efforts to change these structures or policy choices.

Not every stressful social situation for our patients requires a legal analysis or remedy. Sometimes connection to other community resources is sufficient. Other professionals can also play a key role, such as social workers, housing workers, system navigators, or income security health promoters. However, certain problems that our patients face require engaging in a legal process or asserting a legal right to access safe housing, a stable income, personal safety, or many other recognized SDOHs. In these situations, primary care providers can play an essential role in their patients' accessing legal services and, ideally, justice.

"Access to justice" has traditionally been evaluated by the ability to name, blame, and claim justice,[5] although scholars have also emphasized the need to assess the extent to which individuals actually perceive that they are being treated fairly and without discrimination when evaluating the extent to which a society is just.[6] Equitable access to justice is an imperative that legal scholars,[7] the judiciary,[8] and the legal profession[9] in Canada have long identified as an unmet aspiration. One approach to improving access to justice has been to identify and train potential trusted intermediaries to identify legal needs in the population and connect the population to appropriate legal resources.[10] Primary care providers, especially in Canada, where financial means are not explicitly a barrier to accessing health care, are in an ideal position to be trusted intermediaries to further the goal of equitable access to justice.

Facilitating access to justice can, in turn, allow patients to improve their SDOHs. Accepting that equitable access to justice affects health, we propose that equitable access to justice is itself a distinct SDOH, and not merely a means to securing other known SDOHs. The evidence base for the effects on health of accessing justice, specifically through partnerships or formalized pathways, must be established. This evidence base is inherently difficult to establish, given the complexity of the intervention and the difficulty of finding appropriate control groups. Nonetheless, a growing body of research is establishing positive health outcomes for health directly from interventions initiated by health and justice partnerships.[11] Furthermore, other studies have established positive impacts on provider attitudes towards addressing SDOHs[12] and on recognized SDOHs,[13] which can be inferred to indirectly have positive impacts on health. If or when access to justice becomes recognized as a SDOH, broad potential policy implications could follow.[14]

Returning to our cases, the issues facing Malalai, Jim, Jessica, Kim, Angela, Erica, Jamal's father, and Billy are likely to be complex. In fact, they are likely to involve multiple interconnected legal issues. Legal professionals who frequently work with people living in poverty know that their clients frequently bump up against "sharp legal things."[15(p. 1050)] Clinically, patients occasionally present with discrete social problems, but they more commonly present with some form of complex medical, psychological, or social crisis. This text breaks their issues down into individual topics for the purposes of illustration with the hope that you will acquire new tools to understand and address your patients' complex problems.

In doing so, the hope is that health care providers will develop more confidence to meet their responsibility to engage in advocacy, which has been emphasized by the College of Family Physicians of Canada,[16] the College of Nurses of Ontario,[17] and the Canadian Association of Social Workers.[18]

In chapter 1, we provide an introduction to interprofessional health and legal collaboration, including some key tips for issue identification and working effectively with legal professionals. We also provide an overview of legal services in Canada and the health and justice partnership service model.

In chapter 2, Dr. Beth Bilson provides an overview of relevant legal frameworks in Canada, including sources of domestic and international law, with a focus on human rights legislation that requires disability accommodations.

In chapter 3, Christa Big Canoe and Dr. Suzanne Shoush set the context of how and why Indigenous people experience health care in Canada. They begin with an exploration of Indigenous perspectives on medicine, law, and wellness and move on to a review of examples of the adversity and discrimination that Indigenous peoples in Canada have experienced and continue to experience while highlighting the enduring strength of Indigenous communities.

In chapter 4, Dr. Andrew Bond and Benjamin Ries review the various ways in which health affects housing and vice versa. The opportunities and limits of connecting low-income patients with housing problems to legal professionals are also explored, all in the context of a growing housing and homelessness crisis in Canada.

In chapter 5, Nabila F. Qureshi and Dr. Andrew Pinto explore the relationship between health and income through rights at work. They review commonly encountered issues in employment, workplace, and human rights law relevant to primary care in Canada.

In chapter 6, Dr. Gary Bloch, Anu Bakshi, and Louise Simbandumwe further explore the relationship between health and income by reviewing the various income support programs in Canada and how health care providers can provide invaluable support to their patients to navigate these programs, including by engaging legal professional support when necessary.

In chapter 7, Dr. Michaela Beder, Dilan Brar, Dr. Ritika Goel, Dr. Vanessa Redditt, and Jennifer Stone, with Diana Gallego and Luis Alberto Mata advising, explore the relationship between health and precarious or lack of immigration status, with an introduction to immigration and refugee law. This includes viewing immigration status as "the right to have rights" and how primary care providers can best support their patients through these processes.

Chapter 8, by Anita Volikis, Jamie Ahn, and Dr. Kathleen Doukas, explores family law, where destabilization of the family unit commonly engages both legal rights and health, especially when issues of violence, separation, divorce, and custody arise in primary care.

Chapter 9, by Dr. Flora Matheson, Promise Holmes Skinner, and Christine Carthew, focuses on a common issue for noninstitutionalized patients involved in the criminal-legal system, where primary care providers can make a significant impact.[19] They present the extremely high prevalence of traumatic brain injury among justice-involved individuals and walk through the various steps of the criminal justice system and how health care providers can support their patients at each step. This chapter gives particular focus to the overrepresentation of Indigenous people in the criminal justice system.

Chapter 10, by Robin Nobleman, Debbie Rachlis, Ryan Peck, Devan Nambiar, and Dr. Gordon Arbess, reviews the common legal issues facing patients living with HIV, including contexts of discrimination, privacy risks, and risks of criminalization. Given how important access to pharmacotherapy is to patients living with HIV, they also provide a review of the various ways to access medicine regimes currently available in Canada.

Chapter 11, by Dr. Sarah Gander, Lee Ann Chapman, and Melanie Laking, reviews the rights of children to equitable health by exploring key legal issues related to health care decision-making, safety and protection, education, and the youth criminal justice system. They then turn to particular experiences of discrimination, racism, and trauma by Indigenous and 2SLGBTQ+ children and youth. Finally, they review common SDOHs that affect families' ability to care for children, including immigration status, employment, tax-related benefits, income supports, and housing safety and stability.

Chapter 12, by Dr. Naheed Dosani, Edgar-Andre Montigny, and Mercedes Perez, reviews issues most relevant to end-of-life care, including substitute decision-making for an incapable person during that person's lifetime and issues related to small estates and the transfer of property after a person's death.

Chapter 13, by Dr. William F. Sullivan, Mercedes Perez, John Heng, and Paula Hutchinson, reviews a model of solidarity to promote health care decision-making capabilities while mitigating vulnerabilities for people with intellectual and developmental disabilities in primary health care.

We have attempted to foreground the issues facing Indigenous people in Canada in this text in recognition of the massive inequities in health justice that they experience. In addition to the context-setting chapter 3 by Christa Big Canoe and Dr. Suzanne Shoush, chapters 9 and 11 include Indigenous co-authors. Two Indigenous reviewers also provided feedback on chapter 10. In addition, we attempted to recruit Indigenous co-authors for the other chapters and, when that was not possible, we attempted to recruit Indigenous legal experts to provide a reflection on the content of those chapters from an Indigenous perspective. We are grateful for the reflections of Sara Mainville, Douglas Varrette, Caitlyn E. Kasper, and Kate Forget on chapters 5, 6, 8, and 12, respectively. In future editions, we hope to have Indigenous co-authorship of all chapters. We are grateful for the guidance and support of Christa Big Canoe, executive director of Aboriginal Legal Services, a member of our Advisory Committee, and co-author of chapter 3, in these efforts.

A Note on Gladue and Gladue-Type Briefs

Chapter 9 of this text, on health and the criminal justice system, provides an overview of how Indigenous people have come to be over-represented within it. That chapter describes how, in a series of landmark cases, beginning with *R. v. Gladue*,[20] the Supreme Court has taken judicial notice of the unique circumstances of Indigenous Peoples. This is having a growing impact on other areas of law.

Since that decision, criminal courts must take the cultural genocide-related factors described in Chapters 3 and 9 into account when sentencing an Indigenous person.

The principles set out in *Gladue* have been adapted and applied beyond the criminal sentencing context.[21(pp. 1–6)] The ongoing process of colonization affects Indigenous peoples in profound ways that are critical to understanding the issues that bring them before a court or administrative tribunal.

Just as sentencing in the criminal law context necessitates an individualized assessment of each Indigenous person, the "whole-person" approach required in disability appeals (or discretionary

> relief from eviction sought by a tenant) obligates various tribunals to consider how an individual's experience as an Indigenous person has contributed to the scope and depth of their circumstances.[22(p.1)]
>
> We are particularly indebted to a resource, presently unpublished, that guides Ontario's legal aid service providers to ensure that Gladue factors are raised in submissions to administrative tribunals that have delegated discretionary decision-making. This is a relatively newer practice and one we believe is an important development in the commitment to reconciliation.

Importantly, the content of each chapter was co-written by legal and health professionals. The hope is not only to convey expert legal knowledge in a clinically relevant way but also to continue the iterative process of creating a common health justice language to better serve our communities.

Furthermore, we recognize that our patients and clients are often our best teachers; thus, several chapters have integrated lived experience expertise, through co-authorship, consultation, or reflection. We are grateful for their willingness to share their expertise.

By focusing on Indigenous health perspectives, we also want to acknowledge what is missing. Despite some discussion of the over-representation of Black and Indigenous people in Canada's prisons in chapter 9, this text does not give due discussion to the health inequities that flow from anti-Black racism. As well, this text does not tackle the significant barriers to health care and justice faced by the transgender and gender-nonconforming community. We hope future editions will build on this first text of its kind in Canada and foreground these key issues to expand knowledge and improve outcomes.

NOTES

1 Commission on the Social Determinants of Health. Closing the gap in a generation: health equity through action on the social determinants of health. Geneva: World Health Organization; 2008.

2 Pinto A, Bloch G. Framework for building primary care capacity to address the social determinants of health. Can Fam Physician. 2017;63:e476–82.

3 See, for example, Hatef and colleagues, who found that "after adjusting for other factors, patients with housing instability and homelessness had

49% and 34% more encounters with the health care system compared to patients without housing issues ($P<0.00001$)" (Hatef E, Ma X, Rouhisadeh R, et al. Assessing the impact of social needs and social determinants of health on health care utilization: using patient- and community-level data. Popul Health Manage 24[2]. https://doi.org/10.1089/pop.2020.0043).

4 World Health Organization. A conceptual framework for action on the social determinants of health [Internet]. Geneva: World Health Organization; 2010. Available from: https://www.who.int/publications/i/item/9789241500852 f.

5 Felstiner WLF, Abel RL, Sarat A. The emergence and transformation of disputes – naming, blaming, claiming.... Law Soc. 1981;15(3–4):631–54, 883–910.

6 Mosher JE. Lessons in access to justice: racialized youths in Ontario's safe schools. Osgoode Hall Law J. 2008; 46(4):807–51.

7 Mosher notes that "special attention should be paid to how we access the formal doorways of justice and whether the pathways provide adequate accommodation and accessibility to those seeking justice" (Mosher JE. Lessons in access to justice: racialized youths in Ontario's safe schools. Osgoode Hall Law J. 2008; 46[4]:807–51).

8 See, e.g., Wagner R. Access to justice: a societal imperative: remarks of the Right Honourable Richard Wagner, P.C. Chief Justice of Canada [Internet]. Ottawa: Supreme Court of Canada; 4 Oct 2018 [modified 14 May 2019; cited October 2020]. Available from: https://www.scc-csc.ca/judges -juges/spe-dis/rw-2018-10-04-eng.aspx.

9 Canadian Bar Association. Reaching equal justice report: an invitation to envision and act [Internet]. Ottawa: The Association; November 2013 [cited October 2020]. Available from: http://www.cba.org/CBAMediaLibrary /cba_na/images/Equal%20Justice%20-%20Microsite/PDFs/EqualJustice FinalReport-eng.pdf.

10 Law Foundation of Ontario. Part 2 – Trusted help: The role of community workers as trusted intermediaries who help people with legal problems [Internet]. Toronto: The Foundation; 1 May 2018 [last updated 20 July 2021; cited October 2020]. https://lawfoundation.on.ca/download /part-2-trusted-help-the-role-of-community-workers-as-trusted -intermediaries-who-help-people-with-legal-problems-2018/.

11 See, for example, Beardon S, Woodhead C, Cooper S, et al. International evidence on the impact of health-justice partnerships: a systematic scoping review. Public Health Rev. 2021;42:1603976. https://doi.org/10.3389 /phrs.2021.1603976, and O'Sullivan MM, Brandfield J, Hoskote SS, et al. Environmental improvements brought by the legal interventions in the homes of poorly controlled inner-city adult asthmatic patients: a proof -of-concept study. J Asthma. 2012;49(9):911–17.

12 O'Toole JK, Burkhardt MC, Solan LG, et al. Resident confidence addressing social history: is it influenced by availability of social and legal resources? Clin Pediatr. 2012;51(7):625–31.

13 Beck AF, Klein MD, Schaffzin, JK, et al. Identifying and treating a substandard housing cluster using a medical-legal partnership. Pediatr. 2012;130(5):831–38.

14 Nobleman R. Addressing access to justice as a social determinant of health. Health Law J. 2014;21(49):49–74.

15 Wexler S. Practicing law for poor people. Yale Law J. 1970;79:1049–67.

16 Working Group on Curriculum Review. CanMEDS – family medicine [Internet]. Mississauga (ON): College of Family Physicians of Canada; 2009. Available from: https://www.cfpc.ca/CFPC/media/Resources /Care-of-the-Elderly/CanMeds-FM-Eng.pdf.

17 College of Nurses of Ontario. Entry-to-practice competencies for registered nurses [Internet]. Toronto: College of Nurses of Ontario; 2019. Available from: https://www.cno.org/globalassets/docs/reg/41037-entry-to -practice-competencies-2020.pdf.

18 Canadian Association of Social Workers (CASW). CASW scope of practice statement [Internet]. Ottawa: CASW; 2020. Available from: https://www .casw-acts.ca/files/documents/Scope_of_Practice_Statement_2020_1.pdf.

19 The authors have changed the language from "justice system" to "legal system" to acknowledge the existing and historical injustices a number of communities have experienced within the criminal-legal system. They recognize that we must continue to reflect on the language that we use in representing the people, processes, and problems we study and write about.

20 *R. v. Gladue*, [1999] 1 SCR 688. Also see *R. v. Ipeelee*, [2012] 1 SCR 433 at para. 60.

21 Truth and Reconciliation Commission of Canada. Honouring the truth, reconciling for the future: summary of the final report of the Truth and Reconciliation Commission of Canada. Ottawa: The Commission; 2015.

22 Hamilton Community Legal Clinic et al. "The ancestors are with us at all times": helping our community heal through the application of Gladue in administrative tribunals. Ontario Community Legal Clinics training manual, March 2020.

1 Forming Partnerships and Effectively Collaborating with Legal Professionals in the Care of Patients

RAMI SHOUCRI AND JENNIFER STONE

In our introduction, you met several patients. Let's consider three of them in more detail to guide us through the issues covered in this chapter.

- Malalai, a 37-year-old woman, is married to your patient Ali. Both are new to the country and parents to two young children also in your practice. Malalai begins to tell you of conflict in her relationship.
- Jim, a 64-year-old man on social assistance for a chronic mental health condition, is coming in for his routine check-up. He is unaware of the upcoming potentially drastic changes to his financial situation.
- Angela, a 29-year-old woman, might be getting evicted; she fell behind on rent because her partner had a relapse of their addiction.

In this chapter, we elaborate on some common concepts and issues that are important in engaging with the health-harming social problems that may have legal remedies for patients in your practice:

- identification of an issue as a potentially health-harming legal need;
- understanding the system within which your patient might seek legal recourse and what resources might be available to them;
- how you can build partnerships with legal professionals in your community to support the care of your patients (and community);
- what you can and cannot say to your patients about legal problems; and
- how best to communicate with legal professionals, including what kind of information you can and should (and what you cannot or should not) provide to legal professionals in a referral and what to document.

Issue Identification: Responsive, Screening, or Case Finding

Responsive

For Angela, the legal issue of eviction is obvious, and she raises it with you explicitly. The challenge here is not so much identification of the issue but rather having the comfort, the tools, and the knowledge to effectively respond to the health-harming legal issues raised by patients while staying safely within your scope of practice.

Screening

Patients such as Malalai and Jim may not explicitly raise legal issues with their primary care provider; thus, alternative approaches to the identification of legal issues should be considered, such as screening and case finding.

Screening is the identification of an asymptomatic disease, unhealthy condition, or risk factor.[1] In this context, screening would involve asking all patients in a practice the same question or set of questions with the goal of preventing a health-harming legal issue from arising. Advocating for broad screening for health-harming legal needs, or any other asymptomatic disease or risk factor, traditionally requires a strong evidence base.

Several questionnaires are available to identify health-harming social needs that may have legal solutions.[2] However, they have not been validated for use with the general population. That is, the evidence is insufficient to support demonstrable benefit at acceptable cost in asking every patient a question or series of questions to identify potential health-harming legal needs. As the evidence continues to grow for the accessibility, feasibility, and efficacy of early intervention with health-harming legal needs, this calculation may change.

Case Finding

A case-finding approach, however, is reasonable, and several approaches are suggested here. Case finding is a targeted approach to early detection in which only people who are at increased risk are tested. This is a more efficient approach to identifying individuals who may benefit from intervention, and it reduces the risk of harm from false-positive screens and minimizes the burden on practices and providers. We encourage all providers to undergo training in recognizing implicit or unconscious bias when taking this approach.

We discuss two approaches here for identifying populations at higher risk for having health-harming legal needs.

SCREENING FOR POVERTY

The overall benefit-versus-harm profile of screening for poverty is somewhat controversial. The most studied screening question is "Do you (ever) have difficulty making ends meet at the end of the month?" Statistically, this question has been found to have a sensitivity of 98 per cent and a specificity of 40 per cent.[3] The main area of controversy is not so much the specificity of 40 per cent, because it is fairly well accepted that a screening test will be over-inclusive, but that the evidence of long-term benefit for patients in asking this question is not clear.[4] That is, are the interventions or referrals, if any, triggered by a positive screen effective in alleviating poverty (and improving health)?[5]

The evidentiary gap is complicated by the fact that screening for poverty may have unintended harms. For example, a patient or family may feel frustration if the type or quality of resources and services that are available do not meet their needs, and a patient or family may feel stigmatized if the screening is limited to people in particular subgroups. The risk of unintended harm can be minimized through coordination of care, collaboration with service providers, shared decision-making before making referrals, screening the entire practice population rather than subgroups, and acknowledging and building on patient and family strengths.[6]

Please see chapters 5 and 6 for further discussion of the nuances of and options in screening for poverty in your practice.

KEY LIFE EVENTS, FORMS, AND KEY RED- OR YELLOW-FLAG STATEMENTS

Another approach to case finding or identifying higher-risk subgroups for more detailed questioning about health-harming legal needs is to be aware that (1) key life events, (2) particular forms, or (3) red- or yellow-flag statements may indicate a situation that requires further probing or intervention.[7]

Life events that should trigger consideration of further probing or intervention include, for example,

- separating from a partner;
- death or significant illness of a partner;
- losing a job;
- starting to get income support;
- turning age 18 or becoming a senior citizen; or
- being evicted.

Similarly, any forms that the patient brings in to fill out related to any of these processes should trigger consideration of further probing or intervention.

As we know, however, patients often do not present with explicit and well-defined problems. This is particularly true if the patient does not perceive the social issue as health-harming, one that may have a legal remedy, or one that the primary health care provider can assist with. In these situations, it is up to the astute clinician to rely on their active listening skills and to sensitively probe whether their concerns are reasonable. Of course, a clinician's confidence to probe will only increase with increasing knowledge of remediable legal issues and how to access the resources available to support their patients.

If higher risk is identified on the basis of the preceding criteria, a clinician can consider a more structured questionnaire to identify not only the most pressing legal issue but perhaps other concurrent legal issues because they often coexist. Several questionnaires are available that are based on the acronym "iHELP" (Income, Housing, Employment and education, Legal status, Personal and family stability).[8] Alternatively, a referral to a legal professional to complete a more thorough assessment (if available) is certainly acceptable.

An expressed legal need does not necessarily correspond to a significant health-harming risk or necessarily require your intervention. For example, a patient complaining about the work that a contractor has done on their second home is not likely experiencing a significant health impact because of this contractual dispute. Similarly, not all people expressing a legal need require your assistance with connecting to resources or system navigation. If you're not sure, a simple question such as "Have you consulted with a lawyer?" may assuage you.

Returning to our cases, let's consider Jim first. In terms of case finding, several factors in our very brief history should prompt consideration of further questioning. Being on social assistance, he is at higher risk for having an unmet health-harming legal need. Furthermore, he is approaching a key life stage, turning age 65. Depending on which province he lives in and his particular situation, he may or may not be at increased risk of having an unmet health-harming legal need in the near future. For example, if he lives in Ontario and has previously been exempted from paying child support payments by virtue of being on social assistance, he may be at risk for significant loss of income through garnishment because federal income supports, as opposed to provincial income supports, are not protected from outstanding orders or judgments.[9] Chapter 6 includes a review of various income support programs in Canada and associated legal issues that primary care providers may be able to support their patients with.

Similarly, for Malalai, a potential separation certainly qualifies as a key life stage that should give a clinician pause. However, other factors would need to be considered to better assess her risk for having an unmet health-harming legal need in the near future. What is her financial situation? What is her family's immigration status? Is there intimate partner or other abuse in the household? On the one hand, if Malalai is relatively financially secure and socially connected, she might very well be aware that numerous potential legal issues are upcoming and have already consulted a lawyer. However, if she receives social assistance and lives in social housing, chances are that she will have serious unmet, potentially health-harming legal needs in the near future. These issues are explored in more detail in chapter 8.

Legal Services in Canada

Now that you have identified potential health-harming legal needs for Malalai and Jim, what resources are available to them to remedy their problems?

Unlike health care, legal services are primarily in the marketplace. That is, access to legal advice typically requires a person to pay for it. This text primarily focuses on the low-income population because they will most likely require assistance in navigating the legal system. This is not meant to suggest that higher-income people do not experience highly stressful and potentially health-harming legal needs. However, they are more likely than lower-income patients to be able to navigate and access the necessary legal services.

In Canada, the legal profession, much like health care, is regulated provincially. Therefore, across the country, a wide spectrum of systems are in place to support individuals who are unable to afford legal services. In addition to the provincial legal aid schemes set out in Appendix 1, individuals needing legal assistance may also benefit from pro bono, or volunteer, lawyer services. These pro bono programs, although strongly encouraged by provincial law societies that regulate lawyers, vary widely from region to region in terms of accessibility and comprehensiveness. Depending on a patient's province and employment situation, they may be able to benefit from other low-cost or free access to legal services, including through their unions, university-associated legal clinics, or their provincial bar (legal) association.

Appendix 1 summarizes legal aid services provided across Canada's provinces and territories. Subject to financial eligibility requirements, criminal law defence where a sentence could include jail time will always be covered because of the constitutional right to a lawyer when one's liberty is at stake. Child protection and mental health law should similarly be state funded for low-income people.[10] Other legal issues covered vary significantly across Canada's different jurisdictions. Note that these services are all means-tested, with Ontario's income eligibility threshold being higher, at about $19,000 per year, than those of Nova Scotia (about $13,000) and New Brunswick (about $14,000), which have the lowest income eligibility thresholds for legal aid services across the country. This stark reality means that if a person earns more than these amounts, they may not be eligible for state-funded legal help.

Also noteworthy is that Ontario is unique in the country in having a community legal aid clinic system. Legal Aid Ontario funds legal services for low-income Ontarians through duty counsel in courthouses; some specialty staff offices, such as the Refugee Law Offices and Family Law Service Centres; paying private bar lawyers who accept legal aid certificates; and 72 community-governed legal aid clinics across the province.

In chapter 4 of this text, on health and housing, the fundamental characteristics of Ontario's community legal clinics are discussed further. These clinics were historically formed (with the oldest being Parkdale Community Legal Services in 1972) in response to the unique legal needs of people living in poverty. Community legal aid clinics in Ontario are funded by the province through the Ministry of the Attorney General but are accountable to their communities by virtue of being independently governed by community boards of directors. The notion that people with lived experience of poverty can best dictate the scope and priorities of their local legal aid clinic is a proud legacy that continues today. In addition to individual casework in areas defined as clinic law (generally tenant-side housing law, income security law, immigration law, and employment and human rights law), community legal aid clinics approach poverty as a systemic issue and are mandated to also carry out public legal education, community organizing, and law reform initiatives, which include test case litigation. This laudable community resource has, unfortunately, too often been subject to the vagaries of partisan politics. After years of underfunding and a devastating 30 per cent funding cut to Legal Aid Ontario in 2019, some funding increases have in recent years slowly returned to the Legal Aid Ontario system. Notably, the Health Justice Program that the authors are involved with is funded by Legal Aid Ontario.

The exact resources available to Jim, Malalai, and Angela thus depend on which province they live in and specific legal and demographic factors, such as income. It is complicated, and the reality is that health care professionals have their hands full navigating the complex health care system. The best way to learn about the options available to your low-income patients is to reach out to local legal professionals to learn more and consider forming some level of medical–legal or health and justice partnership, as discussed in the next section.

Health and Justice Partnership Model and Adaptations for Canada

Collaboration between medical and legal professionals is not especially novel. What is relatively novel is a formalization of the collaboration with some key common elements, including co-location and a three-part mandate:

1. *Direct legal services to patients*: The cornerstone of a program, this work ideally helps to inform the next two activities.
2. *Education*: This can focus on many groups or stakeholders, including patients, health professionals, and legal professionals.
3. *Advocacy*: This focuses on upstream issues.

It is generally accepted that this formalization can be traced to a medical–legal partnership started in the late 1990s by Dr. Barry Zuckerman in Boston in the United States. There are now more than 450 partnerships (as of 2025) in the United States.[11] An extensive literature documenting the history of this movement[12] and the subsequent impacts of individual partnerships now exists.[13]

As mentioned, a key element of this model is the co-location of legal professionals in the health care setting. The rationale for this is based on the importance of relationships and relationship building, including the long-standing and typically trusting relationships between primary care health providers and their patients as well as the relationships between legal service and health service providers. The primary health care provider–patient relationship of trust facilitates the exploration of significant but potentially sensitive social issues that patients may not know how to pursue or feel comfortable pursuing. The primary health care provider–legal services provider relationship helps facilitate interprofessional capacity building to identify and address issues and transform health and legal institutions to better serve patients. It also allows for collaboration regarding identification of and addressing upstream structural social issues. Nonetheless, if resources or capacity do not allow for co-location of services, relationships and eventually partnerships can certainly be formed through alternative means, including meetings and iterative working relationships.

In Canada, there are a growing number of health and justice partnerships in a variety of settings, including hospital based,[14] urban primary care,[15] and rural primary care.[16]

In terms of building towards your own health and justice partnership, the primary goal is to focus on the need among your patient population and the local resources available (both health and legal) to establish a partnership that works in your setting. It is typically an iterative process that adapts to changing patient population needs and available services (and funding). Broadly speaking, and in no particular order, consider the following three points of departure:

1. Research and reach out to local legal aid or pro bono legal service providers.
2. Review tools, such as draft memoranda of understanding, available from other organizations that support health and justice partnerships: the National Centre of Medical Legal Partnerships – USA,[17] Health Justice Australia,[18] and the Health Justice Partnership Team at University College London in the United Kingdom.[19]
3. Reach out to established health justice partnerships in your jurisdiction (municipal, provincial, or national).

Even if your partnership starts out informally with a phone call or a quick meeting, the idea is that it can grow over time, with the ultimate goals being improved care for Angela, Jim, Malalai, and other patients; better inter-professional support and collaboration for both you and the legal professional; and, as the partnership develops, potential work on upstream issues together.

Legal Information versus Legal Advice

Health care providers are in an ideal position to provide Angela, Malalai, and Jim with legal information. It may be intimidating for non-lawyers to engage with a body of knowledge as complex as the law and the legal system. Clearly, it is important to acknowledge the limits of one's knowledge and expertise. However, this does not mean that you should actively avoid exploring these issues. In fact, considering how critical the social determinants of health (SDOHs) are to your patient's well-being, we argue that it is incumbent on providers to be sensitive to their patient's potential health-harming legal needs.

A useful framework for understanding the limits of what you can do for your patients once health-harming legal issues are identified is distinguishing between legal information and legal advice (Table 1.1).

Legal information can help people understand their legal rights, how legal processes work, and how to get more help. It is well accepted that non–legal professionals such as health care providers can safely and effectively provide legal information, as long as they have relatively

Table 1.1. Legal Information versus Legal Advice

Legal information	Legal advice
Is general	Is specific
Identifies problems as legal	Confidential and protected by solicitor–client privilege
Links to help or resources	–
Who? Anybody with up-to-date knowledge about a particular area of law	Who? Licensed legal professionals

up-to-date knowledge about the issues and the resources. The distinguishing elements of legal information are that it

- is general information about the law – that is, not about an individual's specific situation;
- can help a person understand when a problem is a legal problem; and
- can provide guidance on when a person needs more help and advice and how to find it.[20]

Legal advice, however, guides a person about their specific situation. That is, legal advice interprets legislation, case law, and procedural rules and applies them to a particular situation. Only licensed legal professionals can provide legal advice. To distinguish it from legal information, legal advice

- is specific to an individual's particular situation; people's situations and circumstances are different even when facing the same legal problem and
- provides recommendations to a person about their options, based on an assessment of how the law applies to their specific situation and what the person wants to achieve.

Returning to our patients, one could, for example, safely communicate the following messages:

Angela, you have legal rights during an eviction process. If you haven't spoken to a lawyer yet, I could connect you to X lawyer and/or to Y website that explains your rights and the processes.

Jim, turning 65 might have some important consequences for your financial situation. I could connect you to X lawyer and/or to Y website that explains your rights and the processes.

> Malalai, a separation, especially with children involved, might get compli-
> cated legally. If you haven't spoken to a lawyer yet, I could connect you to
> X lawyer and/or to Y website that explains your rights and the processes.

If they need and agree to referral to a legal professional, some key considerations in the communication and documentation of that process
are reviewed in the following section.

Interprofessional Information Sharing with Different Privacy Regimes

In collaborating with legal professionals, it is also important to be aware
of the applicable rules of professional conduct, legislation governing
health and legal information, and their implications for safe and effective collaboration between these two professions.

It is important to know that legal and medical professionals are regulated provincially; thus, applicable legislation and rules of professional
conduct vary across the country. However, broadly speaking, medical professionals owe a duty of confidentiality to their patients, with
important exceptions that are usually enumerated in provincial legislation or rules of professional conduct. Legal professionals also owe a
duty of confidentiality to their clients. However, the level of protection
for this information is even higher than that for medical information
and is protected under the concept of solicitor–client privilege.[21]

Information Sharing When Making a Referral

Medical professionals should only share information with legal professionals with explicit consent from their patients. This includes even the
most basic identifying information. The patient's signature provides
evidence of consent but is neither necessary nor sufficient to establish
informed consent. More important is a discussion of the implications of
the referral and documentation of the patient's consent to the referral
in a note. This section explores the risks and potential benefits in more
versus less detailed referral notes to legal professionals.

Of note, some partnerships take the position that embedded legal
professionals are within the "circle of care" of health providers and
thus grant unrestricted access to a patient's health records once they
are referred. This approach is not recommended for one-off referrals to
legal professionals and should only be adopted by partnerships after
careful considerations of the risks and the benefits and potentially seeking independent legal advice on this practice.

EFFECTIVE REFERRALS

As noted, patient consent for a referral is a prerequisite. This consent need not be written, but it should be express and documented. It is strongly advised that very little about your thoughts on the actual legal issue be documented and shared in the referral; this is the legal professional's job.

However, the amount of health information included in the referral lies along a spectrum of risk to the health care provider and utility for both the patient and the legal professional and indirectly for you as the referrer. The least risky referral would have no information other than something such as "please see for possible legal issue."

However, we would argue that the potential improvement in the utility of the referral that comes with sharing carefully selected information justifies an extended consent discussion with the patient.

Information that is especially helpful for the receiving legal professional includes (a) health and social supports that the patient already has, which helps in knowing what supports the patient might have in navigating typically complicated legal processes, and (b) how the patient can be accommodated, including a general sense of medical issues that might make navigating systems difficult. Depending on the nature of the issue, a health provider can consider a referral as an ongoing relationship between the provider and the lawyer that is in the best interests of the patient. In such situations, it is necessary to have explicit consent for two-way communication between the professionals. The lawyer would typically require signed consent from the patient on file.

Let's use Jim's situation to consider the strengths and weakness of three possible referrals.

1. "Please see this patient re: possible legal issues around income." This referral is adequate and certainly better than no referral. However, it would benefit from more context, including information about Jim's baseline financial situation, a description of the complexities of his social or medical situation, and how he might be best accommodated.
2. "Please see this 64-year-old man, lives alone in TCHC, wants legal advice about debt issue. Possibly past child support issue. Very difficult to connect with; has relationship with XYZ social worker. Various health issues, including current investigations for possible Alzheimer's. I have received verbal consent from the patient to share this information with you." This referral is ideal. It highlights the complexities of both Jim's personal and health situations and his legal issues. The documentation of the consent is excellent,

and the information about Jim's connection with the social worker would likely prove to be extremely helpful to the legal professional.
3. "Please see this 64-year-old man, lives alone in TCHC. Possible legal issues to do with debt. Various health issues including current investigations for possible Alzheimer's, but patient resistant to engaging with this." This referral is problematic for one important reason, the apparent lack of consent from Jim to share the concerns about his cognitive status, reflected in the statement that he is "resistant to engaging with this." This referral, thus, runs afoul of health information privacy laws. Furthermore, there is a less-than-ideal level of detail about Jim's personal and legal situation.

Please see chapter 10, page 315, for a discussion of releasing health information in the markedly distinct context of requests from external and potentially adversarial parties, such as employers requesting further information for accommodations. We argue here that, with explicit patient consent, the benefits of disclosing relevant health information to a trusted legal professional working in partnership in the interests of your patient justifies selective disclosure of relevant health information.

Self-Referral and Secondary Consultations

Other low-barrier options for patients to access legal advice or benefit from legal information should also be considered in situations in which legal service providers have the capacity to do so, usually in partnership settings.

One option is to create a self-referral or drop-in model that is advertised in the health care setting. These can be supported by notices that simply list the services available or by legal health posters.[22] These have the advantage of eliminating the barrier of either the patient needing to raise the issue with the health care provider or the health care provider having the time to address the issue in a typically short appointment, while also reinforcing the messaging to patients that the issues they are facing affect their health.

Another option is to create the opportunity for secondary consultations between health providers and legal providers. These are intended to be brief conversations between providers to, for example, learn about available resources for a particular patient or determine whether a referral would be indicated.

Documentation in the Chart

Generally, everything relevant to the care of the patient should be documented in the medical chart. However, caution should be used in documenting the nature of legal problems. Given limited knowledge of legally salient facts and interpretation, health professionals are prone to misstating or misrepresenting a patient's situation. This is potentially damaging to a patient's interests if the medical records are subpoenaed in a subsequent legal proceeding.

Similarly, to the extent that the lawyer reports back on the consultation to the medical professional, the provider should for the same reasons be very cautious regarding what to document in the medical chart. Lawyers are typically very guarded about what they share with anybody after a legal consultation, given the sanctity of solicitor–client privilege and the concern about adversely affecting their client's interests. However, as partnerships grow and develop, understandings can be reached in which information that may be relevant to the patient's ongoing health care can safely be shared with the referring provider without necessarily risking a patient's legal interest. Of course, the lawyer would have to ensure patient consent to share any information back to the referring provider.

Effective Letters

A common request of medical professionals in relation to their patient's legal problems is a letter. This can be a daunting task for health professionals. Although the most appropriate content and tone of the letter depends on the letter's exact purpose and the audience, some general tips include the following:

1. Use plain language.
2. Try to remain neutral and objective; be an advocate without appearing to be openly advocating.
3. Explain qualifications and professional experience.
4. Avoid a lengthy summary of the patient's history.

If a patient already has a legal professional involved, it is perfectly acceptable with patient consent to discuss with the legal professional the exact purpose of the letter and to request feedback on drafts. If done with integrity, this does not take away from the independence of your medical opinion of the situation. Throughout this handbook – for example, in chapter 10 (pages 316 and 351) – you will find various examples of template letters for particular purposes, although it is important to note that every circumstance is unique.

See chapter 4, regarding health and housing, for a general discussion of how health care providers can contribute to advocacy by providing expert affidavits, participating in class actions, and contributing to legislative and policy development by way of deputations to government bodies.

Summary

Effective primary care requires seeing patients holistically. This includes understanding the impact of the SDOHs on their well-being. Increasingly, a team-based approach is being recognized as the most effective way to address the myriad problems that may affect a patient's health, including health-harming legal needs. This chapter and those following establish a justification and a foundation for interprofessional health and legal collaboration across Canada. This includes taking a case-finding approach to identifying potential unmet health-harming legal needs; understanding the system within which a patient might seek legal recourse and what resources might be available to them and you; how you can build partnerships with legal professionals in your community to support the care of your patients (and community); guidance on appropriate legal information that can be provided by health care providers to their patients; and guidance on how best to communicate with legal professionals, including what kind of information you can and should (as well as what you cannot or should not) provide to legal professionals in a referral and what to document in your patients' charts when working with a legal partner.

In upcoming chapters, common health-harming legal needs such as those facing Malalai, Jim, and Angela are explored in more depth, with a focus on a practical approach to identifying and addressing them in a primary care setting. First, chapter 2 provides an overview of the legal framework in Canada and chapter 3 provides an Indigenous perspective on wellness, law, and medicine that provides a foundation for the issue-specific discussions in subsequent chapters.

NOTES

1 Cochrane A, Holland W. Validation of screening procedures. Br Med Bull. 1971; 27(1):3–8. https://doi.org/10.1093/oxfordjournals.bmb.a070810.
2 See, for example, Halton Legal Clinic. Legal health check-up [Internet]. Oakville (ON): The Clinic; 2014 [cited Oct 2020]. Available from: https://legalhealthcheckup.ca/en/.
3 Brcic V, Eberdt C, Kaczorowski J. Development of a tool to identify poverty in a family practice setting: a pilot study. Int J Family Med 2011; 2011:812182; Brcic V, Eberdt C, Kaczorowski J. Corrigendum to

"development of a tool to identify poverty in a family practice setting: a pilot study." Int J Family Med 2015; 2015:418125.

4 For a review of the definitions and implications of "sensitivity" and "specificity," please see Shreffler J, Huecker MR. Diagnostic testing accuracy: sensitivity, specificity, predictive values and likelihood ratios. In: StatPearls [Internet]. Treasure Island (FL): StatPearls Publishing; 2024 Jan [updated 6 Mar 2023]. Available from: https://www.ncbi.nlm.nih.gov/books/NBK557491/.

5 Sokol R, Austin A, Chandler C, et al. Screening children for social determinants of health: a systematic review. Pediatrics. 2019;144(4):e20191622. See also Purkey E, Bayoumi I, Coo H, et al. Exploratory study of "real world" implementation of a clinical poverty tool in diverse family medicine and pediatric care settings. Int J Equity Health. 2019;18:200. https://doi.org/10.1186/s12939-019-1085-0.

6 Garg A, Boynton-Jarrett R, Dworkin PH. Avoiding the unintended consequences of screening for social determinants of health. JAMA. 2016; 316(8):813–14.

7 Community Legal Education Ontario (CLEO) Connect. Detecting legal problems [Internet]. Toronto: CLEO; 2024 [cited January 2025]. Available from: https://cleoconnect.ca/wp-content/uploads/2024/11/1.-Detecting-legal-problems5Nov2024.pdf.

8 Marple K. Framing legal care as health care [Internet]. Washington (DC): National Center for Medical-Legal Partnership; 2015 [cited Oct 2020]. Available from: https://medical-legalpartnership.org/mlp-resources/messaging-guide/.

9 Ahn J. Turning 65 and owing child support [Internet]. Toronto: Neighbourhood Legal Services; 2021 [cited 24 Feb 2023]. Available from: http://www.nlstoronto.org/blog/turning-65-and-owing-child-support.

10 See, for example, *New Brunswick (Minister of Health and Community Services) v. G. (J.)*, in which the Supreme Court of Canada ruled that indigent parents have a right to state-funded counsel in child protection cases (*New Brunswick [Minister of Health and Community Services] v. G. [J.]*, [1999] 3 SCR 46).

11 National Center for Medical Legal Partnership. Partnerships [Internet]. Washington (DC): National Center for Medical Legal Partnership; 2025 [cited March 2025]. Available from: https:// medical-legalpartnership.org/partnerships/.

12 See, for example, Zuckerman B, Sandel M, Lawton E, Morton S. Medical-legal partnerships: transforming health care. Lancet. 2008; 372(9650):1615–17.

13 See, for example, Murphy C. Making the case for medical-legal partnerships: An updated review of the evidence [Internet]. Washington (DC): National Center for Medical Legal Partnership; October 2020 [accessed October 2020]. Available from: https://medical-legalpartnership

.org/evidence-of-mlp-impact/, and Beardon S, Woodhead C, Cooper S, et al. International evidence on the impact of health-justice partnerships: a systematic scoping review. Public Health Rev. 2021;42:1603976. https:// doi.org/10.3389/phrs.2021. Beardon et al. conclude that "there is strong evidence that HJPs: improve access to legal assistance for people at risk of social and health disadvantage; positively influence material and social circumstances through resolution of legal problems; and improve mental wellbeing. A wide range of other positive impacts were identified for individuals, services and communities" (p. 1).

14 Pai N, Miller W, Chapman LA, et al. Tipping the scales: a lawyer joins the health care team. Paediatr Child Health. 2011;16(6):336. https:// doi.org/10.1093/pch/16.6.336.

15 Drozdzal G, Shoucri R, Macdonald J, et al. Integrating legal services with primary care: the health justice program. Can Fam Physician. 2019 Apr;65(4):246–48.

16 See, for example, Justice and Health Partnerships. Why are we promoting justice & health [Internet]. Belleville (ON): Community and Advocacy Legal Centre; n.d. [cited 24 February 2023]. Available from: https:// communitylegalcentre.ca/jhp/.

17 National Center for Medical-Legal Partnership. Resources [Internet]. Washington (DC): The Center; 2020 [cited October 2020]. Available from: https://medical-legalpartnership.org/resources. For example, see Marple K, Curran M, Lawton E, Rahajason D. Bringing lawyers onto the health center care team to promote patient & community health: a planning, implementation, and practice guide for building and sustaining a health center-based medical-legal partnership [Internet]. Washington (DC): The Center; 2020. Available from: https://medical-legalpartnership.org /download/health-center-toolkit/.

18 Health Justice Australia. Practice [Internet]. Sydney (NSW): Health Justice Australia; 2020 [cited October 2020]. Available from: https://www .healthjustice.org.au/practitioners/.

19 Beardon S. A brief guide to support the implementation of health justice partnerships [Internet]. London: Health Justice Partnership; 2023. Available from: https://www.ucl.ac.uk/health-of-public/sites/health_of_public /files/hjp_implementation_guide_digital.pdf.

20 Community Legal Education Ontario (CLEO). Clues to reliable legal information and sources for online legal information [Internet]. Toronto: CLEO; 2024 [cited January 2025]. Available from: https://cleoconnect.ca /tools-tips/tip-sheets-and-referral-information/.

21 Technically, there are no exceptions to solicitor–client privilege, but a lawyer may breach it if they reasonably believe someone's life is imminently in danger. See section 3.3-3 of Law Society of Ontario. Rules

of professional conduct [Internet]. Toronto: Law Society of Ontario; 2000 [amended October 2014]. Available from: https://lso.ca/about-lso /legislation-rules/rules-of-professional-conduct/chapter-3.

22 Community Advocacy & Legal Centre. Legal health check-up [Internet]. Belleville (ON): The Centre; 2022. Available from: https:// communitylegalcentre.ca/tcodownloads/legal-health-awareness-poster/.

2 Law 101: An Introduction to the Canadian Legal and Constitutional Framework for Health Care Providers

BETH BILSON

All of us, including health care professionals, carry out our activities within a web of legal rules and obligations. We may not be conscious of this all the time, or even know in detail what legal restraints and obligations bind us, but we still tend to stop at red lights, refrain from breaking our neighbours' windows, and pay our taxes.

In this chapter, I describe some of the major elements of the constitutional and legal framework within which Canadians live their lives. It is clearly impossible in this space to provide a complete manual laying out all the legal and regulatory requirements that are relevant to those who work in the health care sector. Although I allude to some of these requirements, the primary focus here is on human rights and equality law, and I conclude with some practical advice for health care providers who play an advocacy role for patients with disabilities seeking accommodations where they work, study, or access services.

The law clearly intersects with the provision of health care in many ways. If Jessica comes to you in tears because she thinks she might lose her job if she falls ill; if Malalai tells you that she is thinking she will have to leave her husband, but she is not sure what effect that will have on her immigration status; or if Kim says that she thinks her boss fired her from her customer service job because she is transgender, all of these scenarios invoke legal and constitutional principles that may affect the possible options for addressing them.

The Canadian Constitution, Written and Unwritten

Many of Canada's constitutional ideas can be traced to a version of constitutional monarchy that was solidified in the United Kingdom in the seventeenth century, and they are thus firmly rooted in an inherently colonial paradigm. Under this constitutional model, the unilateral authority of the monarch is constrained by the decisions made in a parliament that represents the people. This representation takes a dual form, because the British Parliament includes the House of Commons, in which membership is determined by the electorate, and the House of Lords, whose members represent historic religious and economic interests. The British constitution has not taken a comprehensive written form but is found scattered through a variety of public documents and judicial decisions, as well as in customary ways of making decisions.

When Canada was being established through the joining of four British colonies in 1867, the constitutional arrangements that would govern the new confederation were articulated in the *British North America Act, 1867*,[1] a statute of the British Parliament. This statute, among other things, laid out the shape and membership of the Parliament of the new dominion. This Parliament would have a House of Commons composed of elected members and an analogue to the House of Lords in the Senate, which would represent regional rather than historic interests.

The *British North America Act* also allocated jurisdiction for the federal and provincial governments; within their own specified areas of jurisdiction, the provinces were to exercise complete, rather than subordinate, authority. Although health care was not specifically mentioned, the provinces were given authority over the establishment of hospitals and asylums, property and civil rights, and matters of a local or private nature. These authorities were ultimately interpreted as conferring jurisdiction over most health care to the governments of the provinces. In the ongoing process of give and take that has characterized federal–provincial relations, the authority of the provinces over health care has continued to be respected, although limited authority has been recognized for the federal government to establish national standards and principles to ensure that health care is uniformly accessible and of an acceptable calibre.

In the 1970s, there was growing momentum behind the idea of "patriating" the Canadian constitution. The *British North America Act* was, after all, a British statute, and it could only be amended by the British Parliament. Negotiations both within Canada and between Canada and the United Kingdom led the British Parliament to pass the *Canada Act 1982*,[2] which transferred jurisdiction over the Canadian constitution to Canada. Enacted as Schedule B to this act was the *Constitution Act, 1982*,[3] which incorporated many of the provisions of the *British North America Act*, described the history of amendments and revisions since 1867, and provided a process for future constitutional amendment.

The other – and totally new – part of the *Constitution Act, 1982*, was the *Canadian Charter of Rights and Freedoms*.[4] Canada had had since 1960 a *Bill of Rights* setting out fundamental rights and freedoms,[5] but it was a federal statute; it was subject to amendment or even repeal and did not enjoy constitutional status. Including an entrenched charter of rights in the constitution was controversial. Because the interpretation and enforcement of the rights in the *Charter* would be done through the courts, some premiers and other commentators saw it as enlarging the powers of appointed judges at the expense of elected legislatures.

The *Charter* protected several fundamental freedoms – speech, assembly, association, and conscience – and articulated a number of rights. Some of these were procedural rights, such as the right to a fair and speedy trial or the prohibition of unreasonable search and seizure. The *Charter* also laid out democratic rights, such as the right to vote, and rights related to mobility. Other parts of the *Charter* were designed to protect citizens from discrimination, most notably the equality provisions of section 15, which has perhaps given rise to more interpretive effort than any other part of the *Charter*; this section reads as follows:

1. Everyone has the right to equality before the law and to equal protection of the law without discrimination because of race, national or ethnic origin, colour, religion, age or sex.
2. This section does not preclude any law, program or activity that has as its object the amelioration of conditions of disadvantaged persons or groups.

Other sections of the *Charter* were aimed at reinforcing the rights of women, Indigenous people, multicultural communities, and minority language groups.

Several general features of the *Charter* should be noted. The first of these is that section 52(1) declares the *Charter* to be the "supreme law of the land" and permits the courts to find any law or action inconsistent with it to be "of no force and effect." The enumerated rights and freedoms are thus given first priority, and the *Charter* becomes the primary lens through which all other statements of legal requirements or limitations are viewed.

The statements in the previous paragraph come with some caveats. One of these is that, despite the ring of universality in section 52(1), the *Charter* only applies to public actors. Statutes and regulations passed by Parliament and by provincial legislatures, and the decisions made by judges, statutory tribunals, or public officials, are all caught by the *Charter*; the actions of private entities, such as corporations or individuals acting as private citizens, are not. The line between "public" and "private" is sometimes hard to identify. Most hospitals and other health care organizations are treated as public actors, as are regulatory bodies of the professions (including those in the health sector). Universities, however, are usually treated as falling on the private side of the line.[6]

Another limitation on the reach of the *Charter* is contained in section 1, which states that the guarantees of rights and freedoms are subject to "such reasonable limits prescribed by law as can be demonstrably justified in a free and democratic society." Although, as can be imagined, the determination of what limits are reasonable in these terms is not an easy task, the basic principle is that the rights and freedoms of individuals cannot be absolute and that there may be occasions when a collective interest justifies placing limitations on how individuals are permitted to conduct themselves.

A final limitation on the sweep of the *Charter* is that contained in section 33, known as the "notwithstanding" clause. This provision permits legislatures to pass legislation that they know to infringe constitutional rights by including a statement that they are doing so notwithstanding the *Charter*. This provision was included at the behest of premiers concerned that unelected judges would use their power to interpret and apply the *Charter* to frustrate the legitimate goals of democratically elected governments. Supporters of the *Charter* feared that the clause would be invoked so broadly that it would render the protections in the *Charter* meaningless. In fact – perhaps because of the political risks associated with openly declaring that legislation is known to be inconsistent with constitutional rights – the notwithstanding clause has been used relatively rarely.

As shown here, Canada's written constitution contains two major elements: the legacy of the *British North America Act, 1867*, which sets out the respective jurisdictions of federal and provincial governments, the terms on which new provinces may be admitted to the federation, and the design of government institutions, and the newer *Charter of Rights and Freedoms*, which is now accompanied by a rich body of judicial and academic commentary and which has had an enormous impact on the way Canadians understand constitutional rights.

As the heading of this section suggests, Canada is also still governed by some unwritten constitutional principles, an inheritance of a British constitutional system that did not take the form of a single comprehensive document but grew and changed organically as legislators and courts articulated fundamental principles. The courts have recognized that such things as the independence of judges and the legal profession, the rule of law, the role of the Crown, and the expectations surrounding democratic processes still linger as constitutional principles.

Common and Civil Law

Under the terms of the federation of colonies articulated in the *British North America Act, 1867*, protection was given to certain religious, linguistic, and legal features that characterized what is now the Province of Quebec, and rights were also conferred on francophone residents of other provinces. The idea that constitutional status should be accorded to two founding cultures is being re-examined in light of the claims of Indigenous people to have their laws, languages, and cultural traditions similarly recognized, but biculturalism, bilingualism, and bijuralism have continued as a constitutional theme.

From the time that Britain gained control over the French colony of New France in 1763, the question of the degree to which the legal system inherited from France should be recognized and protected has continued to be an issue of debate.

The legal systems originating in Britain and France differ in important respects, and it is a significant feature of the Canadian legal system that both traditions continue to be part of the legal landscape. The British system of law is referred to as a common law system, and it is in place in many countries that are English speaking or were once part of the British Empire. Under the common law system, the principles of law emerge from the analysis by judges of the factual context in which events occur that become the subject of a legal dispute or challenge. The principles over time are continually refined and sharpened or differentiated in new factual settings. Judges are bound by earlier statements of principle in cases decided by judges who are superior to them in status, but it is always open to a judge to decline to apply a precedent decision that is based on some distinction between that decision and the case before them. Because of the way it operates, the common law is flexible, but change happens slowly, and the law is shaped by whatever cases are presented to judges, not by some coherent set of prior principles.

The system inherited from France is a civil law system, and systems of civil law, stemming from Roman law, are in place in most of the world's countries. Civil law is characterized by legal codes, statements of legal principle that are intended to anticipate and govern all law-related situations that may arise. In its current form in Canada, the central legal text is the *Civil Code of Québec*,[7] passed by the National Assembly in 1991. The role of judges is to interpret the *Civil Code* and to apply it to the factual situations before them.

These two systems have inevitably become intertwined to some extent, although it seems fair to say that the civil law system has had less impact on the common law system than the reverse. From the outset of British rule, the British government saw French criminal law as inferior to British criminal law, and it ordered that the latter prevail in the new colony of Quebec. Over time, principles of public law directed at the decisions of public officials were also made uniform across the country. Federal statutes and regulations apply to Quebec as they do to other provinces, although the operation of federal–provincial relations has meant that some of these statutes include exemptions or modifications with respect to their application.

Although the traditional common law system was founded almost entirely on legal principles invented by judges, in any modern society statute law plays an increasingly important role in defining legal entitlements and obligations. The law relating to the status of immigrants and refugees, for example, is almost entirely dependent on statutes. Like civil law judges, common law judges spend more and more of their time articulating and applying canons of statutory interpretation, and in this respect their tasks are comparable with those performed by civil law judges.

Notwithstanding the similarities between the two systems, and the leakage of common law features into the law in Quebec, the civil law system continues to be distinct and robust, particularly in areas of private law, such as property law, family law, and the law of commercial affairs.

Influence of International Law

After the horrors of World War II and the founding of the United Nations, many countries dedicated themselves to creating a regime of international law that would advance the dignity and welfare of all human beings. The *Universal Declaration of Human Rights*,[8] adopted by the United Nations in 1948, was a statement of basic human rights – rights to be treated without discrimination; to be granted due legal process; to enjoy freedom of thought, expression, assembly, and association; to engage in cultural participation; and so on. The *Declaration* also stated that education, economic security, and access to health care and social programs are basic human rights. Many, although not all, of these rights and freedoms would be familiar to readers of Canada's *Bill of Rights* from 1960 or of the more recent *Charter of Rights and Freedoms*.

In the 1960s, these rights and freedoms were elaborated in the *International Covenant on Civil and Political Rights* and the *International Covenant on Economic, Social and Cultural Rights*.[9] The signatories of the former of these, including Canada, signalled their determination to provide protection for people around the world from discrimination, exclusion from public and political processes, unfair legal procedures, and practices such as slavery. Again, the *Charter* reflects a commitment on the part of Canada as a nation to many of the rights and freedoms listed in the *International Covenant on Civil and Political Rights*.

Canada was also a signatory to the *International Covenant on Economic, Social and Cultural Rights*. As the title suggests, this covenant was far less about participation in a political or legal system and more about how people lead their daily lives. This covenant characterized housing, access to health care, education, social and economic security, family life, work, and economic resources, among other things, as human rights that ought to be available to everyone. Unlike the rights contained in the *International Covenant on Civil and Political Rights*, few of the rights outlined in the *International Covenant on Economic, Social and Cultural Rights* are contained in the *Charter*.

One of the features of international legal instruments is that, with few exceptions, they cannot be directly enforced; their implementation is dependent on passage of legislation by signatory governments in their own jurisdiction. In the case of Canada, the constitutional structure means that it is possible for the federal government to sign on to an international accord without being able to require any government to pass the necessary implementation legislation. The natural criticism of this arrangement is that it makes it easy for Canada to establish a positive reputation by supporting international instruments while knowing that they will likely have no concrete results in Canada itself. In the case of the *International Covenant on Economic, Social and Cultural Rights*, programs to advance most of the rights outlined would fall under the jurisdiction of the provinces over health, education, labour, and property matters.

The inability of the Government of Canada to make international commitments that it can be sure will be implemented in Canada does not mean that international law has had no influence on the evolution of Canadian law. Canadian courts, notably the Supreme Court of Canada, have increasingly drawn on international agreements as a source of moral and interpretive support for decisions on many issues, including extradition, the protection of children, and the status of refugees. In the case of *Baker v Canada (Minister of Citizenship and Immigration)*,[10] for example, the Supreme Court held that a decision to deport Ms. Baker to her country of origin was unreasonable in part because it did not take into account the rights of her children under the United Nations *Convention on the Rights of the Child*.[11] The use of international commitments by Canada has been used to bolster liberal interpretations of rights contained in the *Charter* and in Canadian legislation.[12]

However, the courts have until recently shown little inclination to venture to make constitutional interpretations that would support the recognition of social or economic rights.[13] They have resisted efforts to use the equality provisions in section 15 of the *Charter* where claims are based on differential access to social programs or where upholding the claims would necessitate a significant investment on the part of a government.[14] They have generally explained this as legitimate deference to governments whose extensive fiscal responsibilities require them to make hard choices about funding and who are answerable to the public for the policy priorities they choose. Later in this chapter, I touch on the fairly recent decision of a senior Canadian court (although not the Supreme Court) that may or may not be a sign that this posture of the courts is undergoing a change.

Indigenous Rights

It is not possible here to describe in detail the many ways in which Canadian governments and Canadian society have failed Indigenous people. The history of economic neglect; refusal to recognize legitimate aspirations for self-determination; failure to provide adequate health care, education, and social services; and obliviousness to the toll taken by racism and practices founded in colonialism are well known. Please see chapter 3 for an Indigenous perspective on wellness, law, and medicine and how colonialism has undermined the well-being of Indigenous people and communities.

This chapter attempts to explain how Indigenous rights are understood in the Canadian legal framework, as limited as that may be. It is perhaps useful to make a brief digression here regarding terminology. There has been much discussion in recent decades about what is the appropriate nomenclature to use. At the time the *Charter* was being formulated, the term *Aboriginal* was in use to include First Nations, Métis, and Inuit people. *Indian* was the term used specifically to refer to First Nations people as defined in the *Indian Act*.[15] Because under the *British North America Act, 1867* – incorporated into the *Constitution Act, 1982* – the federal government has jurisdiction over "Indians and lands reserved for Indians," the issue of who falls in the category of "Indians" has continued to be significant. The answer to that question may be affected by whether a person continues to live on a reserve, whether they marry someone who has not been classified as Indian, and whether they are male or female; these issues have all been a source of debate and controversy. The term *Indigenous* is used more commonly now to place Canada's Indigenous people in the context of an international community and to recognize the diversity of Indigenous cultures and identities.

Indigenous organizations and allies pressed strongly for the recognition of Indigenous rights in the *Charter*, and two provisions were included that expressly protected historic Indigenous rights.

Section 25 of the *Charter* contains the following statement:

> 25. The guarantee in this Charter of certain rights and freedoms shall not be construed so as to abrogate or derogate from any aboriginal, treaty or other rights or freedoms that pertain to the aboriginal peoples of Canada.

This provision guarantees recognition of both historic and traditional rights and rights that may be acquired through mechanisms such as land claims agreements. Although this section speaks to the priority of Aboriginal rights in the *Charter* itself, section 35 of the *Constitution Act, 1982* (of which the *Charter* is a part), reiterates this guarantee as part of the new constitutional order. In combination with the equality guarantees in section 15, these statements of Indigenous rights have been the foundation of new approaches to issues involving Indigenous people. The wheels of the common law system move slowly, and there are many who are critical of the pace and range of the efforts of courts, governments, and other players to effect necessary change. Nonetheless, the constitutional changes of 1982 are, at least in part, responsible for movement in the direction of making room for Indigenous culture, languages, knowledge, and legal traditions in public discussion and decision-making. The recognition by the Supreme Court of Canada of a duty to consult Indigenous people about proposed projects or programs that will affect their land or their communities, for example, has led to the inclusion of this kind of consultation as a matter of course for resource companies and others planning major initiatives. A richer understanding of the nature of traditional Indigenous use of the land and of legal traditions surrounding concepts of property has emerged from the consideration of Indigenous claims in the context of the constitutional guarantees I have alluded to.

In their fight against historic discrimination, Indigenous organizations have also sought support in international forums. An international coalition of Indigenous people successfully pressed the United Nations to formulate the *Declaration on the Rights of Indigenous People* that was adopted in 2007.[16] At the time, Canada was one of four countries (the others being the United States, New Zealand, and Australia) voting against the *Declaration*. The representatives of Canada cited concerns about the implications of the language in the *Declaration* about

Indigenous claims to land and resources and about the broadness of the concept of consent. In 2021, the Government of Canada changed course, signing on to the *Declaration* and passing a statute, the *United Nations Declaration on the Rights of Indigenous Peoples Act*,[17] intended to bring the *Declaration* into force in Canada. The government declared a renewed commitment to pursuing policies that would build more fruitful relationships with Indigenous people. This wholesale adoption of an international instrument as part of Canadian law, although not unheard of, was an unusual occurrence.

A recent case concluded in the Federal Court of Canada in 2021 illustrates how Canadian courts are starting to draw together many approaches to addressing Indigenous issues – from international law, from Canadian human rights legislation and the *Charter*, and from Indigenous traditions and culture.[18] In 2007, the First Nations Child and Family Caring Society filed a complaint of discrimination against the federal government under the *Canadian Human Rights Act*.[19] The complaint alleged that the federal government's failure to adequately fund family services for First Nations children had led to the consignment of many of those children to foster care, with resulting estrangement from their communities and cultures and damage to their families.

In their representations before the Canadian Human Rights Tribunal, the First Nations Child and Family Caring Society drew on a variety of international instruments, including the *Convention on the Rights of the Child*; the *International Covenant on Economic, Social and Cultural Rights*; and the *Declaration on the Rights of Indigenous Peoples*. They also cited treaties and other commitments made by the Canadian government to Indigenous people.

In addition, they pointed to Jordan's Principle, which had been enshrined in a Parliamentary resolution in 2007. As discussed in more detail in chapter 11, Jordan's Principle arose from a case in which a First Nations child with complex medical needs had spent his entire short life in hospital; this was attributed to the dispute between various levels of government over whose responsibility it was to finance his transfer to specialized foster care. The resolution articulated the principle that the funding should be provided by whichever government agency was the point of first contact, and the ultimate question of responsibility for funding could be decided later.

The Canadian Human Rights Tribunal upheld the complaint of the First Nations Child and Family Caring Society, and this finding was approved in 2021 by the Federal Court of Canada when the decision was appealed. Although the federal government commenced an appeal to the Supreme Court of Canada, the parties were able to reach an agreement before the appeal was heard. Under the settlement agreement, the government agreed to invest $40 billion, partly to compensate individuals and families whose lives had been affected by existing policies and partly to improve child and family services for First Nations.

In October 2023, after a further period of negotiation between the federal government and the First Nations Child and Family Caring Society, a Federal Court judge approved the final settlement.[20] The terms of the settlement included $23 billion as compensation for families who had been adversely affected by the existing system and $20 billion to bring about reforms. The total amount slightly exceeded the sum originally awarded by the court.

Because the case was resolved before the Supreme Court had an opportunity to consider it, there is no way of knowing how the court would have reacted to a decision that seemed to be a significant departure from earlier cases in which the courts declined to interfere with fiscal decisions made by governments on the basis of human rights claims.

The other thing that should be noted is that the size of the sum committed by the federal government should allow First Nations communities to make meaningful progress on creating their own systems of child protection and family services. First Nations representatives and organizations have always seen this as crucial to their claim that they deserve recognition as a self-determining level of government, comparable with federal and provincial governments, with jurisdiction over specific issues.

The most recent development with respect to the child and family services settlement is the rejection of the settlement by the Assembly of First Nations on 24 October 2024. There has to date been no announcement of any renewal of negotiations aimed at a revised settlement.[21]

In the area of child and family services, as in other areas such as land claims, hunting and fishing rights, and resource agreements, it is hard to accurately assess what impact the *Charter* and international agreements have had on the legal recognition of the positive rights of Indigenous people and on their right to be treated without discrimination. It seems safe to say, however, that the articulation of rights in those documents have lent important support to the legal analysis that has resulted in increasing recognition of the claims of Indigenous people to historic and cultural identity, economic security, and political participation.

Human Rights Legislation and the Duty to Accommodate

In the early to mid-1970s, all Canadian jurisdictions, provincial and federal, passed human rights legislation prohibiting discrimination based on listed grounds, such as sex, race, and disability. Although the legislation varied from one jurisdiction to another, there were some common features.

Unlike the *Charter*, human rights legislation applies to the private sector as well as to public actors, and it specifically prohibits discrimination in many contexts, such as education, employment, provision of goods and services, and accommodation. Although human rights statutes are not part of the constitution as such, they have been described by the courts as "quasi-constitutional"; that is, other statutes and the actions of individuals or organizations should be assessed using these statutes as an interpretive tool. For example, the Supreme Court of Canada has suggested that labour arbitrators considering collective agreements between unions and employers should interpret those agreements as though the relevant human rights statutes were incorporated into them.

The common model put in place to enforce this legislation was composed of a human rights commission, as well as an adjudicative body known as a tribunal (or, in some provinces, a board of inquiry). Under this model, the human rights commission served as a gatekeeper, receiving, screening, and investigating complaints of discrimination. The commission might decide that a process of mediation would be appropriate for a complaint or that it should be referred to adjudication by a tribunal. If a complaint was referred to the tribunal, the human rights commission would represent the complainant during the proceeding.

Human rights legislation gives human rights tribunals power to order a range of remedies, including orders that the discrimination cease, orders that respondents engage in training, and orders that damages be awarded for harm to the dignity of the complainant.

When a person believes they have experienced discrimination, they should ideally receive legal advice as soon as possible because there are often strict deadlines for starting a human rights complaint. In many provinces, free public legal education resources on human rights are available online.[22] Some provinces have also publicly funded legal aid clinics or clinics associated with law schools that can offer free legal advice.[23] Individuals may also be able to obtain a referral to a lawyer who can provide brief summary advice for free or at a reduced cost through their provincial or territorial lawyer referral service.[24]

If the discrimination or harassment happened in an area that falls under federal jurisdiction, the Canadian Human Rights Commission (CHRC) is the appropriate place to start a complaint. The CHRC has online tools to help potential complainants determine whether it is the right forum for their complaint.[25] Most complaints related to housing, education, medical services, retail, and other service providers fall under provincial or territorial jurisdiction (although there are exceptions). Complaints that fall under provincial or territorial jurisdiction should be directed to the appropriate provincial or territorial human rights agency. These agencies are specialized bodies that adjudicate human rights disputes and enforce the jurisdiction's human rights statute. Some provinces and territories, as well as the federal human rights system, operate under a "gatekeeper" model, which means complaints are first assessed by an independent investigator at a human rights commission who decides whether the complaint is a valid human rights issue and can proceed to the tribunal. If a complaint is allowed to proceed, the tribunal may hold a hearing at which both sides present their case to an independent adjudicator. In other provinces and territories, complainants can make a complaint to the tribunal directly. In Ontario, it is also possible to bring a human rights claim in civil court if it accompanies another type of civil claim (e.g., wrongful dismissal).[26]

The other significant function laid out for human rights commissions was public education about human rights. The legislation of the 1970s was based on the premise – perhaps naive – that supplying the public with information about the harm done by discrimination would lead them to change their behaviour. The limited resources made available to human rights agencies made it difficult for those bodies to maintain a vigorous educational program; although human rights commissions still engage in educational activities, they have become a less prominent feature of the human rights regime over time.

Over the past several decades, the processes arising from complaints of discrimination before human rights tribunals, labour arbitrators, and the courts have generated a rich literature concerning the meaning and implications of discrimination and equality laws. Perhaps no product of these processes has had as much significance in the daily lives of Canadian workers, students, and consumers as the duty to accommodate.

Although there is no specific mention of the duty to accommodate in many human rights statutes or in the *Charter*,[27] the concept has been expressed as a corollary of the ideas of equality that have been articulated by the courts and human rights agencies. When human rights statutes and the *Charter* were first being interpreted, and equality was first being defined, the courts were faced with a choice between a concept of equality based on treating everyone the same (formal equality) and a concept of equality taking into account the inherent differences between people (substantive equality). The second of these has been the prevailing and most important influence on concrete ways of advancing equality as a value.

The idea of substantive equality supposes that people will come into any environment with differing capacities and that their backgrounds will have conferred on them a range of advantages and disadvantages – skills, capacities, and historic treatment. A regime of laws or actions that presumes all people to be the same – and able to derive equal benefit in any given situation – does not take into account those different capacities and levels of advantage. Only a concept of equality that recognizes that people are differently situated and makes some correction for that will put everyone on a genuinely equal footing.

The duty to accommodate represents a way of translating the grand idea of substantive equality into concrete strategies for accommodating people who are identified as experiencing one of the prohibited grounds of discrimination listed in human rights statutes or in the *Charter*. These grounds include sex, family status, religion, and sexual orientation, but it is the duty to accommodate disability that is likely to have the most relevance for physicians. I use disability as the example in the following outline of the duty to accommodate, but similar principles would apply to a complaint based on another ground, such as religion or family status.

Discrimination means unequal or different treatment causing harm. Only some types of unequal treatment are considered illegal discrimination. It may be helpful to think about illegal discrimination through this equation:

Social area + protected ground + negative outcome – defence = illegal discrimination.[28]

Each human rights law lists certain social areas in which it applies, such as services, housing, and employment. In every jurisdiction, human rights laws apply to the provision of health care services. Human rights laws do not apply outside of the areas listed in any given human rights statute, such as in private interpersonal interactions.

Each statute also lists certain protected characteristics, or grounds, that are protected from discrimination in each social area, such as race, ancestry, sexual orientation, gender identity, gender expression, age, family status, and disability. The protected grounds vary in each province or territory, and some grounds are protected only in a certain social area (e.g., record of offences is a protected ground in the Ontario *Human Rights Code* in the area of employment, but not in other social areas). General unfairness not connected to one of the listed grounds is not considered illegal discrimination. Human rights laws also prohibit harassment based on certain grounds in specific social areas. *Harassment* means engaging in a course of upsetting comment or conduct that is unwelcome.

To establish discrimination, a person must show, on a balance of probabilities (i.e., that it is more likely than not) that

- they have a protected characteristic;
- they experienced a negative outcome in a covered social area; and
- their protected characteristic was a factor in that negative outcome.

It is not necessary to prove that there was an intent to discriminate, only that there was a negative effect on the person claiming discrimination. There are certain defences that the person or organization accused of discrimination can raise if discrimination is proven (e.g., undue hardship, which is explained later).

Discrimination can be direct or indirect (called "adverse effect" discrimination). Both are prohibited under human rights law.

People may also face complex discrimination based on intersecting personal characteristics. An example of intersectional discrimination is found in a British Columbia case in which the human rights tribunal found that a hotel discriminated against an Indigenous woman by evicting her. Although they had other Indigenous guests and other female guests, the tribunal found that the hotel relied on particular stereotypes about an Indigenous woman renting a room alone (specifically, they assumed she was a sex worker) and found discrimination based on a combination of her race and sex.[29]

The *Canadian Charter of Rights and Freedoms* also prohibits discrimination. The *Charter* is part of the Constitution of Canada, the highest law of the land. It applies to all other laws passed by federal, provincial, and territorial governments and to all actions by the state. It does not apply to non-government actors unless they are carrying out a government program. The *Charter* protects certain fundamental rights. This includes the right, in section 15 of the *Charter*, to equality before and under the law, as well as to equal protection and equal benefit of the law, without discrimination based on various grounds. Some of these grounds are listed explicitly in the *Charter* (e.g., sex, race, religion, disability), but section 15 also includes other grounds that courts have determined are similar (e.g., sexual orientation).

In 2017, Statistics Canada calculated that 6.8 million people, or roughly 22 per cent of Canadians, have at least one disability that affects their daily activities.[30] Some of these effects are less serious than others, but these numbers make it clear that every group of people, however small, is likely to include someone with limited ability to participate in activities that are arranged on the premise that everyone will be equally abled.

All social actors – employers, businesses, educational institutions, providers of health care and other public services, governments, landlords, professional firms – are subject to the duty to accommodate and must seek ways of ensuring that persons who have physical, psychological, or cognitive disabilities can work, study, or obtain goods and services on an equal footing with others. Human rights adjudicators, labour arbitrators, and judges have interpreted the concept of the duty to accommodate as imposing serious obligations on those who provide employment or services, obligations that are only exhausted if they occasion undue hardship. As a defence to a complaint that an employer or service provider has discriminated by not appropriately accommodating a disability, what is put forward as undue hardship must be more than inconvenience or the need to make complicated changes; *undue hardship* refers to expense, organizational adjustments, or effects on other people that are so significant that it would be unreasonable to ask an employer or service provider to undergo them. Thus, for example, it may be expected that an employer will reconfigure job duties for a disabled employee so it is possible for them to perform effectively, to move an employee to a different part of the workplace or renovate the space they work in, to invest in modifications of machinery, or to negotiate with a union to deviate from provisions of a collective agreement. An employer would not be expected, however, to create a whole new job for an employee, to provide them with busy work that does not make a meaningful contribution to the enterprise, or to permit unlimited absences from work. See Table 2.1 for some distinguishing features a tribunal may consider if the requested accommodation would lead to undue hardship.

As the understanding of the duty to accommodate has evolved, there has been an increase in the extent to which employers and service providers are expected to take positive steps to anticipate what employees, students, or clients may require to make full participation possible in the context of different kinds of disabilities.[31] In the case of some kinds of disabilities, such as those imposing restrictions on mobility, it is possible to make provisions that are generic – installing a wheelchair-accessible washroom, for example, will serve the needs of a number of employees and clients, present and future. It is important to note, however, that the duty is to accommodate individuals, not just take steps that will meet some lowest-common-denominator standard. A set of workplace arrangements, a program of study, or a health care plan must be tailored to give an individual disabled person the optimal opportunity to participate on a basis as close to equal as possible. The situations of persons with physical or psychological challenges are enormously

Table 2.1. Distinguishing Features Regarding Undue Hardship in Accommodations

Factors likely considered undue hardship	Factors likely not considered undue hardship
Excessive cost	High cost
Creation of new job	Significant modification of existing job or combination of parts of existing jobs
Absenteeism with no prospect of correction	Significant or erratic absenteeism
Construction of entire new working environment	Relocation of employee or renovation of working environment
Changes that affect other employees to an unacceptable degree	Changes that other employees can be expected to absorb to accommodate a co-worker
Renegotiation of major provisions of collective agreement	Negotiation of reasonable exceptions or waivers of collective agreement clauses for purposes of accommodation
Accepting all features of employee's preferred accommodation	Making good faith efforts to identify a reasonable package of accommodation measures

variable, and accommodative responses to them may be more or less complex. It is often relatively straightforward, for example, to devise an adequate accommodation for someone who will be recuperating from surgery for a limited time, whereas it may be more difficult to come up with a suitable plan for someone who is subject to periodic unpredictable bouts of psychiatric illness or who is dealing with a substance addiction.

The types of accommodation that may be considered are virtually limitless, although some common responses to disability can be given as examples. An educational institution, for example, may grant students with cognitive limitations more time to write exams, or it may use forms of assessment that do not entail a written examination. An employer may modify the duties assigned to employees so that they can avoid heavy lifting, alter the ventilation system to assist those with scent sensitivities, permit employees to take extra breaks or absences, or arrange their work environment so they have limited interaction with other employees. A court may arrange to have interpreters for persons with hearing impairments or permit advisors other than lawyers to be present in legal proceedings with participants who face psychological issues.[32]

The obligations imposed by the duty to accommodate are relevant to physicians in several ways. To start with, physicians themselves are under such a duty towards their employees and patients. In the settings in which they practice, physicians must be alert to any features of the physical space, the procedures they use, or the protocols they lay down that will constitute barriers for persons with different forms of disability. Ensuring that there is elevator access to an office, that patients who experience acute stress in the presence of others can be placed in a quiet space, or that arrangements are made to provide oral versions of documentation or print-magnifying technology for employees with limited vision are all measures that can be anticipated as being necessary to accommodate employees or patients. It is a requirement of the duty to accommodate that those on whom the duty rests try to anticipate what kinds of limitations will be faced by people in their patient or employee populations. In addition, however, physicians must be prepared to devise accommodations that will meet conditions they may not have anticipated and to modify their procedures and spaces accordingly. It must be remembered that the standard of undue hardship is an onerous one, requiring imagination and serious effort to formulate a strategy for accommodation; only when it can be demonstrated that accommodation will impose unreasonable costs or disruption is the duty exhausted.

The other important role for physicians is as advocates for patients who are seeking to be accommodated by their employers, by their educational institutions, or by others providing them with goods and services. Judges and other adjudicators have placed an increasing burden on employers and others who have a duty to accommodate; they have viewed this duty as requiring proactive steps to identify those who require accommodation and to offer options to them. The person seeking accommodation also has a responsibility, however, which is to cooperate in the process of arriving at an appropriate accommodative regime. See the box for a summary of the responsibilities of each party.

Responsibilities in the Accommodation Process

The person with a disability is required to:

- make accommodation needs known to the best of their ability, preferably in writing, so that the person responsible for accommodation can make the requested accommodation
- answer questions or provide information about relevant restrictions or limitations, including information from health care professionals
- take part in discussions about possible accommodation solutions

- co-operate with any experts whose assistance is required to manage the accommodation process, or when an expert is required to provide more information about the disability
- meet agreed-upon performance standards and requirements, such as job standards, once accommodation is provided
- work with the accommodation provider on an ongoing basis to manage the accommodation process.

The accommodation provider is required to:

- be alert to the possibility that a person may need an accommodation even if they have not made a specific or formal request
- accept the person's request for accommodation in good faith, unless there are legitimate reasons for acting otherwise (i.e. do not assume a person is being dishonest because you do not perceive them to have a disability)
- get expert opinion or advice where needed (but not as a routine matter)
- take an active role in ensuring that alternative approaches and possible accommodation solutions are investigated, and canvass various forms of possible accommodation and alternative solutions
- keep a record of the accommodation request and action taken
- communicate regularly and effectively with the person, providing updates on the status of the accommodation and planned next steps
- maintain confidentiality
- limit requests for information to those reasonably related to the nature of the limitation or restriction, to be able to respond to the accommodation request
- consult with the person to determine the most appropriate accommodation
- implement accommodations in a timely way, to the point of undue hardship
- bear the cost of any required medical information or documentation (for example, the accommodation provider should pay for doctors' notes, assessments, letters setting out accommodation needs, etc.)
- bear the cost of required accommodation.

Source: This list is taken from part 8 of the Ontario Human Rights Commission. Policy on ableism and discrimination based on disability [Internet]. Toronto; The Commission; 2016. Available from: https://www3.ohrc.on.ca/sites /default/files/Policy%20on%20ableism%20and%20discrimination%20based%20 on%20disability_accessible_2016.pdf. Internal citations have been omitted.

In the case of persons with disabilities, this requires that an employee, student, or client provide enough medical information to make it possible to determine what accommodation might be required. Although employers or service providers are not entitled to have access to sensitive medical information or details about a diagnosis, they must have enough information about how an individual's performance is likely to be affected by their medical situation to support sensible decision-making about accommodation. They look to physicians for reliable information about what limitations on an individual's performance should be taken into account. It is difficult to assess the value of the individual's own account of what is required, and having expert input is important.

It is not helpful to the process of developing options for accommodation to have a physician provide a note that says something such as "This employee should avoid lifting heavy weights" or "This employee should be placed in a less stressful environment." An employer or service provider must consider many factors in devising an accommodation that will meet the needs of the person being accommodated, often for a long time, and the more information that can be brought to bear on this decision, the sounder the accommodation plan is likely to be.

It would be helpful if physicians reminded themselves of the following questions when drafting documents to support a request for accommodation:

- What is the nature of the limitations the patient faces because of the disability?
- How might these limitations affect particular tasks or duties to be performed by the patient?
- Is the disability permanent? If not, what would be the expected duration of the disability?
- Will the effects of the disability fluctuate over time?
- Will the limitations faced by the patient change over time, and how will those changes affect the patient's ability to perform tasks or duties?
- What kinds of events or experiences might trigger negative developments related to the disability?
- Will the patient require physical modifications to be made to a work or study space?
- What are the characteristics of a location that would be an optimal environment for the patient?
- Are there issues of safety that would be of concern in the patient's workplace, educational institution, or other environment?
- How will the patient's disability affect, or be affected by, interaction with other people?

- Is the disability such that it requires regular medical monitoring or testing? How can the patient's physician collaborate with the employer or service provider on this?
- Will the patient require absences from work or study, and, if so, what would be the likely length and frequency of these absences?
- What training might be necessary for the supervisors, instructors, or colleagues of the patient?
- What capacity does the patient have to manage the disability or anticipate changes?

The ideal situation would be one in which the patient's medical team could collaborate with representatives of the organization providing accommodation to the patient. In some cases, the patient may be able to retain their own lawyer, or they may be represented by a union, and it may be preferable for the physician to work through these representatives. It seems likely that this would result in an accommodation plan more directly suited to the needs of the patient, without the complications that arise from false starts and misunderstandings over the nature and implications of the disability. Being able to recruit expert medical input when the accommodation plan is being formulated would assist a patient trying to function in the world on an equitable footing and an employer or service provider trying in good faith to treat the patient fairly.

Throughout this text, you will find draft template letters regarding accommodation requests in specific scenarios; see, for example, the "Supporting People Living with HIV in Requesting Accommodation" section of chapter 10 for the application of these issues in the context of people living with HIV.

Access to Justice

In theory, the legal system is equally available to all Canadians as a mechanism for resolving their law-related problems and disputes. In practice, many people are unable to access the legal services they need at the times in their lives when they need them most. This is largely because, unlike health care, legal services are primarily provided by the private sector. Although there is considerable public investment in courts, administrative agencies, and law enforcement, there is very little public funding directed to legal representation.

Every jurisdiction has some form of public legal aid system. See Appendix 1 for a summary of the services available in each province and territory. These services are generally inadequately funded, and their eligibility requirements tend to exclude anyone whose income exceeds social assistance levels. In any case, the scope of these programs is often restricted to representation on criminal charges and some limited family law issues. People who need services for other kinds of legal issues – including immigration or refugee matters, family law issues, or property concerns – will find themselves unable to qualify for assistance from legal aid programs in most of Canada. Notably, in Ontario the community legal aid clinic system provides broader poverty law services relating to housing, immigration, and social assistance matters.

Most lawyers regard it as part of their professional obligation to provide some of their services pro bono, but this kind of service, as valuable as it is, cannot be expected to create a systematic or reliable foundation for a truly accessible legal system.

The rising costs of the private legal services on which most Canadians must rely have generated what many perceive to be a crisis in access to the legal system. In particular, two high-profile reports, one from the Canadian Bar Association and the other from the National Action Committee on Access to Justice in Civil and Family Matters,[33] outlined in harsh terms the problems that individuals and families have in obtaining legal representation for the most fundamental matters. These important reports have generated a national conversation about access to justice, and they have given rise to a number of experiments and innovations. Some lawyers have redefined themselves as "legal coaches" and work in partnership with their clients to find functions associated with legal proceedings that the clients can do for themselves.[34] Some provincial justice ministries have been experimenting with online dispute resolution forums as a means of lowering the costs of legal proceedings and making them more convenient for the participants,[35] or they have looked at ways to license practitioners, often referred to as paralegals, to perform a limited range of legal services. Although the COVID-19 pandemic was a dismal experience in many ways, it can be given some credit for accelerating the thinking of the courts and administrative tribunals about the possible uses of technology, and this may ultimately have some effect in making these fora more accessible to litigants. This is, of course, notwithstanding the deep digital divide we have also seen emerge – with low-income and older persons and persons with disabilities struggling to access legal processes that have gone online because of a lack of access to technology, Internet services, and digital know-how.

It should be noted that several projects are underway to train and support trusted intermediaries such as librarians and social workers to play a greater role in directing their patrons and clients to relevant legal information or services.[36] Health professionals themselves, particularly those who work in institutional contexts such as hospitals, may be suited to play a role as trusted intermediaries who could act as a channel for interactions between their patients and lawyers, employer representatives, government agencies, or community-based organizations that may have some involvement in the legal or human rights interests of the patient.

These initiatives are all worthwhile and are likely to make some contribution to improving the accessibility of the legal system. It is likely, however, that without dramatic changes in public policy – and levels of public investment – there will continue to be significant disparities in the degree to which the justice system is available and helpful to Canadians.

Parting Thoughts

I have tried in this brief space to describe the legal and constitutional framework in which physicians and other providers of health care carry out their professional responsibilities. I have in particular focused on the way that evolving constitutional and human rights regimes have transformed the obligations that rest on all of those who employ, train, shelter, or provide goods and services to others. Many of the actions of individuals and organizations in both the public and the private spheres are now assessed against a backdrop of robust interpretations of constitutional instruments and human rights legislation. These interpretations support the rights of all Canadians to be treated equally and to be free from discrimination, and they have been translated into requirements for concrete and continuing modifications of systems, facilities, and processes to move these aims forward. Those who provide health care are expected to be partners in these endeavours.

NOTES

1 *British North America Act, 1867*, 30–31 Vict c 3 (UK).
2 *Canada Act 1982* (UK), 1982, c 11.
3 *Constitution Act, 1982*, being Schedule B to the *Canada Act 1982* (UK), 1982, c 11.
4 *Canadian Charter of Rights and Freedoms*, Part I of the *Constitution Act, 1982*, being Schedule B to the *Canada Act 1982* (UK), 1982, c 11.
5 *Canadian Bill of Rights*, SC 1960, c 44.
6 See, for example, *University of Alberta Pro-Life v Governors of the University of Alberta*, 2020 ABCA 1; *Longueépée v University of Waterloo*, 2020 ONCA 830.
7 c 64 *CCQ (1980)*.

8 UN General Assembly, *Universal Declaration of Human Rights*, 10 December
   1948, 217 A (III).

9 UN General Assembly, *International Covenant on Civil and Political Rights*,
   19 December 1966, United Nations, Treaty Series, vol. 999; UN General
   Assembly, *International Covenant on Economic, Social and Cultural Rights*, 16
   December 1966, United Nations, Treaty Series, vol. 993.

10 *Baker v Canada (Minister of Citizenship and Immigration)*, 1999 CanLII 699
    (SCC), [1999] 2 SCR 817. Available from: https://canlii.ca/t/1fqlk.

11 UN General Assembly, *Convention on the Rights of the Child*, 20 November
    1989, United Nations, Treaty Series, vol. 1577.

12 For examples of Canadian courts referring to international accords
    and recognizing the impact of international tribunals, see *Saskatchewan
    Federation of Labour v Government of Saskatchewan*, 2015 SCC 4 (in reference
    to international agreements on labour rights); *Charles Chitat Ng v Canada*,
    CCPR/C/49/D/469/1991, United Nations Human Rights Committee, 7
    January 1994; and *Reference re Ng Extradition*, [1991] 2 SCR 858 (which both
    refer to proceedings concerning the extradition of an accused to the United
    States under circumstances in which he might face the death penalty).

13 *Canada (Attorney General) v First Nations Child and Family Caring Society of
    Canada*, which is discussed later, is an example of a different approach by
    a court (*Canada (Attorney General) v First Nations Child and Family Caring
    Society of Canada*, 2021 FC 969 [CanLII], [2022] 2 FCR 614. Available from:
    https://canlii.ca/t/jjblh).

14 Examples of this prior approach are *Auton (Guardian ad litem of) v British
    Columbia (Attorney-General)*, 2004 SCC 78, and *Gosselin v Québec (Attorney-
    General)*, 2002 SCC 84.

15 *Indian Act*, RSC 1985, c I-5.

16 UN General Assembly, *United Nations Declaration on the Rights of Indigenous
    Peoples*, resolution adopted by the General Assembly, 2 October 2007,
    A/RES/61/295.

17 *United Nations Declaration on the Rights of Indigenous Peoples Act*, SC 2021, c14.

18 *Canada (Attorney General) v First Nations Child and Family Caring Society of
    Canada*, 2021 FC 969 (CanLII), [2022] 2 FCR 614. Available from: https://
    canlii.ca/t/jjblh.

19 *Canadian Human Rights Act*, RSC 1985, c H-6.

20 Major D, Stefanovich O. Judge approves historic $23B First Nations child
    welfare compensation agreement. CBC News [Internet]; 2023 October 24.
    Available from: https://www.cbc.ca/news/politics/judge-approves-23
    -billion-first-nations-child-welfare-agreement-1.7006351.

21 Indigenous Services Canada. First Nations leadership vote on the final
    agreement to reform Child and Family Services [Internet]. Ottawa:
    Government of Canada; 18 October 2024. Available from: https://www

.canada.ca/en/indigenous-services-canada/news/2024/10/first-nations
-leadership-vote-on-the-final-agreement-to-reform-child-and-family
-services.html.

22 See Canadian Human Rights Commission. Other human rights agencies
[Internet]. Ottawa: The Commission; n.d. Available from: https://www.chrc
-ccdp.gc.ca/en/complaints/provincial-territorial-human-rights-agencies.

23 In Ontario, the HIV & AIDS Legal Clinic Ontario (HALCO; https://www
.halco.org) provides free legal services to people living with HIV in Ontario
on human rights and many other areas of law; BC Human Rights Clinic
(https://bchrc.net/) and Ontario's Human Rights Legal Support Centre
(http://www.hrlsc.on.ca).

24 See, for example, Manitoba Community Legal Education Association
(http://www.communitylegal.mb.ca/programs/law-phone-in-and
-lawyer-referral-program/), Law Society of Saskatchewan (https://www
.lawsociety.sk.ca/for-the-public/finding-legal-assistance-saskatchewan/),
and Law Society of Ontario (https://lso.ca/public-resources/finding-a
-lawyer-or-paralegal). See also JusticeNet (https://www.justicenet.ca/) to
find lower-cost legal services.

25 Canadian Human Rights Commission. Complaints: am I in the right place
[Internet]. Ottawa: The Commission; n.d. [cited 20 July 2022]. Available
from: https://www.chrc-ccdp.gc.ca/en/complaints/am-i-the-right-place.

26 *Human Rights Code*, RSO 1990, c H19, s 46.1.

27 One exception is the *Ontario Human Rights Code*, RSO 1990, c H.19, ss 11
and 17.

28 Thank you to Community Legal Education Ontario for this helpful
framing of discrimination.

29 *Frank v AJR Enterprises Ltd. (c.o.b. "Nelson Place Hotel")*, (1993), 23 C.H.R.R.
D/228 (BCCHR).

30 Statistics Canada. New data on disability in Canada, 2017 [Internet]. Ottawa:
Statistics Canada; 2018 [modified 28 Nov 2018]. Available from: https://
www150.statcan.gc.ca/n1/pub/11-627-m/11-627-m2018035-eng.htm.

31 For a discussion of this positive obligation, see *British Columbia (Public
Service Employee Relations Committee) v British Columbia Government Service
Employees' Union (Meiorin)*, [1999] 3 SCR 3.

32 For some examples of how the duty to accommodate is understood and
applied, see *Toronto District School Board v Canadian Union of Public Employees*,
2021 CanLII 55830 (ON LA); *Martin v Carter Chevrolet Oldsmobile*, 2001
BCHRT 37 (duty to inquire); *Fraser Health Authority v Health Employees'
Union*, 2019 CanLII 104261 (BC LA); and *Inland Kenworth v International
Union of Operating Engineers*, 2020 CanLII 89929 (BC LA) (continuing duty).

33 Canadian Bar Association. Reaching equal justice: an invitation to envision
and act. Ottawa: The Association; 2013, and National Action Committee

on Access to Justice in Civil and Family Matters. A roadmap for change. Ottawa: The Committee; 2013. See also Cromwell TA, Anstis S. The legal services gap: access to justice as a regulatory issue. Queen's LJ. 2016; 42(1).

34 See, for example, the website of Lana Wickstrom, a Saskatoon lawyer: https://www.lanawickstrom.com/.

35 For example, the online civil resolution tribunal in British Columbia (https://civilresolutionbc.ca/).

36 For example, the work of the Saskatchewan Access to Legal Information project housed in the CREATE Justice centre at the University of Saskatchewan (https://www.lawsociety.sk.ca/initiatives/access-to -justice/saskatchewan-access-to-legal-information/). See also Law Foundation of Ontario. Trusted help: the role of community workers as trusted intermediaries who help people with legal problems [Internet]. Toronto: Law Foundation of Ontario; 2018. Available from: https:// lawfoundation.on.ca/download/part-1-trusted-help-the-role-of -community-workers-as-trusted-intermediaries-who-help-people-with -legal-problems-2018/.

3 Health, Law, and Indigenous People

CHRISTA BIG CANOE AND SUZANNE SHOUSH

This chapter is designed to provide context for how Indigenous people experience health care, including the adversity and discrimination that occur in health systems and delivery of health services in Canada.

The context is intended to highlight the strength of Indigenous communities and practices, not just to focus on the deplorable health outcomes experienced by many Indigenous people. Covering some of the worst examples of how the health care system is failing Indigenous populations is necessary to develop the context of why change is required to improve systems and provide the knowledge and awareness to do better. It is our hope that the message this chapter makes clear is that knowledge of Indigenous people and their culture, practices, and solutions are key to ensuring equitable, fair, and better outcomes for Indigenous people who seek health care in Canada.

Note that this context-setting chapter on Indigenous health perspectives lays the groundwork for many of the chapters in this text. Chapters 9 and 11 include Indigenous co-authors. Sara Mainville, Douglas Varrette, Caitlyn E. Kasper, and Kate Forget provide their perspectives as Indigenous people in chapters 5, 6, 8 and 12, respectively. Two Indigenous reviewers also provided feedback on chapter 10.

We are two professional Indigenous women, one who practices medicine and one who practices law. In our own lived experience, we have faced racism, discrimination, and inequitable treatment and therefore speak from a place of truth. We are also both dedicated advocates for change who have used our expertise to promote understanding, demand equitable treatment of Indigenous people in health care, and seek health justice for Indigenous people. Our goals in writing this chapter are to provide an overview of Indigenous understandings of wellness, law, and medicine and to discuss the context of racism against Indigenous people in the health care system and ways to promote anti-racist approaches and best practices moving forward.

The first point to highlight is that there is a diversity of Indigenous people in Canada. When we use the term *Indigenous*,[1] we include First Nations, Inuit, and Métis people. This chapter does not delve into the nuances and history of each of these distinct groups. We encourage you to learn more about each group and to specifically learn about the Indigenous people who originate or reside in the area in which you practice medicine and health care. Knowledge of Indigenous people in the territory wherein you are practicing is crucial to learning how to provide better health care and combat stereotypes, systemic racism, and misapprehensions about the circumstances of any Indigenous patients you may be serving.

The parts in this chapter have both Anishinabemowin and English headings.[2] In each part we explain the Anishinaabe (Ojibwe) words. We hope that this demonstrates that plurality of beliefs and practices can coincide successfully, but we also do this to recognize the language of one of the original peoples in the territory we are writing from and do our work in.

This chapter is designed to raise issues and topics as a foundation of knowledge and context and does not deeply explore each area. It covers the following topics:

1. *Mino Bimaadiziwin – the good life through Indigenous law and medicine*: In this section, we explain fundamental Indigenous world views of Indigenous law and medicine. We situate the way in which Indigenous people approach wellness and how they work towards or try to walk the road of "the good life."
2. *Maanadamon, Bibikwadamon – the reality*: This section looks at the realities that Indigenous people have historically and currently experience in terms of health outcomes and measurements and what impacts colonial interference has created. It discusses the resounding imprint this interference has left on Western health care.
3. *Qwayakotam – hear the truth*: In this section, we use real case studies and experiences to highlight the issues of systemic harm towards Indigenous people and the cost to health and life racism causes Indigenous people.
4. *Aandaakonige – changing practices*: Here we address how Indigenous practices in medicine and law, along with supporting Indigenous-based practices, are integral to ensuring substantive equity in health access and promotion of wellness. We also discuss the need for accountability. Accountability to Indigenous patients must occur

across all health services on the part of each practitioner and each institution in the entire health and wellness system.

Mino Bimaadiziwin – The Good Life through Indigenous Law and Medicine

According to the *Ojibwe People's Dictionary*, *mino bimaadiziwin* translates to "the good life" in English.[3] The phrase that captures this philosophy is "to live the good life." For the Anishinaabe, it is part of being and part of our laws. Elder Benson Benai would explain that living the good life is a gift that we have all received, but throughout our lives it is a choice. The choice to live and follow the principles of *mino bimaadiziwin* has been interrupted by colonial practices and marginalization of Indigenous people, but there continue to be people and communities who practice these laws, and a large resurgence in implementing these laws and principles is happening. In his article, *Anishinaabe Inaakonigewin: Principles for the Intergenerational Preservation of Mino Bimaadiziwin*, Kekek Jason Stark explains,

> The foundational principles embedded in Anishinaabe law are derived from the ancestral link tying together the generations through language, traditional stories, and our continuous inter-relationship with the earth. In this process it has established how these foundational principles of Anishinaabe law are utilized to live a good life in harmony with all of creation and how the seven sacred laws of the creation – the seven grandfather teachings consisting of the principles of wisdom, love, respect, bravery, honesty, humility, and truth are utilized as foundational values for achieving harmony and implementing Anishinaabe law principles.[4(p. 337)]

If we break down this statement, we can see how Anishinaabe *Inaakonigewin* (law) guides the wellness of each person, community, and all creation. First, the foundational principles embedded in Anishinaabe law are derived from the ancestral link tying together the generations through language, traditional stories, and our continuous inter-relationship with the earth. We believe that the lessons of those who came before us are instructive in living healthy and respectful ways. We need to teach our own and future generations about these practices and understandings to achieve a good life. Loss of language, through assimilative policies and genocidal practices, such as forcibly removing children from their families, languages, and cultures,[5] has been the biggest interruption to Indigenous people being able to practice *mino bimaadiziwin*.

Second, these foundational principles of Anishinaabe law are used to live a good life in harmony with all creation. Our law instructs us to treat ourselves and others in a way that respects life and creation. This is a holistic approach that is gaining more and more uptake by health practitioners. More recently, Western medicine has recognized that a person's health goes beyond physical wellness and treatment of illness and also includes internal factors such as mental wellness and external factors such as the reciprocal affective relationship between the person's health and the health of the environment.

Third, the Seven Sacred Laws of creation, often referred to as the seven grandfather teachings, consist of the principles of wisdom, love, respect, bravery, honesty, humility, and truth, and they are used as foundational values for achieving harmony and implementing Anishinaabe law principles. If these same laws and principles governed all interactions between patients and health providers, not only would there be better relationships, there would also be an acknowledgment that this more holistic approach can achieve better outcomes that could address the distrust between Indigenous people and the health care system.

John Borrows and Aaron Mills explain in *Revitalizing Anishinaabe Inaakonigewin (Law): Aadizookaanag Biboon* that

Anishinaabe law has long looked to the natural world to understand how to live better as human beings. Lessons about how to encourage and regulate behavior and resolve disputes, as learned from the natural environment are embedded in stories, language, songs, ceremonies, treaties, and community stories.[6]

To understand Indigenous perspectives on health and wellness, it is important to understand that most Indigenous cultural and belief systems see the person as a whole being situated in all creation of the living world. This means that all aspects of being are interconnected with one another internally in each person, and each person is also interconnected with all other living things. Internal connection and being has four components: Spirit/Spiritual, Mind/Mental, Physical/Body, and Emotion/Emotional. This can be seen in medicine wheels, which have quadrants that represent both internal and external connections. Figure 3.1 is an example of a basic medicine circle diagram (Anishinaabe wheel).

For Indigenous people there is an inseparable connection between law and medicine. For example, *minaadendamowin*, or the law of respect for self and others, one of the seven sacred teachings, requires us to see the relationships among all living things and to understand the independence, reliance, and reciprocal nature of every relationship.

Figure 3.1. A Basic Medicine Circle Diagram (Anishinaabe Wheel)

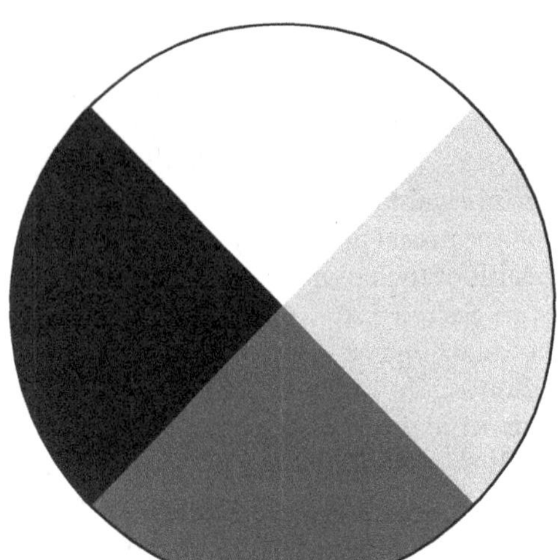

Traditional Indigenous practices in both law and medicine are part of the solution to providing anti-racist approaches to health services. Recognizing the value of holistic Indigenous approaches to well-being and living the good life will combat racism, stereotypes, assumptions, and dangerous practices that undervalue Indigenous health, wellness, and lives.

Maanadamon, Bibkwadamon – The Reality

According to the *Ojibwe People's Dictionary*, *maanadamon* translates to "it (road or trail) is bad, is poor,"[7] and *bibikwadamon* translates to "it is a bumpy road" (see note 4).[8] These phrases encapsulate philosophies and Indigenous perspectives about how life is treated as a pathway, such as a road, river, or trail, and those pathways can be bad, poor, and bumpy. In reality road blockages have occurred and trails have been burned down because of the imposition of colonial laws, policies, and systems, including health care systems. The reality is that the way Indigenous people are treated in health care is appalling.

When we look at practices of Western medicine on Turtle Island (the Americas), we see exclusion; unfair distribution of resources; refusal to provide services or unequal provision of services; services geographically distant from the populations that require assistance; and, most tragically, a history in which modern medicine has used Indigenous people as test subjects for research in the advancement of disease treatment and pharmaceutical medicines. Medical colonialism is the systematic harm inflicted by health care providers and the health care system on Indigenous people and entire Indigenous communities. This includes Indian hospitals; the intentional spreading of infectious diseases, such as smallpox and tuberculosis, as a strategy to clear land for settlement; forced or coerced sterilization of Indigenous women and girls; and large-scale nutritional experiments conducted without consent on entire communities. This is in addition to the large-scale medical violence conducted against Indigenous children throughout the Indian residential school system (IRSS) and the role that health care providers have played and continue to play in the Sixties Scoop[9] and in removing Indigenous children from their families on the basis of medical assessments of lack of fitness to parent. These events are not so far in the past as to be outside the consciousness of Indigenous people. In fact, Indigenous people continue to face discrimination and assumptions even when accessing basic medical assistance.[10]

Since colonization there has been a purposeful, systematic violation of the fundamental rights of Indigenous people. Institutions, policies, laws, markets, and entire structures of governance have been established to benefit colonial life and values at the deliberate exclusion and expense of Indigenous life and values. This has led to a centuries-long process of devaluing Indigenous life. Anti-Indigenous racism and associated negative stereotyping of Indigenous people remains insidious and inescapable in Canada.[11]

It is not surprising that Indigenous people distrust a system that was not created with their interests in mind. Indeed, the very concepts of social determinants of health (SDOHs) do not include an Indigenous vision of wellness, nor do they factor in key elements required for an Indigenous person to feel healthy. There has been little room for Indigenous concepts and practices of wellness, including using food to heal, traditional herbal medicines, and respect and reciprocity for and with the earth and all our relations (human, animal, plant, and natural), nor for the critical importance of kinship, language, and ceremony. Often these practices have been ridiculed as simple or ineffective approaches to medicine that do not have any true healing value. Ironically, we are seeing a shift towards holistic practices for the whole well-being of individuals, but assumptions remain from a Western point of view that Indigenous practices are not helpful or are nonsensical.

What is most troubling is that anti-Indigenous racism and institutional racism prevail in Canadian health care systems, with long-standing stereotypes about the prevalence of alcoholism and substance use disorders among and poor health choices of Indigenous people that are void of the recognition of the historical impacts these discriminatory systems have created.[12] Both historical and existing racism cause harm to Indigenous people, and each health professional should acknowledge that "racism and intersecting forms of discrimination shape Indigenous peoples' experiences in the health care system, and must be considered determinants of health for Indigenous peoples."[13(p. 4)]

A starting point is to learn the history of the treatment of Indigenous people in Canada and then take an anti-racist approach to providing services. Structures of racism rooted in Canadian law and policy have played a fundamental role in generating the health and social disparities seen today, including gaps in well-being, safety, and health.[14] Centuries of aggressive stereotyping were a key element of the devaluation of Indigenous people so that settler colonialism could establish itself; these biases have been deeply woven into the fabric of Canadian society and culture. A pervasive belief that Indigenous people have inherently less value allowed land to be confiscated, children to be apprehended on a mass scale during the IRSS, and Indigenous people to face the alarming gaps in health outcomes still seen today. Learning about those structures and the impact they have is key to achieving better outcomes and better services for Indigenous people.

Structures of Racism – Law, Policy, and Institutional Practices of Harm

To understand anti-Indigenous racism in Canada, one must understand its colonial history. For some it is a challenge to understand why events that occurred many hundreds of years ago continue to affect lives and outcomes in the present day, yet this understanding is fundamental to understanding why Indigenous and non-Indigenous people have strikingly different privilege, power, influence, and societal outcomes.

THE LAW

Race and ethnicity are protected human rights grounds in Canada's Constitution and *Charter of Rights and Freedoms*,[15] along with various human rights codes in provinces and territories. One cannot legally discriminate against an individual on the basis of these traits. Of course, intentional acts of individual racism and hate are illegal and should never go ignored or uncorrected. Structural racism, however, is extremely nuanced. It undercuts all Canadian society, regardless of how "not racist" an individual is. It includes everything that perpetuated the current status quo, in which resource, wealth, power, influence, and health are hoarded in some communities and denied in others.

Structural racism is the outcome of historical cultural devaluation based on colonial stereotypes of Indigenous inferiority that were subsequently fashioned into laws ensuring settler rights and superiority. Racial segregation, absence of education about the dignity and rights of Indigenous people, and the whitewashing of crimes committed against Indigenous people throughout Canadian history has led to learned and ongoing social, political, and economic exclusion of Indigenous people from power.

Law and policies by the Canadian government and their colonial predecessors were designed to eliminate Indigenous people to clear lands to create the new Dominion and space for newcomers. Many of the laws are based on a foundation of racist theory that has long been debunked as inaccurate but was only recently addressed in a statement by the Catholic Church in March 2023 that repudiated the legal and political "doctrine of discovery."[16] The Prime Minister also acknowledged genocidal acts and practices during the ceremonial launch of the final report of the National Inquiry into Missing and Murdered Indigenous Women and Girls (MMIWG) in June 2019.[17] The National Inquiry into MMIWG also released a supplementary report on genocide.[18] For many years the language commonly used to describe law and policy about Indigenous people included the term *assimilation*. More recently there has been an uptake in understanding that the language of assimilation does not adequately characterize the acts against Indigenous people or the truth. *Genocide* more accurately describes how law, policy, and Canadian society have treated Indigenous people.

Despite recent acknowledgments, there are long-standing effects of law and policies that were built on eliminating Indigenous people. The legal concept of *terra nullus*, or "vacant lands," and the Doctrine of Discovery perpetuated colonial powers' ability to take up lands and displace Indigenous people and their basic rights. The Doctrine of Discovery provided a legal, ethical, and moral framework to legitimize the colonial powers' seizure and exploitation of Indigenous people and land. Indigenous people were seen as less than others – as non-human entities with no more rights to land than deer or other animals. Under Canadian law First Nations people became wards of the federal government and were forcibly relocated to reserves. Métis people were forced into the fringes, such as through road allowances, and their communities pared down. The Inuit people were forced to geographical communities that were counterintuitive to their lifestyle and food security so that the country could claim settled sovereignty over lands in the north. In 2023, in response to immense public pressure, the Vatican repudiated the Doctrine of Discovery – distancing itself from the catastrophe of colonization. Repudiation of the doctrine is different from rescinding it: the legal framework remains intact.

The law not only provided a way to displace Indigenous people, but it also controlled all aspects of their daily lives and created inequity. Law allowed the mass race-based apprehension of Indigenous children into Indian residential schools and day schools and their apprehension and placement in child protection as part of the Sixties Scoop and the Millennial Scoop. Indigenous children are now removed from their families and culture at a greater rate than at the height of the Indian residential school era.[19] Law and policies have been dismantling Indigenous family structures and communities since the imposition of colonial laws on the land and on the people of the land.

It is resoundingly our position that Canadian law is the catalyst creating lasting and ongoing harm to Indigenous people. Anti-Indigenous legislation included the *Gradual Civilization Act* of 1857, which predated confederation and granted rights to Indigenous people only if they pledged to "live as white." The *Gradual Enfranchisement Act* of 1869 further legislated assimilation and control of "Indians." These two pieces of legislation merged into the *Indian Act* of 1876, which remains active law in Canada.[20]

The fact that this law still exists – that in a free and democratic society, we still have a race-based act that knowingly discriminates against First Nations people – is appalling and internationally embarrassing. The fact that all Canadians do not learn the depth and impact of this law is also surprising. In a country as diverse as Canada, with many races, cultures, and backgrounds, it seems unfathomable that anyone would support or stand for a race-based act that treats one group as fundamentally different from any other. The reality is that it does, and it has caused many of the current egregious disparities Indigenous people face.

Although the *Indian Act* has undergone amendments over the years that are seen as less discriminatory, great discrimination remains in the act and the policies to implement the act. Historically, the law (to name a few examples)

- defined who was Indian on the basis of a nonsensical registration system that followed male lineage (resulting in gender discrimination that continues despite legislative amendments);
- removed traditional structures of Indigenous government (forcing a governance structure across all First Nations);
- banned and made illegal spiritual practices of ceremony and all ceremonial objects, languages, cultural practices, and celebrations;

- controlled commerce and all hunting and fishing practices, including sustenance hunting and fishing on reserve;
- allowed for the enforcement of apprehension of children for education (children were mandated to attend the IRSS – one of the most egregious structures of racial violence in Canadian history); and
- governed the gathering and movement of Indians off reserves, with a pass system overseen by Indian agents, who controlled the movement of Indians on and off reserve.

The impacts of control over First Nations communities and people, including extreme violence, continues to ricochet through generations as intergenerational trauma. The fact that the law has created spaces to oppress and control Indigenous people is a contemporary reality within law and policy.

The Connection between Structures of Racism and Racism in Health Care

In early colonization, physicians played a role in propagating illness among Indigenous communities, contributing to a massive depopulation of the Americas, opening land for settlement. Entire communities of Indigenous people, segregated and under total control of European settlers by way of the *Indian Act*, were subject to mass starvation so physicians could study the long-term impacts of malnutrition.

Famously, Indian residential schools had astronomically high rates of preventable deaths of children, which Dr. Peter Bryce contemporaneously stated to be between 24 per cent and 69 per cent. The Bryce report,[21] dated 1907, clearly stated that the federal government was directly responsible for the conditions that caused these deaths. Despite knowing the clear harms, the residential school system continued for another 89 years.

In addition to the IRSS, we have seen a legacy of medical violence against Indigenous people carried out in government-funded, often church-run Indian hospitals. These hospitals were designed for segregation and were rife with medical abuse, from surgical experimentation to forced sterilization. Structural racism in health care is an ongoing legacy of these systems. Issues of forced sterilization continue to be addressed in our government today.

Many resources are available to examine and understand the health discrepancies faced by Indigenous people in Canada. To contextualize statistical and known discrepancies in health outcomes, it is important to consider the fundamental concept of wellness and SDOHs. There are social determinants critical to wellness for Indigenous people that

Table 3.1. Examples of Health Access and Outcome Discrepancies for Indigenous People in Canada

Access issues	Health outcome
Poor access to primary health services	The First Nations population admitted to the emergency department for acute illness is roughly double the population of the rest of Ontario seeking the same or similar services from the emergency department.
	Roughly 10%–20% of First Nations people use the emergency department more than 6 times in a 2-year span, in comparison with roughly 1% of the rest of the Ontario population that does so.
	First Nations people have a much more difficult time obtaining diagnoses for chronic diseases. Of the Inuit population in Ottawa older than age 50 y, 23% reported having a screening.
Prejudice, discrimination, and lack of trust	First Nations children are less likely to be admitted to the hospital than non-native children, and maternal and child mortality rates are higher because of concurrent illnesses.
	The infant mortality rate among the Inuit is 4 times the national average.
Long waiting lists, especially for health services for children	Rates of asthma and chronic ear infections are 2 times as high as among the non-Indigenous population; 22% of Indigenous parents are worried about their children's development.
	The prevalence of tuberculosis among First Nations people is 184 cases per 100,000 people, which is 38 times higher than the national average.
Jurisdictional issues	Jordan's principle (see chapter 11 on paediatric issues for a full discussion of Jordan's principle)

may not be considered fundamental SDOHs, such as language, connection to land, kinship strength, and access to traditional ways of knowing.

Some examples from Our Health Counts of health access and outcome discrepancies for Indigenous people in Canada are summarized in Table 3.1.[22]

Qwayakotam – Hear the Truth

According to the *Ojibwe People's Dictionary qwayakotam* translates into "s/he hears the right thing, finds out the truth."[23] This is different from the Anishinabemowin word *debwewin*, which simply means "truth."[24] We have chosen to "hear the truth" because the truth of circumstances has always existed, but it is past time for service providers to actually listen to the truth Indigenous people experience.

Colonialism resulted in the hoarding of resources in non-Indigenous communities. Land and resources in Canada are unequally distributed because of colonialism, depriving Indigenous communities of medical and other resources. This enforcement of privilege and societal value deeply affects health and social status. In Canada, there is an unequal distribution of access to opportunity, resources, information, political influence, and socio-economic power. Political influence and economic power are critical factors in wellness at both the individual and the population levels, because these traits influence one's privilege or value in society and hence influence resource distribution. Power and privilege are what enable a group to live a comfortable, safe, healthy life, and Indigenous people in Canada are historically and contemporaneously excluded from having power and privilege.

Not only do power and privilege skew the distribution of resources, but the privileged group also defines what it means to be healthy through the SDOHs. The SDOHs are deeply intertwined with specific values of each culture and directly correlate to one's value, or privilege, within a society. In a multicultural society like Canada's, a dominant culture will emerge and will have the strongest influence on defining wellness and will control resource distribution. The most influential SDOHs are colonial and therefore exclude Indigenous indicators of wellness. SDOHs are defined by the dominant culture in Canada and may not consider critical factors that non-dominant cultural groups require for wellness. For Indigenous communities, this includes the use of language, connection to the land, and time with Elders. Without these factors, an Indigenous person may feel they lack wellness and good health regardless of their income, housing, education, or social status.

Differences in world views and cultural values are integral to the explanation of how and why children are removed, or stolen, from Indigenous homes and communities. The Western world view determines resource allocation and typical health care decisions, such as investments in palliative care as opposed to resuscitation. Palliative care is seen as a way to manage the symptoms of illness, most commonly for people of old age, whereas age is not the primary factor for Indigenous communities, who recognize the need for their Elders. Resuscitation became of greater importance with severe acute respiratory syndrome and COVID-19, when the most affected population was older people.

Without an understanding of Canada's colonial history, it can become commonplace to blame Indigenous people for poor wellness outcomes that were intentionally designed through a long process of disenfranchisement. Such instances contextualize contemporary issues of institutional racism, overt racism, and discriminatory practices.

Lived Experience and Case Studies

Anti-Indigenous racism and the accompanying negative outcomes in health, wealth, well-being, housing, incarceration, education, and more are outlined in detail in several landmark national reports, including the Truth and Reconciliation Commission Report, the final report of the National Inquiry into MMIWG, and the Royal Commission on Aboriginal Peoples.

Two specific well-known examples of Indigenous people who died as a direct result of anti-Indigenous racism in a health care setting are Brian Sinclair and Joyce Echaquan.

Brian Sinclair was an Indigenous man whose death in a Winnipeg hospital was attributed directly to racism. He was pronounced dead in his wheelchair on 21 September 2008, at only 45 years old, after a 34-hour wait in the emergency department in which he was not seen or medically assessed. He had been sent to the hospital directly by his family physician, who was concerned about uro-sepsis. While in the emergency department he began to deteriorate dramatically, becoming unresponsive. And yet, despite several bystanders raising concerns, he was never medically assessed. Health care workers assumed that he was "drunk and sleeping it off," that he was homeless and "only inside to avoid the cold," or that he had been discharged and was sitting in the emergency department because he had "nowhere else to go." These racist biases directly resulted in the preventable death of Mr. Sinclair. After more than a day waiting to be cared for, Mr. Sinclair was found by another visitor to be dead in his wheelchair, with rigour mortis already setting in.

He silently died a preventable death in the waiting room of the emergency department of the Health Sciences Centre in Winnipeg, Manitoba, alone and unseen. Sinclair's story reflects the manner in which Indigenous communities receive health care in Canada and the discrimination that happens in health services, as well as the negative health consequences of racism.[25]

Indigenous people in Canada continue to face systemic anti-Indigenous biases and stereotypes that cause delay and avoidance in seeking health care. As witnessed in the devastating viral social media video of Joyce Echaquan's death in a Nova Scotia hospital amid horrific racial abuse and medical neglect, there continue to be serious trauma and racism in health care. This incident brought immediate awareness of the poor treatment of Indigenous women seeking medical health care because nurses used racial and sexual slurs at Joyce, who was clearly in medical distress and died without the adequate care she deserved. Indigenous people continue to face astonishingly high rates of premature and preventable death and illness due to systemic barriers in accessing health care services, adequate housing, clean drinking water, and more. A lack of culturally safe health care in which the threat of stereotyping is actively minimized contributes to the ongoing status quo of poor health outcomes for Indigenous people.

The National Inquiry into MMIWG (the final report was released in May 2019) noted that addressing systemic racism requires coherent, systematic action. Uprooting Indigenous-specific racism in health care requires shifts in governance, leadership, legislation and policy, education, and practice. The 24 Recommendations provide a coherent and comprehensive approach to achieving these changes.

Calls for Justice for All Governments: Health and Wellness

3.1   We call upon all governments to ensure that the rights to health and wellness of Indigenous Peoples, and specifically of Indigenous women, girls, and 2SLGBTQQIA people, are recognized and protected on an equitable basis.

3.2   We call upon all governments to provide adequate, stable, equitable, and ongoing funding for Indigenous-centred and community-based health and wellness services that are accessible and culturally appropriate, and meet the health and wellness needs of Indigenous women, girls, and 2SLGBTQQIA people. The lack of health and wellness services within Indigenous communities continues to force Indigenous women, girls, and 2SLGBTQQIA people to relocate in order to access care. Governments must ensure that health and wellness services are available and accessible within Indigenous communities and wherever Indigenous women, girls, and 2SLGBTQQIA people reside.

3.3   We call upon all governments to fully support First Nations, Inuit, and Métis communities to call on Elders, Grandmothers, and other Knowledge Keepers to establish community-based trauma-informed programs for survivors of trauma and violence.

3.4   We call upon all governments to ensure that all Indigenous communities receive immediate and necessary resources, including funding and support, for the establishment of sustainable, permanent, no-barrier, preventative, accessible, holistic, wraparound services, including mobile trauma and addictions recovery teams. We further direct that trauma and addictions treatment programs be paired with other essential services such as mental health services and sexual exploitation and trafficking services as they relate to each individual case of First Nations, Inuit, and Métis women, girls, and 2SLGBTQQIA people.

3.5   We call upon all governments to establish culturally competent and responsive crisis response teams in all communities and regions, to meet the immediate needs of an Indigenous person, family, and/or community after a traumatic event (murder, accident, violent event, etc.), alongside ongoing support.

3.6   We call upon all governments to ensure substantive equality in the funding of services for Indigenous women, girls, and 2SLGBTQQIA people, as well as substantive equality for Indigenous-run health services. Further, governments must ensure that jurisdictional disputes do not result in the denial of rights and services. This includes mandated permanent funding of health services for Indigenous women, girls, and 2SLGBTQQIA people on a continual basis, regardless of jurisdictional lines, geographical location, and Status affiliation or lack thereof.

3.7   We call upon all governments to provide continual and accessible healing programs and support for all children of missing and murdered Indigenous women, girls, and 2SLGBTQQIA people and their family members. Specifically, we call for the permanent establishment of a fund akin to the Aboriginal Healing Foundation and related funding. These funds and their administration must be independent from government and must be distinctions-based. There must be accessible and equitable allocation of specific monies within the fund for Inuit, Métis, and First Nations Peoples.

Calls for Justice for All Governments: Human Security

4.1   We call upon all governments to uphold the social and economic rights of Indigenous women, girls, and 2SLGBTQQIA people by ensuring that Indigenous Peoples have services and infrastructure that meet their social and economic needs. All governments must immediately ensure that Indigenous Peoples have access to safe housing, clean drinking water, and adequate food.

4.3   We call upon all governments to support programs and services for Indigenous women, girls, and 2SLGBTQQIA people in the sex industry to promote their safety and security. These programs must be designed and delivered in partnership with people who have lived experience in the sex industry. We call for stable and long-term funding for these programs and services.

Source: National Inquiry into Missing and Murdered Indigenous Women and Girls: Reclaiming Power and Place: The Final Report of the National Inquiry into Missing and Murdered Indigenous Women and Girls. Volume 1b. Ottawa: National Inquiry into Missing and Murdered Indigenous Women and Girls; 2019.

Aandaakonige – Changing Practices

Aandaakonige translates to "they change something: a plan, rule, a law, a policy."[26] *Aandaakonige* occurs when there is a need for change, but it is done in a planned way so that everyone knows what is happening and why. Clearly, the entire health care system needs to set into motion massive change to address the systemic harms Indigenous people have faced and that it causes to Indigenous Peoples.

Increasing Knowledge and Cultural Understanding to Combat Racism, Assumptions, and Stereotypes

Challenges may be encountered when providing comprehensive care to people who are culturally, economically, and geographically diverse, yet physicians, nurses, and all health care providers in Canada are mandated by the colleges who license them to do exactly that. As per the Canadian Medical Protective Association, physicians have a fiduciary duty that requires them to act with "good faith and loyalty towards the patient."[27] Physicians and other health care providers must exercise "reasonable and acceptable standards of care, competence, and skill in attending upon the patient"[28(p. 10)] and prevent patients from experiencing undue harm or injury. Health care providers are legally, morally, and ethically responsible for the health outcomes that occur to the people in their care. Patients are extraordinarily diverse; therefore, health care providers must become culturally competent when aware of the risks involved in treating people who are culturally different from themselves.

Cultural safety and cultural competency are fundamental to a physician's ability to practice medicine in the manner mandated by the law and our colleges. Practices must take into account equitable treatment of Indigenous people with a focus on anti-racism and the means to combat implicit bias.[29]

> Understanding the principles of cultural safety will help health care institutions and providers to practice from an anti-racist and anti-discriminatory stance. In tandem with trauma- and violence-informed principles, cultural safety is about mitigating the potential harms, traumas and lack of safety that people may experience as they seek help at any given health care setting. (p. 13)
>
> Although the word "cultural" is used, cultural safety is not the same as cultural sensitivity. Instead, cultural safety is about counteracting the everyday impacts of racism and other forms of discrimination on peoples' lives. Key features of cultural safety are that it:

- Locates the primary problem in health practices and policies – not with cultural issues/practices/barriers
- Focuses on strategies to mitigate the harmful effects of interacting with health systems, practices and policies
- Actively counteracts racism, stigma and others forms of discrimination by working against power differentials, stereotypes, and structural violence
- Draws attention to the often-harmful effects of "cultural sensitivity" training, which can further entrench stereotypes. (p. 14)

Trauma- and violence-informed care means that the responsibility for the physical, cultural and emotional safety of the person accessing care or services rests with the organizations and professionals providing care. This can be thought of as a universal approach to ensuring that individuals do not suffer further harm when seeking care and are helped in ways that are based on their strengths and capacities and offer meaningful choice and collaboration. This is differentiated from trauma-specific services, where interventions are provided to those identified with trauma symptoms, and expands on trauma-informed practice, where the focus is on individual-level traumatic experiences and responses. TVIC includes explicit attention to structural and systematic violence, with a focus on people's life conditions as well as their trauma and violence experiences. (p. 9)[30]

Health authorities, government sectors, organizations and institutions cannot view training programs as stand-alone programs; commitments to addressing anti-Indigenous racism and improving health care for Indigenous people will require full-scale policy and organizational transformations.... Any and all training must be embedded as part of broader system transformation. This requires multiple approaches, policy directives, accountability mechanisms, and interventions that can be maximally disruptive of systemic racism and stigmatizing discourses about Indigenous peoples. (pp. 14–15)

Conclusion

Acknowledging Indigenous practices in medicine and law is key to creating *aandaakonige*-changing practices for all health care services.

Indigenous cultural safety training that is evidence based and proven to reduce negative outcomes in health related to anti-Indigenous racism must be mandatory for all health care providers.

Health care workers must have training in managing implicit bias, understanding how emotional prejudice affects decision-making, and mitigating the harmful impact of stereotyping on health and criminal justice outcomes.

In September 2024, the Canadian Medical Association (CMA) apologized for its role, and the role of the medical profession, in past and ongoing harms to First Nations, Inuit, and Métis Peoples in the health system.[31] The CMA acknowledged harms such as the Indian hospital system and forced sterilizations as specific examples of racism and maltreatment caused by medical professionals.[32] This demonstrates progress and acknowledgement. But to be truly lasting and effective, the CMA's stated commitment to accountability, and to working with Indigenous Peoples to do better in the spirit of humility and reciprocity, must be followed up with action that demonstrates meaningful change and better health outcomes for Indigenous people.

Acknowledgment

Ms. Big Canoe and Dr. Shoush thank the law students who assisted them in research and formatting of this chapter, including Hannah Wilson, Rhea Murti, and Elisia Wong.

NOTES

1 *Indigenous* is a term of preference for the inclusive collective of peoples. Often groups prefer to be named by their specific nation, collective, or Inuit region. It is best to ask individuals how they define themselves rather than to assume their background. Past terms of preference and use have included terms such as *Aboriginal*, *Eskimo*, *half-breed*, and *Indian*. The last three are unacceptable, derogatory, and racist names for Indigenous people. *Indian* should only be used if referring to the legislative context of race (this is discussed in the context of the *Indian Act*).

2 *Anishinabemowin* is the native name used by the Anishinaabe peoples to refer to their languages. It literally means "original people's language." Because *Anishinaabe* is a general term used by several Algonquian speaking tribes of the Great Lakes and prairie regions, *Anishinabemowin* can sometimes be used to refer to more than one distinct language, such as the Ojibwe, Algonquin, Ottawa, Oji-Cree, or Potawatomi languages. These languages are all related but are not identical, similar to the Romance languages of Spanish, French, Portuguese, and Italian. Our use of *Anishinabemowin* refers to Ojibwe words and understanding (Native Languages of the Americas. Anishinabemowin [Internet]. Minneapolis [MN]: Native Languages of the Americas; 2015. Available from: http://www.native-languages .org/definitions/anishinabemowin.htm).

3 The *Ojibwe's People's Dictionary* is an online resource that translate Anishinabemowin (Ojibwe) into English and vice versa. It should be noted that there are varying dialects of Anishinabemowin; this is just one resource (Livesay N, editor; Nichols JD, linguistic editor]. Ojebwe people's dictionary. 2021. Available from: https://ojibwe.lib.umn.edu/).

4 Stark KJ. Anishinaabe Inaakonigewin: principles for the intergenerational preservation of Mino-Bimaadiziwin. Montana L. Rev [Internet]. 2021;82(2):293–41. Available from: https://ssrn.com/abstract=4205937.

5 McKenzie HA, Varcoe C, Browne AJ, Day L. Disrupting the continuities among residential schools, the sixties scoop, and child welfare: an analysis of colonial and neocolonial discourses. Intern Indig Policy J. 2016; 7(2):4.

6 Borrows J, Mills A. Revitalizing Anishinaabe Inaakonigewin (law): Aadizookaanag Biboon 2016–17: interim and final report [Internet]. Montreal: Pierre Elliott Trudeau Foundation; 19 July 2017. Available from: http://www.fondationtrudeau.ca/sites/default/files/aadizook aananproject-finalreport.pdf.

7 Both *maanadamon* and *babikwadamon* are inanimate intransitive verbs (Livesay N, editor; Nichols JD, linguistic editor. Ojebwe People's Dictionary. 2021; Available from: https://ojibwe.lib.umn.edu/).

8 Livesay N, editor; Nichols JD, linguistic editor. Ojebwe people's dictionary. 2021. Available from: https://ojibwe.lib.umn.edu/.

9 "The term *Sixties Scoop* was coined by Patrick Johnston, author of the 1983 report *Native Children and the Child Welfare System*. It refers to the mass removal of Aboriginal children from their families into the child welfare system, in most cases without the consent of their families or bands … The Sixties Scoop refers to a particular phase of a larger history, and not to an explicit government policy. Although the practice of removing Aboriginal children from their families and into state care existed before the 1960s (with the residential school system, for example), the drastic overrepresentation of Aboriginal children in the child welfare system accelerated in the 1960s, when Aboriginal children were seized and taken from their homes and placed, in most cases, into middle-class Euro-Canadian families. This overrepresentation continues today" (First Nations & Indigenous Studies, University of British Columbia. Sixties scoop [Internet]. (BC): The University; 2009. Available from: https:// indigenousfoundations.arts.ubc.ca/sixties_scoop/).

10 Browne A, Smye V, Rodney P, et al. Access to primary care from the perspective of Aboriginal patients at an urban emergency department. Qual Health Res. 2011;21(3):333–48.

11 Turpel-Lafond ME. In plain sight: addressing Indigenous-specific racism and discrimination in B.C. health care. Addressing Racism Review Full Report. Victoria: Government of British Columbia; 202.

12 Allan B, Smylie J. First peoples, second class treatment: the role of racism in the health and well-being of Indigenous peoples in Canada. Toronto: Wellesley Institute; 2015.

13 Written Submissions of Expert Witness Dr. Annette J. Browne, PhD, RN, FCAHS, FCAN, dated 28 May 2021, to the Quebec Coroner's public inquiry into the death of Joyce Echaquan [Internet]. 2021. Available from: https://www.faq-qnw.org/wp-content/uploads/2021/05/Dr.-Annette-J.-Browne-Expert-Witness-Written-Submission-May-28-2021.pdf.

14 McKenzie HA, Varcoe C, Browne AJ, Day L. Disrupting the continuities among residential schools, the sixties scoop, and child welfare: an analysis of colonial and neocolonial discourses. Intern Indig Policy J. 2016;7(2):4.

15 The *Constitution Act*, 1982, being Schedule B to the *Canada Act 1982* (UK), 1982, c 11, which came into force on April 17, 1982.

16 Joint Statement of the Dicasteries for Culture and Education and for Promoting Integral Human Development on the "Doctrine of Discovery," 30.03.2023. Rome: Holy See Press Office; 2023. Available from: https://press.vatican.va/content/salastampa/en/bollettino/pubblico/2023/03/30/230330b.html. See also Assembly of First Nations. Dismantling the doctrine of discovery. Ottawa: The Assembly; January 2018. Available from: https://www.afn.ca/wp-content/uploads/2018/02/18-01-22-Dismantling-the-Doctrine-of-Discovery-EN.pdf.

17 Tunney C. Trudeau says deaths and disappearances of Indigenous women and girls amount to "genocide." CBC News. 4 June 2019. Available from: https://www.cbc.ca/news/politics/trudeau-mmiwg-genocide-1.5161681. See also the Prime Minister's comments in 2021, in which he reiterated the National Inquiry into MMIWG report's findings on genocide (Alhmidi M, Canadian Press Staff. Trudeau's acknowledgment of Indigenous genocide could have legal impacts: experts. CTV News. 5 June 2021. Available from: https://www.ctvnews.ca/canada/trudeau-s-acknowledgment-of-indigenous-genocide-could-have-legal-impacts-experts-1.5457668#:~:text=Amid%20growing%20outrage%20and%20grief,what%20happened%20amounts%20to%20genocide.%22).

18 National Inquiry into Missing and Murdered Indigenous Women and Girls. A legal analysis of genocide: Supplementary report of the National Inquiry into Missing and Murdered Indigenous Women and Girls [Internet]. Vancouver: Privy Council Office; 4 June 2019. Available from: https://www.mmiwg-ffada.ca/wp-content/uploads/2019/06/Supplementary-Report_Genocide.pdf.

19 Blackstock C. The long history of discrimination against First Nations children. Policy Options/Options politiques. 6 October 2016. Available from: https://policyoptions.irpp.org/magazines/october-2016/the-long-history-of-discrimination-against-first-nations-children/.

20 The *Indian Act*, RSC 1985, c I-5.

21 Bryce PH. Report on the Indian schools of Manitoba and the Northwest Territories [Internet]. Ottawa: Government Printing Bureau; 1907. Available from: https://publications.gc.ca/collections/collection_2018/aanc-inac/R5-681-1907-eng.pdf.

22 Our Health Counts Toronto. Adult access to health care [Internet]. Toronto: Well Living House; 2018. Available from: http://www.welllivinghouse.com/wp-content/uploads/2022/06/Access-to-Health-Care-OHC-Toronto_1June2022.pdf.

23 Livesay N, editor; Nichols JD, linguistic editor. Ojebwe people's dictionary. 2021. Available from: https://ojibwe.lib.umn.edu/.

24 Livesay N, editor; Nichols JD, linguistic editor. Ojebwe people's dictionary. 2021. Available from: https://ojibwe.lib.umn.edu/.

25 Manitoba Provincial Court. In the Provincial Court of Manitoba. In the matter of: *The Fatality Inquiries Act* and In the Matter of: Brian Lloyd Sinclair, deceased. Winnipeg: The Court; 2014. Available from: https://www.manitobacourts.mb.ca/site/assets/files/1051/brian_sinclair_inquest_-_dec_14.pdf.

26 Livesay N, editor; Nichols JD, linguistic editor. Ojebwe people's dictionary. 2021. Available from: https://ojibwe.lib.umn.edu/.

27 Canadian Medical Protective Association (CMPA). Duty of care [Internet]. Ottawa: CMPA; 2023. Available from: https://www.cmpa-acpm.ca/en/education-events/good-practices/medico-legal-matters/duty-of-care.

28 Canadian Medical Protective Association (CMPA). Medico-legal handbook for physicians in Canada, version 9.0. Ottawa: CMPA; May 2021; revised October 2024. Available from: https://www.cmpa-acpm.ca/en/advice-publications/handbooks/medical-legal-handbook-for-physicians-in-canada.

29 Indigenous Physicians Association of Canada; Royal College of Physicians and Surgeons of Canada. Promoting culturally safe care for First Nations, Inuit and Métis patients: a core curriculum for residents and physicians. Ottawa: Indigenous Physicians Association of Canada; 2009. See also Browne AJ, Varcoe C, Lavoie J, et al. Enhancing health care equity with Indigenous populations: evidence-based strategies from an ethnographic study. BMC Health Serv Res. 2016; 16(1):544, and Sukhera J, Gonzalez C, Watling CJ. Implicit bias in health professions: from recognition to transformation. Acad Med. 2020;95(5):717–23. The following quotes are from Annette J. Browne's submission to the public inquiry into Joyce Echaquan's death (Written Submissions of Expert Witness Dr. Annette J. Browne, PhD, RN, FCAHS, FCAN, dated 28 May 2021, to the Quebec Coroner's public inquiry into the death of Joyce

Echaquan [Internet]. 2021. Available from: https://www.faq-qnw.org
/wp-content/uploads/2021/05/Dr.-Annette-J.-Browne-Expert-Witness
-Written-Submission-May-28-2021.pdf).

30 This quote is from Canas E, Pradhan S, Wathen N. Development of a
core trauma- and violence-informed care e-learning curriculum. In CN
Wathen, C Varcoe, eds. Implementing trauma- and violence-informed care:
a handbook. Toronto: University of Toronto Press; 2023: 295–309, as cited
in Written Submissions of Expert Witness Dr. Annette J. Browne, PhD,
RN, FCAHS, FCAN, dated 28 May 2021, to the Quebec Coroner's public
inquiry into the death of Joyce Echaquan [Internet]. 2021. Available from:
https://www.faq-qnw.org/wp-content/uploads/2021/05/Dr.-Annette
-J.-Browne-Expert-Witness-Written-Submission-May-28-2021.pdf.

31 Canadian Medical Association (CMA). An apology for harms to
Indigenous Peoples [Internet]. Ottawa: CMA; 2024. Available from:
https://www.cma.ca/our-focus/indigenous-health/apology-harms
-indigenous-peoples.

32 Larsen K. CMA apologizes for harms to First Nation, Inuit and Métis
Peoples. CBC News, 18 September 2024. Available from: https://www.cbc
.ca/news/canada/british-columbia/cma-indigenous-peoples-apology
-1.7326213.

4 Health and Justice Partnerships for Health and Home

ANDREW BOND AND BENJAMIN RIES

Throughout their practice, primary health care providers are confronted with the reality that the health and housing status of their patients, individually and collectively, are intimately intertwined.

Health care providers fundamentally understand this and frequently encounter patients who contend with housing issues that arise because of their health as well as patients whose health conditions are directly affected by their housing situation. Assistance for individuals with these vulnerabilities presents a unique and multidimensional challenge wherein health care and housing law intersect.

The three goals of this chapter are as follows:

1. *To identify common challenges*: This chapter aims to help health care providers recognize the common housing challenges that their low-income patients may face, including understanding both the potential for and the limitations of legal assistance in resolving these issues.
2. *To understand the context*: This chapter provides a definition of housing law, illustrates the particular ways low-income and vulnerable tenants experience the law of residential tenancies and related policies, and analyses the reciprocal nature of the relationship between human health and housing inadequacy, homelessness, or the possibility of either.
3. *Engagement and advocacy*: Finally, the chapter identifies ways health care providers can become agents of change by getting involved in health and justice partnerships (HJPs) and discusses how engaging in advocacy can create broad-based changes in systems and policies that will benefit low-income patients.

To illustrate these complex dynamics, this chapter follows a dual case study approach:

- The first case highlights how an individual tenant's medical status can negatively affect their tenancy and how substandard housing conditions can further exacerbate the tenant's medical condition. This case serves to demonstrate the challenges and opportunities involved in leveraging medical–legal support for individual patients.
- The second case pivots to underscoring the challenges and opportunities for medical–legal supports at the policy level. By highlighting advocacy efforts at larger scales, this vignette illustrates how systemic change that would benefit many low-income patients simultaneously can be achieved.

Case Vignettes

Case Vignette 1

Mrs. VH is a 74-year-old woman living alone in a large, dense community housing complex. She is well-known to you and your urban family practice. A retired kindergarten teacher, Mrs. VH has no children of her own and lost her husband to prostate cancer 10 years ago. Uncharacteristically, she has not attended her appointments with you for the past six months. Before that, she had complained of a progressive decline in her short-term memory, which you had confirmed with a series of clinical assessments. Thankfully, you were able to connect her with a community worker. With the appropriate consents already in place, you reached out to the worker, who informed you that Mrs. VH has become increasingly withdrawn, keeps to herself, and only comes out of her unit when necessary and that she is increasingly fearful for her personal safety. You are able to arrange a home visit with the support of the community worker.

You enter a building that has for several decades been struggling to overcome challenges of substance use and human trafficking, unit takeovers, and poor conditions in units and shared spaces. The complex is also home to many multigenerational families, including those with young children.

In Mrs. VH's unit, you find debris and strewn garbage, as well as largely uncleaned physical and functional spaces. Additionally, she has very little food in her refrigerator. You also find that the housing supervisor has issued an eviction notice to Mrs. VH on the grounds that her unit conditions are unsafe and a fire hazard and that she has consistently interfered with others' peaceful enjoyment of their homes. On further investigation, you learn that Mrs. VH's fears of being unsafe have led her to be increasingly suspicious that the person in the neighbouring unit is following and observing her. Subsequently, she has begun vocalizing loudly at night in perceived self-defence. She has also on occasion confronted her neighbour about her concerns, much to their confusion.

Case Vignette 2

You are a nurse finishing up your sixth emergency department (ED) shift in January and are concerned about the number of patients that you have treated for cold-exposure conditions such as frostbite. Several patients reported to you that they were sleeping in a nearby park until municipal staff and police destroyed their tents and forced them to leave. You consult with your department's social worker and learn that because the local public health unit only declares a cold weather advisory when the temperature is below −15°C, there are no warming centres open when most cold injuries are presented to the ED. You already know that when attempting to complete shelter referrals upon ED discharge, staff spend hours on hold until they are typically advised that either (a) the municipality's existing shelters are already over capacity or (b) the patient in question has been prohibited from returning to the shelter because of past behaviour. You wonder, "How did we get to this situation, and what can I do?"

Homelessness, Social Determinants, and Health

What Would Happen If Mrs. VH Became Homeless?

Homelessness has been characterized as a form of multiple,[1] compounded,[2] and clustered social disadvantages[3] and one of the most potent determinants of health. It reduces the average age at mortality by more than 30 years[4] and has profound impacts on chronic mental and physical health.[5] The causes, experiences, and impacts of sheltered versus unsheltered homelessness are sharply divergent,[6] as are those of Indigenous Peoples,[7] youth,[8] elderly individuals,[9] newcomers,[10] and those living with a chronic physical or mental illness[11] or cognitive disability,[12] all of which are compounded by gendered differences.[13]

Table 4.1. Overview of 2018 World Health Organization *Housing and Health Guidelines*

Topic	Recommendation	Strength of recommendation
Crowding	Strategies should be developed and implemented to prevent and reduce household crowding.	Strong
Indoor cold and insulation	Indoor housing temperatures should be high enough to protect residents from the harmful health effects of cold. For countries with temperate or colder climates, 18°C has been proposed as a safe and well-balanced indoor temperature to protect the health of general populations during cold seasons.	Strong
	In climate zones with a cold season, efficient and safe thermal insulation should be installed in new housing and retrofitted in existing housing.	Conditional
Indoor heat	In populations exposed to high ambient temperatures, strategies to protect populations from excess indoor heat should be developed and implemented.	Conditional
Home safety and injuries	Housing should be equipped with safety devices (e.g., smoke and carbon monoxide alarms, stair gates, and window guards), and measures should be taken to reduce hazards that lead to unintentional injuries.	Strong
Accessibility	On the basis of the current and projected national prevalence of populations with functional impairments and taking trends in aging into account, an adequate proportion of the housing stock should be accessible to people with functional impairments.	Strong

You know that Mrs. VH is especially vulnerable given her isolation, gender, and elderly status, as well as her emerging cognitive impairments and mental illness.

The intersectionality of causes, experiences, and consequences of homelessness[14] are deepened by the relationship between health and housing, wherein health status,[15] low income, housing affordability, racialized poverty, disability status, and justice system involvement, among others,[16] are significant drivers of homelessness. The reciprocal corrosive[17] relationship between homelessness and health status predisposes people experiencing homelessness to entrenched income deprivation and housing instability, with an attendant and profound impact on individual and community health and health systems performance.[18] The World Health Organization has developed helpful *Housing and Health Guidelines* to support health-informed approaches to housing conditions (Table 4.1).[19]

Homelessness is one of the most daunting policy problems across high-income countries,[20] affecting more than 235,000 Canadians annually.[21] As with all "wicked problems,"[22] homelessness faces the combined challenges of changing and conflicting definitions; non-linear causality; and an enormous range of types, patterns of experiences, and emergent properties.[23] The policy complexity of homelessness is exacerbated by its being quadri-jurisdictional, with municipal, provincial, federal Canadian, and Indigenous governments playing fundamental and distinct roles.[24] Achieving effective alignment across infrastructure, urban planning, health, social care, fiscal policy, economic and disability entitlements, and immigration and legal status for effective homelessness policy and practice requires collaborative and collective action in an area heavily shaped by the contours of partisan politics.[25]

Housing Law: A Functional Scope

Before turning to how we can assist Mrs. VH, we begin by elaborating on what we mean by *housing law*. Our proposed definition may be narrower than the law that technically affects everyone's housing and often broader than the set of individual landlord–tenant disputes that may typically be handled by legal services providers. This working definition of housing law is intended to prioritize the needs of individuals, groups, and communities whose housing threatens their health or whose health threatens their housing.

In many ways, the Anglo-American common laws of property, land titles, mortgages, and real estate have home ownership as their dominant, if not paradigmatic, form. Although we cannot entirely exclude each of these areas of law and regulation for the purposes of discussing housing and health, the discussion will not be assisted by a definition of housing law that centres the form of housing enjoyed by middle- and upper-class Canadians. Nor will it be assisted by a definition of housing law that looks to the most common interventions, tasks, and conflicts for which Canadians might seek legal services in relation to their homes (as in the manner that one might typically conceive of family law).

Rather, it is the powerful relationships between human health and threats to housing – housing inadequacy, homelessness, or the looming possibility of each – that direct our attention to the law of residential tenancies. This is not to deny that the size, quality, or potential loss of an owned home may have relevant health dimensions. Nevertheless, two points generally overshadow such concerns: (a) the significantly greater total income and net worth of homeowners relative to tenants[26] means that owners will more frequently have the financial ability to

Figure 4.1. The Housing Continuum

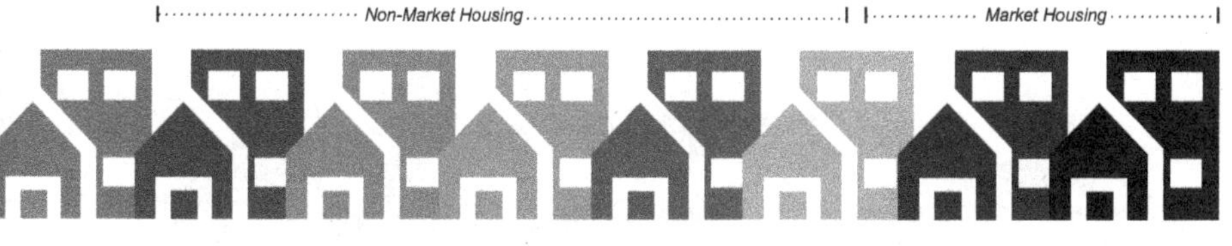

Source: Adapted from Whitzman C, Flynn A, Gurstein P, et al. The municipal role in housing. Toronto: Institute on Municipal Finance & Governance, University of Toronto; 2022. Available from: https://imfg.org/report/the-municipal-role-in-housing/.

resolve housing-related threats to their health and (b), perhaps as a result, the law largely treats the adequacy and security of owned housing as primarily economic concerns. Owners get as much and as good housing as they pay for; mortgage regulation attempts to ensure that they have a level of income that will allow owners to pay back whatever they have borrowed.

The housing continuum is a concept now commonly referenced by governments and researchers in Canada, as reflected in Figure 4.1.

Modern residential tenancy law departs, to an extent, from a purely financial approach to housing because although renting may be the obvious alternative to home ownership, homelessness is a much less acceptable alternative to renting from the standpoint of social and international legal norms.[27] The law's departure from traditional property and contract principles to protect the quality and security of housing for tenants reflects a remedial concern that simply treating tenancies like other contracts, or other forms of property, would lead to unacceptable human consequences – homelessness and unhealthy housing conditions being the most obvious.

For these reasons, we define housing law as it most relates to health as the legislation, regulation, policy, and adjudicative and juridical decisions centring on (a) evictions, security of tenure, and rent control and (b) tenant rights (within housing) and maintenance standards. These central areas are concerned not only with an up-to-date codification of the rules in each province, but the background common law of property, contract, and tort – combined with certain questions

Figure 4.2. Selected Interconnected Aspects of Modern Housing Law and Practice

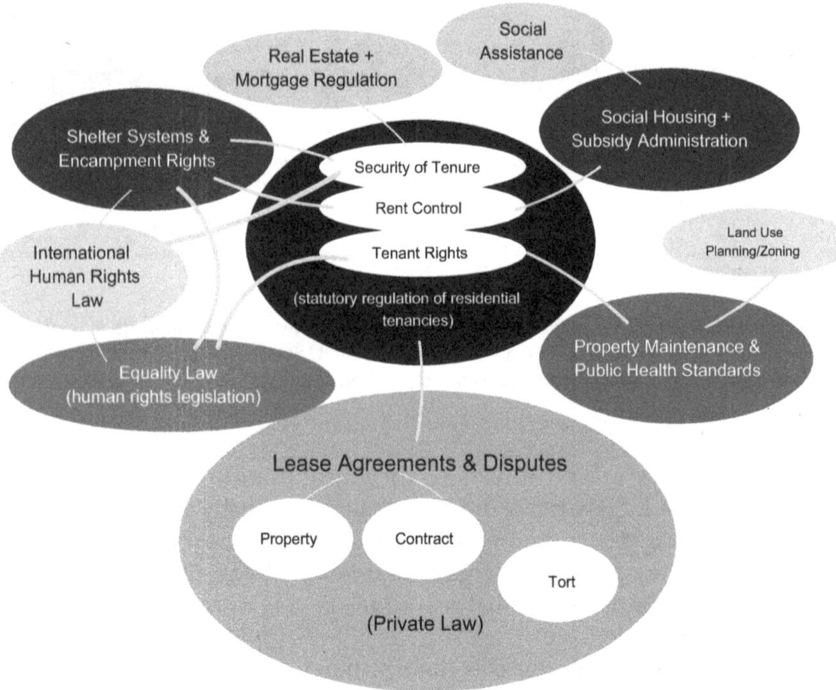

of administrative law and civil procedure, constitutional law, Indigenous law, and international human rights law. See Figure 4.2 for a graphical representation of these interconnected aspects of modern housing law and practice.

Housing law is also very much enmeshed with other areas of legal practice and poverty law – some of which are more fully addressed by other chapters of this text. For example, rent-geared-to-income rules in social housing are a form of social assistance, beyond which social assistance programs typically feature rules about the amount of money one might receive for housing costs. Human rights and equality play a particularly important role in housing, whether in the context of racial segregation or ableism (as further examples). Criminal and family law systems each enjoy two-way relationships with housing law.

A useful definition of housing law does not exclude these areas of overlap, nor can it ignore other areas of law that affect the available supply and form of housing: social housing investment, land use planning, municipal law and property standards, property taxation, building

Table 4.2. Canadian Tenant Protection Laws by Province and Territory (as of 2023)

Province	Security of tenure	Rent control	Statutory tenant rights
British Columbia	Yes	Within tenancies	Yes
Alberta	No	No	Yes
Saskatchewan	No	No	Yes
Manitoba	Yes	Yes	Yes
Ontario	Yes	Within tenancies	Yes
Quebec	Yes	Yes	Yes
New Brunswick	Limited	Within tenancies	Yes
Nova Scotia	No	No	Yes
Prince Edward Island	Yes	Yes	Yes
Newfoundland and Labrador	No	No	Yes
Yukon	No	No	Yes
Northwest Territories	Yes	No	Yes
Nunavut	Yes	No	Yes

Note: This table is highly generalized; each province and territory has a unique legal framework for renters, with numerous exceptions to these descriptions. Consult with a licensed legal professional in your jurisdiction for an up-to-date, accurate summary of local tenant rights.

codes, electrical and fire safety codes, and utility price regulation. Similarly, this functional scope of housing law is increasingly concerned with legal conflicts that arise from housing deprivation: shelter access and standards; criminalization of begging and loitering; and the collision of parks by-laws, trespass laws, and constitutional rights arising from informal encampments.

That these secondary and tertiary components of housing law are sourced and decided in three different branches of government (legislative, executive, and judicial) and at all three levels of government in Canada reflects a more basic observation about poverty and the law. We have proposed that the health of owner-occupiers in Canadian housing is an issue normatively founded in finance, not law (with notable exceptions in population health, such as drinking water, air quality, proximity of food and exercise, etc.), and, as a result, the law treats owned housing in a manner not radically different than an owned car, truck, or boat: as market goods. Owner-occupiers' housing-related interactions with the legal system are traditionally isolated and simpler than the relatively tangled nature of a poorer person's legal interactions.[28]

Every province in Canada has specialized legislation that treats residential tenancies somewhat differently than commercial tenancies and other forms of property and contract (Table 4.2).

Calling in Legal Support: Housing and Health

The legal support available for Mrs. VH will vary, sometimes drastically, depending on which province she lives in. Appendix 1 provides an overview of legal aid, pro bono, law school clinic, and sliding scale options for free or low-cost legal services across Canada.

In relation to tenants in Ontario, the community legal aid clinic system provides housing law advice and representation to select low-income renters across the province. Many related legal aid services include a specialty clinic to advance pro-tenant law reforms and a tenant duty counsel system offering more limited legal advice to the larger audience of all self-represented tenants involved in proceedings at the province's housing tribunal. Although British Columbia has taken steps towards the creation of several community legal clinics, the limited scale of these initiatives likely places them closer to the limited advice services offered in other provinces on a pro bono or grant-funded basis.

Most major urban centres in Canada either contain or are proximate to public universities that host law schools. Most of those, in turn, host (or are affiliated with) clinical programs in which law students offer either legal advice or representation to low-income tenants.

However, health care providers struggling to connect their patients with local organizations that provide free housing law assistance – especially outside of Ontario – may reach the unfortunate conclusion that no such organization exists for their patients. For example, this would appear to be true in Newfoundland and Labrador, where the province's legal aid system offers only criminal and family law help, and the absence of a law school implies there is no student legal clinic. Even in Ontario where many housing law services exist, tenants are overwhelmingly self-represented in legal proceedings against their housing providers because of either lack of low-income eligibility for legal aid clinic services or lack of service capacity on the part of their local clinic.

For these reasons, tenant associations and tenant unions – organized independently or through larger groups such as the Association of Community Organizations for Reform Now (ACORN) Canada – can become vital resources for peer legal support in housing disputes. Similarly, local housing help centres and other publicly funded supports such as rent banks may be best placed to provide up-to-date referral lists for legal support. Finally, national advocacy groups such as the Canadian Centre for Housing Rights may be prepared to collaborate with community health care providers on grant-funded partnerships to meet patients' housing law needs.

Table 4.3. Housing Law Issues by Collective versus Individual Orientation

Community needs that may be met by neighbourhood or student clinics, poverty lawyers, or tenant unions	Individual needs that may require pro bono service, advice-only hotlines, or paid legal representation
Evictions	Disputes with other tenants
Illegal lockouts	Disputes concerning the political governance of non-profit housing cooperatives
Interference with vital services	
Harassment by housing provider or provider's employees	Social housing wait-list priority or transfer
Disputes over rent control or RGI rent calculation	
Disputes concerning maintenance and repair	
Discriminatory denial of housing	
Emergency shelter access and encampment support	

Note: RGI = rent geared to income.

To help anticipate the possible available support and reception from legal colleagues, health care providers should briefly consider, as best they are able, how the nature of their patients' legal needs may or may not be compatible with the legal needs of similarly situated patients and their communities before attempting legal referrals, because such considerations inform the type of complaint and possible legal supports (individual vs. community) that may be available (see Table 4.3). This will help to ensure that referrals are more likely to result in meaningful support and reduce the understandable client and provider frustration and moral distress that may be experienced through the completion of referrals that would be legally inactionable.

These lists are non-exhaustive and may differ for each legal service provider or community organization. Health care providers will note that potentially health-harming legal needs appear in both categories in Table 4.3, and in that respect these categories may not differ in the extent of the urgent importance with which these needs may present. We elaborate on this nuanced but important distinction in the next section.

Understanding Collectivized Housing Law Practice and Referral Pitfalls

Legal aid clinics (largely in Ontario) were historically formed in response to, and based on, the claim that poverty radically changes the nature of law and legal practice.[29] In part because of the lived experiences of poor community members working in clinics,[30] those clinics came to define areas of practice with the explicit understanding that (a) the ways in which law is organized and practiced by the rest of the legal profession are an inadequate fit for poor communities and must be set aside and (b) approaching poverty as a systemic rather than an individualized concern means organizing one's approach to legal problems in terms of how they align with the collective interests of poor communities.[31] This approach identifies housing as a key type of clinic law in jurisdictions that have clinics, neighbourhood law offices, or both. As a further result, medical–legal partnerships involving poverty lawyers may need to navigate the occasional disconnect between individual medical treatment and community lawyering.

Looking back through our proposed scope and ordering of housing law for the purposes of this chapter, we can add another organizing principle that cuts across the topography of housing-related legal spheres. We have identified a field of housing law centred on eviction defence and tenant rights as a kind of "goldilocks" zone between the law practiced for owner-occupiers (whose problems are often reduced to purely financial solutions) and the law practiced for homeless persons (whose legal problems frequently escape the boundaries of a single property dispute). We have further identified several related areas of law – subject to decision-making in different branches and at different levels of government – inextricably connected to the same needs for secure and adequate housing. But the final inventory of available housing law interventions for a community lawyer must exclude disputes that are essentially between similarly situated individuals.

In fact, we might categorize housing law services for low-income people along the following spectrum: (a) advancement of explicitly shared concerns on behalf of an organized community (e.g., against housing providers or governments), (b) advancement of implicitly shared concerns on behalf of individuals or households (e.g., not against other non-owners), and (c) advancement of individual concerns against other non-owners. Consistent with well-developed concepts of democratic and community lawyering,[32] poverty lawyers often aspire to the first of these services while offering the second and refusing the third. Typical conflict-of-interest rules for lawyers mean that, having assisted a person or group on one side of a dispute, the same lawyers cannot assist persons or groups on the other side of that dispute (or in any dispute against their own clients). Poverty law services organized or funded as shared community services will naturally seek to avoid holding a race to see which party to a neighbour-on-neighbour dispute can get to the free lawyer first.

Health providers seeking partnership with low-income housing lawyers must therefore appreciate the ways in which providing health care to their own patients rarely generates a professional conflict between patients in the way that community lawyering with two potential clients often can. Traditional health care delivery models – much like traditional paid lawyering – allow a form of complete loyalty to the individual and complete concern for the individual's needs and problems, limited only by the specialized expertise of the care provider. Individual patients may not immediately distinguish between the harassment they face from their landlord and the harassment they face from another tenant; low-income housing lawyers likely know how to pursue the neighbouring tenant's eviction. However, because low-income housing lawyers are engaging in a shared community service, they would likely decline making a case against the other tenant.

Special Considerations for Social Housing

Social housing – largely built across Canada during the second half of the twentieth century through a variety of federal funding programs under the *National Housing Act* and operated under a series of federal–provincial agreements – gives rise to a more consistent set of legal issues. Because the rent-geared-to-income (RGI) subsidy associated with social housing projects in Canada will typically ensure a household pays no more than 30 per cent of its gross income on rent, the demand for the subsidy has steadily increased. However, this increase, combined with effectively no new supply of social housing beyond the early 1990s, has resulted in tremendous backlogs and inflated waiting lists. For persons in need of this type of assistance, legal determinations as to their eligibility for certain priority categories and their need for units of a certain size can play a significant role in how soon they can be offered RGI housing as well as the suitability, location, and accessibility of that housing.

For households already living in social housing and receiving an RGI subsidy, similar legal determinations control their ability to transfer between buildings or units without losing their subsidy and going to the back of the line on the waiting list. Additionally, legal problems and disputes associated with the calculation of the RGI subsidy, a household's continuing eligibility for that subsidy, or both mirror many of the legal problems associated with social assistance: whether a household has complied with periodic income and asset reporting requirements, what counts as income, and who counts as a member of the household (as opposed to a frequent guest) are all determinations that can cause a household's payable rent in social housing to increase suddenly and trigger eviction proceedings if and when the household does not pay the increased amount.

Poverty lawyers and legal services providers can view legal needs arising from social housing in varying ways that influence service offerings. On the one hand, a household's place on a waiting list or internal transfer list may appear to change only to the benefit or detriment of other community members in need – meriting less dedication of scarce, shared legal aid resources. On the other hand, many priority categories reflect other targeted justice concerns (canvassed in this text) such as family, age, disability, and domestic violence. In any event, the significant value of the RGI subsidy to its recipients – compared with an increasingly unaffordable private housing market – makes the prospect of eviction from social housing (and categorical loss of the RGI subsidy) appear more catastrophic and dangerous than other evictions.

In the context of HJP referrals, collaboration and follow-up between health care and legal services providers is often desirable. See chapter 1 for an explanation of why express consent is required from the patient to share information with a legal professional, who is outside the circle of care. Similarly, legal professionals would require the individual's signed consent to disclose privileged information to a health care provider and would rightly caution against charting this information. Chapter 1 also canvasses the rationale for other options for low-income patients to access a partnering legal professional directly, in a low-barrier way.

Calling (Back) in Health Care Support: Individual Patients

Beyond spotting legal issues and making timely referrals to appropriate legal services providers, primary health care providers and allied health professionals can play an important and ongoing role supporting professional legal advocacy, particularly by providing expert medical evidence. The following examples highlight general principles that medical professionals may consider when doing so.

In jurisdictions that provide security of tenure (see Table 4.2), the eviction process often gives legal decision-makers the ability to exercise discretion over whether, or how quickly, to remove a person from their home – or, alternatively, on what terms and conditions to allow the person to avoid eviction and remain in their home. This stage of the eviction process can often be most critical for low-income people because it is a chance for them to present evidence about the extent to which they would be at risk of homelessness if evicted. Medical evidence may highlight particular vulnerabilities or related risks, including those arising from a household member's disease or disability, to be weighed against the grounds for eviction.

Similarly, behavioural evictions (e.g., alleging that a member of the renting household has breached the law or the conditions of their lease) may involve a tenant's argument that their disability should be taken into account, under human rights and equality law, when considering eviction, as well as conditional refusal of eviction pursuant to a mediated agreement. For example, a person in need of a service animal may require exemption from no-pets rules (in jurisdictions where such rules are otherwise lawful); a person who experiences hallucinations may require relief from eviction for causing undue noise. Medical evidence should confirm diagnoses, enumerate symptoms, and (where relevant) identify reasonable treatment goals to which the patient has agreed.

In cases in which a person alleges that their housing provider has breached a duty to provide vital services (such as heat or electricity) or has failed to maintain their housing in a good state of repair, medical evidence can help confirm when those problems appeared to exist and advise as to the effect of those problems on the individual's state of health. Most often, confirming a health professional's independent assessment and opinion (where possible) will be far more useful than simply parroting what the patient has told their health care providers.

Returning to our first case vignette, Mrs. VH is an elderly woman with a mental disability who is at risk of losing her rental unit because of excessive clutter, unsafe conditions in her unit, and disturbing behaviour that interferes with other tenants' reasonable enjoyment. Considering her vulnerabilities, Mrs. VH would benefit from (a) a letter from you as her health care provider confirming her disability and the associated impairments, restrictions, and needs that are relevant to her landlord's demands; (b) documentation or correspondence characterizing her eligibility for assisted living, supportive housing, both, or lack thereof; (c) a referral (in jurisdictions where available) to a community legal clinic offering eviction defence services; and (d) a commitment to provide supportive testimony along the lines set out in the documentation referenced, if and when called upon during eviction proceedings. Clearly identifying Mrs. VH's disability-related needs and limitations – and possible solutions, where available – helps trigger the landlord's duty to accommodate her disability under provincial human rights legislation (see chapter 2 for further details on this framework). Setting out her other housing options if evicted – or dispelling potential myths about the availability of state-provided or otherwise institutional care – helps underscore (for a decision-maker) the need to grant relief from eviction, if possible, and to make every effort to support Mrs. VH in her current housing. Connecting Mrs. VH with legal representation helps give her the chance to have these facts and arguments clearly explained to her landlord and a legal decision-maker in the eviction process. Being ready to testify within that process makes it far more likely that the facts relating to Mrs. VH's health are taken seriously and understood within the legal process.

In retrospect, you wonder whether you could have intervened earlier. Did she ever complain about a neighbour that she perceived to be threatening? Did she show signs of progressive disorganization that might have provided clues to a deteriorating living situation? Did she stop filling her medication prescriptions, which might have indicated a change in her financial situation? Although early intervention is obviously ideal, the reality is that clinical practice is busy and, furthermore, supports are not often readily available or easy to engage. You vow, however, to learn from Mrs. VH's case, research the legal resources available for low-income people in your community, and schedule a meeting with a similarly partnership-minded local legal professional. As noted in the Introduction to this text, rarely do these legal issues exist in isolation. One way to conceptualize the interconnectedness of these issues centring housing is shown in Figure 4.3.

Moving Upstream Together: Public Health Evidence and Legal Advocacy

Recall Case Vignette 2. What can the concerned ED team do? One approach might be to join efforts by other advocates and health care providers to change the city's Warming Centre Protocol. In the City of Toronto, for example, at the time of writing, warming centres were only open during an Extreme Cold Weather Alert, defined as when temperatures were −15°C or colder or if there was a wind chill of −20°C or colder. These thresholds created highly dangerous situations for the unhoused population. Furthermore, with only four warming centres in the city with a total capacity of 134 people, many were turned away for lack of space even if the temperature threshold was met. In response to advocacy efforts, the city lowered its threshold to −5°C in its 2023/24 winter services plan and increased capacity to 170 spaces.

Of course, this policy issue is very specific, but there are numerous legal or policy situations in which health care expertise is critical to the advancement of claims that go beyond individual legal advocacy. This section focuses on the role of health care expertise in the context of

Figure 4.3. Potential Intervention Points to Prevent Homelessness for Individuals

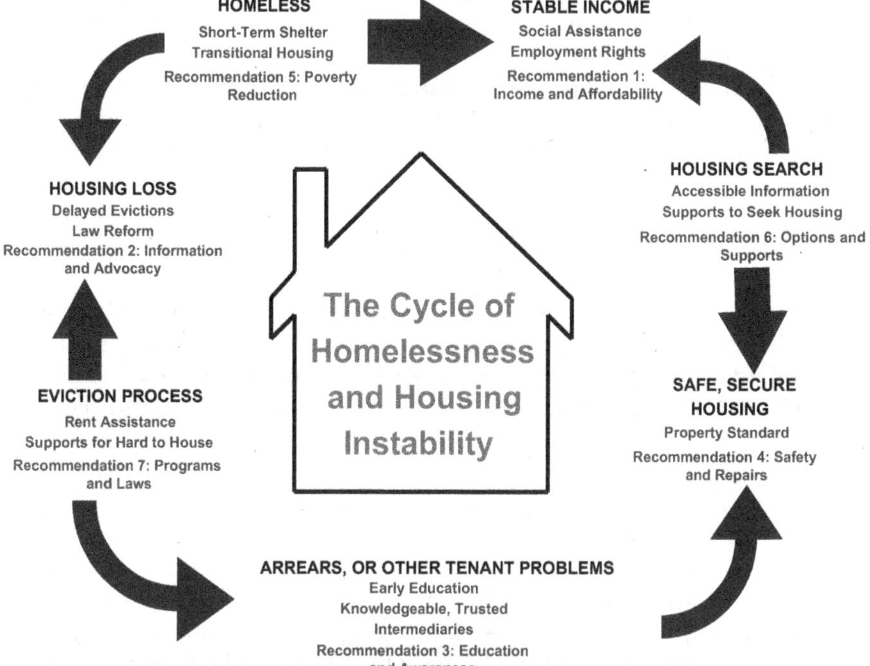

Source: Adapted from Community Advocacy and Legal Centre. Spinning in the cycle of homelessness: call to action on affordable housing & poverty reduction. Belleville (ON): The Centre; 2013. Available from: https://communitylegalcentre.ca/wp-content /uploads/2018/03/Spinning-in-the-Cycle-of-Homelessness.pdf.

legal proceedings or policymaking processes, which may involve *Charter* rights, class action suits, human rights tribunals, reliance on international treaty obligations, and legislative processes.

Role of the *Charter of Rights and Freedoms*

Charter rights claims against governments respecting people who are homeless or vulnerably housed could involve section 7 (life, liberty, and security of person), section 8 (unreasonable search and seizure), section 12 (cruel and unusual treatment or punishment), or section 15 (equality). In the context of homelessness and underhousing, recent cases turn on whether existing government legislation or policy infringe on these sections and, if they do, whether they are acceptable under section 1 (which specifies that only those infringements that are reasonably justified in a free and democratic society will be permitted). The *Charter* section 1 test for policies that are rational and minimally infringing of other *Charter* rights may be a critical space for health care within constitutional advocacy, because the infringement of rights may be incontrovertibly established while still being legal and permitted under the *Charter* for reasons that extend well beyond the sphere of individual health.

Homelessness Law and the International Right to Housing

Although Canada is a signatory to a variety of international human rights treaties purporting to guarantee a universal right to an adequate standard of living that includes shelter – commonly referred to as a "right to housing" – there has been little success in Canada in securing domestic realization and enforcement of those rights. Without fully canvassing the legal and political barriers to enforcement of the right to housing in Canadian domestic law, we simply note that as of the time of this writing, Canadian courts have only enforced the international right to housing by interpreting the *Charter of Rights and Freedoms* to temporarily override certain municipal by-laws prohibiting overnight encampment in public parks, as long as the relevant municipalities offer fewer overnight shelter beds than required by their homeless population.[33]

However, in most cases, courts have accepted that where the homeless population does not clearly exceed emergency shelter supply, municipalities may freely enforce by-laws prohibiting homeless encampments (the forced removal of which are considered contrary to international human rights norms). In the context of the COVID-19 pandemic, courts refused to even temporarily restrain encampment evictions in the face of clear medical evidence of the increased risks of infection and death in the shelter system.[34] Courts have also refused to permit a case arguing that inadequate social housing supply, RGI subsidy availability, and other policy failures together comprise a violation of the right to housing – and, in so doing, have largely denied that a right to housing exists in Canadian law.[35]

Politically, several elected governments have claimed to recognize and even legislate a "right to housing," both at the federal level and in several municipalities. In neither jurisdiction has this right meant anything resembling a guarantee that no person will be homeless, that every person will receive public assistance to secure housing to any standard of adequacy (much less emergency shelter), or that no person will be forcibly removed from their home. These are not only thought to form the content of the right to housing in international law, they are also what Canadians might justifiably think the word *right* means. Instead, governments have claimed a "rights-based approach" that "aspires" to someday provide housing for all; federally, a housing commissioner has been created to investigate and report on homelessness and inadequate housing in Canada.

For housing lawyers practicing domestically in Canada, the right to housing now functions as a theoretical requirement of minimum overnight emergency shelter beds in each municipality, coupled with the possibility of future incremental advancement in response to similar confrontations between governments and people experiencing homelessness. Such attempts require highly coordinated, resource-intensive litigation efforts in the face of substantial risk of failure.

Specific Roles and Advice for Health Care Providers Participating in Advocacy

Expert Opinions through Affidavits

Health care providers are often sought out to provide expert statements in the form of affidavits that particularly speak to the health implications of the issue under consideration on section 1 grounds. Under the section 7 life dimension, risk to the reasonably foreseeable impact on mortality is paramount,[36] whereas the "security of person" can pertain to risk to health and well-being and may not necessarily rise to the level of reasonably foreseeable mortality risk.[37] Evidence from published studies, direct experience, and medical reasoning are given weight, the latter in particular when the health care provider is an established subject matter expert.[38]

Affidavits must be factual, as detailed as possible, and delivered in a non-judgmental manner. Not uncommonly, when an affidavit has a strong personal or professional tone of impassioned perspective or lacks a nuanced analysis reflective of the complexity of the issue at question or when the writer is an established public advocate, the opinion may be disregarded, at times explicitly noting the concern for potential bias or partisanship.[39] This is a complex issue for health care advocates, who often feel as though their other public advocacy is grounded entirely in their professional perspective and commitment. The difference here mostly reflects the legal demand for fact-based submissions based on expertise that requires disclosure of contradictory and competing evidence and has challenges in the existing base of knowledge and the strength of various types of evidence.

Conclusions are only advocated for by the legal representatives of corresponding parties and decided upon by judges, neither of which is the place of the health care professional in this sphere of legal advocacy.

Note that any individual providing an affidavit to support litigation can and often will – if their testimony is compelling or challenging – be summoned to be cross-examined on their opinions by opposing counsel. As with *Charter* advocacy, the objectivity, integrity, and credibility of the expert health care provider may be challenged, and fact-based advocacy is strongly encouraged to provide the best possibility of contributing meaningfully to the proceedings.

The health care expert should be professionally and psychologically prepared for the challenge of cross-examination, which can be extremely challenging for the unprepared provider and have a significant impact on a provider's professional reputation and on future employment. This is not to detract from the value and significance of providing expert testimony – quite the contrary – but to highlight the unique challenges and importance of preparation, training, and support from within the health justice partnership relationships that a provider has developed.

Class Actions

Class actions are civil suits that involve numerous people (the "class" or category of person) for whom civil damages are claimed with a corresponding demand for damages, restitution, or both. Class action suits can be taken against both private (corporate) and public (government or public agency) entities. In the context of housing and homelessness, class action suits can involve either groups of tenants making claims against housing providers or those providing work on their behalf or claims against governments regarding actions taken against groups of homeless or underhoused individuals with respect to the implementation of a policy or a practice that has led to alleged collective harms.

This is another area in which a health care provider might serve as an expert witness (by way of affidavit or a report) for either the plaintiff (the class suing) or the defendant (the entity being sued).

Legislative and Policy Development

A last area of advocacy to be considered here for health care providers pertains to legislation and policy development. Municipal, provincial or territorial, and federal governments each have unique and often complex processes to create by-laws, codes, legislation, and policy. Most such processes involve steps in which public engagement is explicitly involved, creating opportunities to influence democratic decision making. Because homelessness and housing are quadri-jurisdictional, being aware of the various processes and opportunities for engagement is important to shape housing as a social determinant of health and a core element of a just society. Much that affects housing and homelessness in Canada, however, occurs at the municipal level, such as public by-law enforcement, police services and public safety, and shelter and community housing. Learning to engage the municipal policy and budgeting process is an important point of intervention and often involves deputations before municipal councils, committees, and Boards of Health that are connected to local municipalities through their public health units. Although the details of each legislative and policy process are beyond the scope of this chapter, it is important to consider the value and significance of working collectively within coalitions to advance housing and housing-related health rights. Health care providers are an important voice, and at times a critical one, but they are only one along with many others who often have less privilege and power; being mindful and attending to one's social position and location are critical in effective advocacy, particularly with respect to coalition building. This is another dimension in which medical–legal partnerships are so constructive, because they provide a space, language, and process for the knowledge of both legal advocates and health care providers and their respective communities to whom they are accountable to come together in a common cause that is rigorous, evidence informed, interdisciplinary, and effective.

Returning to Case Vignette 2, an ED team concerned about the impact that the local public health cold weather policy has on vulnerable and unhoused patients could draft a petition, letter, or report or conduct a study on the medical repercussions or complications faced by patients for direct submission to the local public health department (which, in many jurisdictions, is led by a physician). The question of which public cold weather supports are most appropriate at what temperatures is, in part, a matter of biomedical expertise: identifying the temperatures at which prolonged exposure presents health risks to a given percentage of the population. Medical professionals have the power to articulate these facts and standards free and clear of the political and fiscal considerations that governments may also consider.

Beyond the question of whether cold weather exposure constitutes a threat to the public health triggering legal powers or even duties for public health officials, the same objective health evidence can support municipal and provincial policy change or a constitutional challenge to police removal of encamped individuals as a breach of their *Charter* rights. An ED director could work with community advocates and pro bono lawyers to advance political and legal advocacy that relies on medical opinion as to the health risks faced by encamped individuals when not permitted to shelter themselves and the adequacy (or lack thereof) of locally available alternative sources of shelter and warmth.

Towards an Ecology of Health and Justice Partnerships: Recovery and Resilience

Although there is a lack of definitive clarity about the most effective interventions for homelessness[40] – mostly because homelessness is a diverse phenomenon and requires highly tailored interventions grounded in intersectional awareness – it has been established that any potentially effective intervention must address homelessness as an ecological problem rather than one of individual knowledge, attitude, or behaviour.[41] The definiteness of this conclusion is important because there remain significant political and public narratives that homelessness and poverty are matters of individual responsibility. Although there is truth in the statement that individual autonomy and correlated responsibilities matter, all are always situated in the broader social context of power, privilege, position, and unequal resources that constitute the social tissue that makes individual autonomy possible and responsibility matter. With respect to housing and homelessness, to be successful solutions must focus on availability, accessibility, affordability, and quality, particularly with a view towards service support needs and adequate available income supports.[42]

There has also recently been renewed debate about the role of mental illness and addiction versus affordable housing availability in homelessness.[43] The fact that homelessness rates in communities with similar mental illness and substance use rates vary by affordable housing availability largely settles the debate in favour of ecological causation.[44] This debate, however, misses another problem, which is the narrowing of causal thinking towards singular causes, as opposed to the preponderance of evidence favouring complex causality.[45] We know definitively, for example, that case navigation through existing systems of support fails,[46] as does isolated clinical treatment without supportive housing interventions.[47] Effective solutions must thus be not only ecological but multiple and complex so as to support recovery from homelessness.[48]

With the social complexity of the causation and consequences of homelessness and underhousing in mind, we hope that this chapter has both helped in understanding the role of HJPs in ecologies of recovery and resilience and provided helpful frameworks and tools for thinking about, and engaging with, the powerful space that exists at the intersection of health, rights, and the law.

Acknowledgment

The authors thank Marie Fiedler, a law student who assisted them in research and formatting this chapter.

NOTES

 1 Cornes M, Joly L, Manthorpe J, et al. Working together to address multiple exclusion homelessness. Soc Policy Soc. 2011;10(4):513–22.
 2 Stafford A, Wood L. Tackling health inequities for people who are homeless: start with the social determinants. Int J Environ Res Public Health. 2017;14(12):1535. https://doi.org/10.3390/ijerph14121535.
 3 Wolff J, de Shalit A. Disadvantage. Oxford: Oxford University Press; 2013.
 4 Hwang SW. Mortality among men using homeless shelters in Toronto, Ontario. JAMA. 2000;283(16):2152–7; Roncarati J, Baggett T, O'Connell J, et al. 2018. Mortality among unsheltered homeless adults in Boston, Massachusetts, 2000–2009. JAMA Intern Med. 178(9):1242–8.
 5 Fazel S, Geddes J, Kushel M. The health of homeless people in high-income countries: descriptive epidemiology, health consequences, and clinical and policy recommendations. Lancet. 2014;384(9953):1529–40; Aldridge R, Story A, Hwang S, et al. Morbidity and mortality in homeless individuals, prisoners, sex workers, and individuals with substance use disorders in high-income countries: a systematic review and meta-analysis. Lancet. 2018;391:241–50.
 6 Roncarati J, Baggett T, O'Connell J, et al. 2018. Mortality among unsheltered homeless adults in Boston, Massachusetts, 2000–2009. JAMA Intern Med. 178(9):1242–8.
 7 Thistle J, Smylie J. Pekiwewin (coming home): advancing good relations with Indigenous people experiencing homelessness. CMAJ. 2020;192(10):257–9.
 8 Embleton L, Lee H, Gunn J, et al. Causes of child and youth homelessness in developed and developing countries: a systematic review and meta-analysis. JAMA Pediatr. 2016;170(5):435–44.
 9 Brown R, Hemati K, Riley E, et al. Geriatric conditions in a population-based sample of older homeless adults. Gerontologist. 2017;57(4):757–66.
10 Kaur H, Saad A, Magwood O, et al. Understanding the health and housing experiences of refugees and other migrant populations experiencing homelessness or vulnerable housing: a systematic review using GRADE-CERQual. CMAJ Open. 2021;9(2):E681–92.

11 Fazel S, Geddes J, Kushel, M. The health of homeless people in high-income countries: descriptive epidemiology, health consequences, and clinical and policy recommendations. Lancet. 2014;384(9953):1529–40.

12 Topolovec-Vranic A, Schuler A, Godzik A, et al. The high burden of traumatic brain injury and comorbidities amongst homeless adults with mental illness. J Psychiatr Res. 2017;87:53–60.

13 Schwan K, Versteegh A, Perri M, et al. The state of women's housing need & homelessness in Canada: a literature review (Hache A, Nelson A, Kratochvil E, Malenfant J, editors). Toronto: Canadian Observatory on Homelessness Press; 2020.

14 Giannini A. An intersectional approach to homelessness: discrimination and criminalization. Marquette Benefits Soc Welf Law Rev. 2017;19(1):27–42.

15 Balasuria L, Buelt E, Tsai J. The never-ending loop: homelessness, psychiatric disorder and mortality. Psychiatr Times. 2020;37(5):12–4; Buccieri K, Oudshoorn A, Frederick T, et al. Hospital discharge planning for Canadians experiencing homelessness. Hous Care Support. 2018;22(4):1–12; City of Toronto. Street needs assessment. Toronto: City of Toronto; 2021.

16 Nicholls L, Latimer E, Godzik A, et al. Profiles of criminal justice system involvement of mentally ill homeless adults. Int J Law Psychiatry. 2016;45:75–88.

17 Wolff J, de Shalit A. Disadvantage. Oxford: Oxford University Press; 2013.

18 Fitzpatrick S. Explaining homelessness: a critical realist perspective. Hous Theory Soc. 2005;22(1):1–17.

19 World Health Organization. WHO housing and health guidelines [Internet]. Geneva: The Organization; 2018 [cited 2024 Dec 2]. Available from: https://www.who.int/publications/i/item/9789241550376.

20 Aldridge R, Story A, Hwang S, et al. Morbidity and mortality in homeless individuals, prisoners, sex workers, and individuals with substance use disorders in high-income countries: a systematic review and meta-analysis. Lancet. 2018;391(10117):241–50.

21 Gaetz S, Dej E, Richter T, et al. The state of homelessness in Canada. Toronto: Canadian Observatory on Homelessness; 2016.

22 Rittel H, Webber M. Dilemmas in a general theory of planning. Policy Sci. 1973;4:155–69.

23 Plsek P, Greenhalgh T. The challenge of complexity in healthcare. BMJ. 2001;323(7313):625–8; Cornes M, Joly L, Manthorpe J, et al. Working together to address multiple exclusion homelessness. Soc Policy Soc. 2011;10(4):513–22; Clark M, Cornes M, Whiteford M, et al. Homelessness and integrated care: an application of integrated care knowledge to understanding services for wicked issues. J Integr Care. 2022;30(1):3–19.

24 Cornes M, Joly L, Manthorpe J, et al. Working together to address multiple exclusion homelessness. Soc Policy Soc. 2011;10(4):513–22; Dej E. A complicated exile: homelessness, exclusion and a call for inclusion. Vancouver (BC): UBC Press; 2020; Thistle J, Smylie J. Pekiwewin (coming home): advancing good relations with Indigenous people experiencing homelessness. CMAJ. 2020;192(10):257–9; Phillips B, Ngo D, Harrison N, et al. Rough sleeping in Ontario: managing Ontario's encampment crisis [Internet]. Policy Options/Options politiques; 2022 June 9. Available from: https://doi.org https://policyoptions.irpp.org/magazines/june-2022 /sleeping-rough-solutions/.

25 Suttor G. Still renovating: a history of Canadian social housing policy. Montreal: McGill-Queen's University Press; 2016; Segel-Brown B, Liberge-Simard R. Federal program spending on housing affordability in 2021. Ottawa: Office of the Parliamentary Budget Officer; 2021.

26 Statistics Canada. "To buy or to rent: the housing market continues to be reshaped by several factors as Canadians search for an affordable place to call home" [Internet]. Ottawa: Statistics Canada; 2022. Available from: https://www150.statcan.gc.ca/n1/daily-quotidien/220921/dq220921b -eng.htm.

27 United Nations (General Assembly). International covenant on economic, social and cultural rights [Internet]. Treaty Series. 1966;999:171. Available from: https://www.ohchr.org/en/instruments-mechanisms/instruments /international-covenant-economic-social-and-cultural-rights.

28 Wexler S. Practicing law for poor people. Yale Law J. 1970; January: 1049–67. Available from: https://openyls.law.yale.edu/handle/20.500.13051/15325.

29 Mossman MJ. Community legal clinics in Ontario. Windsor Yearb Access Justice [Internet]. 1983;3:375–402. https://digitalcommons.osgoode.yorku .ca/scholarly_works/1539/.

30 Blazer M. The community legal clinic movement in Ontario: practice and theory, means and ends. J Law Soc Policy [Internet]. 1991;7:49–72. Available from: https://digitalcommons.osgoode.yorku.ca/jlsp/vol7/iss1/2/.

31 Abramowicz L. The critical characteristics of community legal aid clinics in Ontario. J Law Soc Policy [Internet]. 2004;19(1):70–81. Available from: https://digitalcommons.osgoode.yorku.ca/jlsp/vol19/iss1/5.

32 Piomelli A. The lawyer's role in a contemporary democracy, promoting access to justice and government institutions, the challenge of democratic lawyering. Fordham L Rev [Internet]. 2009;77(4):1383–1408. Available from: https://ir.lawnet.fordham.edu/flr/vol77/iss4/9.

33 *Victoria (City) v Adams*, 2009 BCCA 563 (CanLII). Available from: https:// canlii.ca/t/26zww;*Waterloo (Regional Municipality) v Persons Unknown and to be Ascertained*, 2023 ONSC 670 (CanLII). Available from: https://canlii .ca/t/jv6dc.

34 *Black et al. v City of Toronto*, 2020 ONSC 6398 (CanLII). Available from: https://canlii.ca/t/jb937;*Poff v City of Hamilton*, 2021 ONSC 7224 (CanLII). Available from: https://canlii.ca/t/jk6c3.

35 *Tanudjaja v Canada (Attorney General)*, 2014 ONCA 852 (CanLII). Available from: https://canlii.ca/t/gffz5.

36 *Carter v. Canada (Attorney General)* 2015 SCC 5, [2015] 1 SCR 331, para. 62. https://scc-csc.lexum.com/scc-csc/scc-csc/en/item/1937/index.do. Available from: https://scc-csc.lexum.com/scc-csc/scc-csc/en/item/14637/index.do.

37 *Suresh v. Canada (Minister of Citizenship and Immigration)*, [2002] 1SCR 3, 2002 SCC 1, paras. 53–55. Available from: https://scc-csc.lexum.com/scc-csc/scc-csc/en/item/1937/index.do.

38 *St. Clare's Multifaith Housing Society v. Crossman*, 2023 ONLTB 63451.

39 *Black et al. v City of Toronto*, 2020 ONSC 6398 (CanLII) [Internet]. Available from: https://canlii.ca/t/jb937 at para 37.

40 Wickham S. Effective interventions for homeless populations: the evidence remains unclear. Lancet Public Health. 2020;5(6):304–5.

41 Hwang S, Burns T. Health interventions for people who are homeless. Lancet. 2014;384(9953):1541–7; Stafford A, Wood L. Tackling health inequities for people who are homeless: start with the social determinants. Int J Environ Res Public Health. 2017;14(12):1535. https://doi.org/10.3390/ijerph14121535.

42 Aubry T, Bloch G, Brcic V, et al. Effectiveness of permanent supportive housing and income assistance for homeless individuals in high-income countries: a systematic review. Lancet Public Health. 2020;5(6):342–60; Pottie K, Kendall C, Aubry T, et al. Clinical guideline for homeless and vulnerably housed people, and people with lived homelessness experience. CMAJ. 2020;192(10):e240–54; Zhao J, Williams C, Palepu A, et al. New Leaf Project: direct cash transfer pilot (final report). Vancouver (BC): Foundations for Social Change; 2020.

43 Quinones S. I don't know that I would even call it meth anymore. *The Atlantic*, 2021 Apr 18; Resnikoff N. How the Atlantic's big piece on meth and homelessness gets it wrong [Internet]. San Francisco: UCSF Benioff Homelessness and Housing Initiative; 2021 Nov 15. Available from: https://homelessness.ucsf.edu/blog/how-atlantics-big-piece-meth-and-homelessness-gets-it-wrong; Schellenberger M. San Fransicko: how progressives ruin cities. New York: Harper; 2021; Schwan K, Versteegh A, Perri M, et al. The state of women's housing need & homelessness in Canada: a literature review (Hache A, Nelson A, Kratochvil E, Malenfant J, editors). Toronto: Canadian Observatory on Homelessness Press; 2020; Segel-Brown B, Liberge-Simard R. *Federal program spending on housing affordability in 2021*. Ottawa: Office of the Parliamentary Budget Officer; 2021.

44 Resnikoff, N. San Fransicko is incorrect about housing affordability and homelessness [Internet]. San Francisco: USCF Benioff Homelessness and Housing Initiative; 2022 Jan 5. Available from: https://homelessness.ucsf.edu/blog/san-fransicko-incorrect-about-housing-affordability-and-homelessness.

45 Fitzpatrick S. Explaining homelessness: a critical realist perspective. Hous Theory Soc. 2005;22(1):1–17; Balasuria L, Buelt E, Tsai J. The never-ending loop: homelessness, psychiatric disorder and mortality. Psychiatr Times. 2020;37(5):12–4.

46 Finkelstein A, Zhou A, Aubman S, et al. Health care hotspotting: a randomized control trial. New England J Med. 2020;382(2):152–62.

47 Aubry T, Bloch G, Brcic V, et al. Effectiveness of permanent supportive housing and income assistance for homeless individuals in high-income countries: a systematic review. Lancet Public Health. 2020;5(6):342–60; Pottie K, Kendall C, Aubry T, et al. Clinical guideline for homeless and vulnerably housed people, and people with lived homelessness experience. CMAJ. 2020;192(10):e240–54.

48 Stafford A, Wood L. Tackling health inequities for people who are homeless: start with the social determinants. Int J Environ Res Public Health. 2017;14(12):1535. https://doi.org/10.3390/ijerph14121535; Clark M, Cornes M, Whiteford M, et al. Homelessness and integrated care: an application of integrated care knowledge to understanding services for wicked issues. J Integr Care. 2022;30(1):3–19.

5 Work and Health

NABILA F. QURESHI AND ANDREW PINTO

When we come to you
Our rags are torn off us
And you listen all over our naked body.
As to the cause of our illness
One glance at our rags would
Tell you more. It is the same cause that wears out
Our bodies and our clothes.
The pain in our shoulder comes
You say from the damp: and this is also the reason
For the stain on the wall of our flat.
So tell us:
Where does the damp come from?

– Bertolt Brecht, "A Worker's Speech to a Doctor"

Although written almost 100 years ago, these lines of poetry will resonate with most health providers today who work with individuals from communities made vulnerable by social and economic policies. The upstream causes of illness, disease, disability, and death are what are referred to as the social determinants of health, the conditions in which people live, work, and play that are shaped by the distribution of money, power, and resources.[1] Employment status and working conditions have powerful effects on people's health at the individual, community, and population levels.

Throughout this chapter, we use three cases to illustrate how employment status and working conditions can affect people's health, the importance of worker rights, and the potential role of legal services:

- Maya has worked at a marketing firm for several years, and she has consistently received excellent performance reviews and praise from her customers and managers. She recently had a child and is now pregnant with her second child. She applies for a promotion, but it is awarded to a newer male colleague whose performance reviews are comparatively weak.

- Jasper is a supervisor at a not-for-profit organization. He was involved in a serious car accident that led to the loss of vision in one eye and impaired vision in the other. As a result, he has difficulty reading documents, and staring at screens for prolonged periods causes eyestrain and headaches.
- Khadeejah works on an assembly line at an automotive parts factory. She identifies as Muslim and normally wears a hijab draped over her hair. Her manager tells her that she cannot wear the hijab because it is a safety risk – the cloth may become caught in machinery. However, Khadeejah cannot remove the hijab because she believes her faith requires her to wear it.

In this chapter, we provide a brief overview of work as a key social determinant of health before turning to employment, workplace, and human rights law in Canada. We discuss common problems that patients may encounter at work and some of the ways in which health providers can support patients with work-related health challenges, including key questions to ask patients and effective medical documentation to support disability-related accommodation requests. Throughout, we highlight some of the barriers to decent work and good health experienced by low-wage and precarious workers.

Work as a Key Social Determinant of Health

A large body of evidence has identified key threats to health posed by precarious work. A study of more than 90,000 men and women in Finland who were followed for more than a decade found that mortality was significantly higher among temporary workers compared with permanent workers. Moving from temporary to permanent employment was associated with a lower risk of death.[2] A study of 331 families in Toronto found that families living in market-rent households experienced a significant decrease in food insecurity if an adult gained full-time employment.[3] A study of temporary workers showed a rate ratio of 2.94 for non-fatal occupational injuries and of 2.54 for fatal occupational injuries.[4] Precarious work has consistently been found to have adverse effects on psychological morbidity.[5] A study of 5,679 temporary and permanent workers in Spain found a strong gradient association between the degree of employment precariousness and poor mental health, even after adjusting for age, immigrant status, socio-economic position, and previous unemployment.[6] In a study of 4,174 British civil servants followed for an average of 8.6 years, job insecurity was associated with a 1.42 times greater risk of incident coronary heart disease, controlling for socio-demographic variables and physiological and behavioural risk factors.[7]

In contrast to precarious work, decent work is work that is productive; delivers an income that provides social protection; ensures security in the workplace; leads to personal development and social integration; allows people to express their concerns, organize, and participate in decision-making that affects their work; and provides equality of opportunity across gender, race/ethnicity, age, and sexual orientation.

The health sector can play a role in supporting patients and communities towards the goal of decent work. As discussed later in this chapter, health providers develop close connections to patients and create a safe space in which it is possible to discuss challenging topics, including unemployment, workplace hazards, and precarious employment. Health providers can support patients who are experiencing legal challenges, such as unfair dismissal, abuse, or unfair treatment. Health organizations can be a place to support individuals in obtaining employment, often in close collaboration with employment experts.[8] Finally, networks of health providers can be a powerful voice in advocacy to advance decent work, such as the Decent Work and Health Network.[9]

Much of this chapter focuses on workplace rights and common workplace problems that may affect a patient's health. We acknowledge, however, that not all workplace-related health problems will have an origin or solution related to the law. Patients may experience health problems in relation to their work for which there is no legal recourse, or they may develop health problems in relation to workplace situations that are perfectly legal. For example, patients may develop mental health challenges and distress because of feelings of general disrespect within the workplace. This disrespect could take the form of not feeling valued at work or feeling that their work is not recognized. Often, such disrespect does not meet the legal definition of harassment or discrimination, and it is not illegal. However, patients nevertheless experience real effects on their mental health, and they are equally deserving of the care and support of their health providers.

Key Aspects of Workplace Law in Canada

A number of key terms used throughout this chapter require definition:

- *Employee*: an employee is a person who normally works for a supervising employer and is subject to their control and direction in the manner in which they perform their work. Employees in Canada are covered by the employment standards legislation of their province or territory or by the *Canada Labour Code* if they work in a federally regulated industry. Under such legislation, they are usually entitled to various rights, such as the minimum wage, vacation time, statutory holidays, job-protected parental leave, and overtime pay.
- *Independent contractor*: an independent contractor is a person who is considered to work for themselves. They generally maintain control and direction over the manner in which they perform their own work. Independent contractors are not covered by employment standards legislation in Canada. Many people who are actually employees are illegally misclassified as independent contractors by their employers, which can result in denial of their entitlements under employment standards and other legislation.
- *Worker*: in this chapter, we use the term *worker* as a neutral term that refers to anyone who performs work. This term includes employees, independent contractors, and people who have been misclassified as independent contractors but who are actually employees.

Overview of Workplace Laws in Canada

Employment and working conditions in Canada are regulated by a range of legislation, including provincial and territorial employment standards legislation; the federal *Canada Labour Code*; occupational health and safety legislation; Employment Insurance and workers' compensation legislation; and provincial, territorial, and federal human rights legislation. We provide some basic information about workers' rights under these various statutes, as well as common workplace problems that your patient may encounter.

Employment Standards Legislation

Most workers in Canada are provincially or territorially regulated. Each province and territory has its own employment standards statute that sets out minimum rights and entitlements for employees who work in that province or territory, including their rights concerning the minimum wage, vacation time, hours of work and overtime pay, parental leave and other types of leave, statutory holidays, severance entitlements if they are fired, and filing complaints against employers who may have violated their legal obligations to employees. For example, in Ontario the *Employment Standards Act, 2000* provides that employees have the right to take up to 18 months of job-protected parental leave, subject to certain conditions.[10]

Approximately 6 per cent of workers in Canada work in federal industries, such as banking, telecommunications, or inter-provincial trucking.[11] These workers are regulated by a single federal statute, the *Canada Labour Code*. Similar to provincial and territorial employment standards legislation, the *Canada Labour Code* sets out minimum rights and entitlements for employees.

Workers who are unionized have additional laws and protections that apply to them, compared with non-unionized workers. Employment lawyers generally do not have jurisdiction to advise unionized workers, who must work through their union. The most notable difference between unionized and non-unionized workers is, perhaps, the obvious: unionized workers have a union that can represent them in grievances against their employer and that bargains a collective agreement concerning all union members' entitlements in the workplace. By way of contrast, non-unionized workers are on their own or must hire a representative (such as a lawyer or paralegal) if they want assistance with addressing problems in the workplace.

Although every jurisdiction in Canada has legislation to protect the rights of employees, many employers do not comply with those legal obligations. Some employers do so deliberately, whereas others do so by mistake or because of a lack of knowledge about their legal obligations towards their employees. This can result in serious employment rights violations for employees, such as illegal pay reductions, refusals to pay the minimum wage or overtime pay, withholding of wages or other types of payments, termination without pay, refusing to permit an employee to take a job-protected leave of absence to which they are legally entitled, and illegal reprisals or retaliations against employees who attempt to assert their rights.

Low-wage workers, especially those employed in precarious work, most often experience these violations of their rights.[12(p. 43)] They are disproportionately women, racialized and Indigenous, newcomers or migrants with precarious immigration status, and persons with disabilities.[13(p. 27)] Sometimes they are aware of their rights and violations, but often they are not. Many have language barriers to understanding what their rights are and to communicating with their employer. Those workers who are aware of workplace rights violations often refuse to speak up for fear of reprisal, including getting harassed or fired, or the threat of deportation. Although such reprisal is illegal, many employers do it.

These types of workplace violations can have significant impacts on a worker's health. The denial of wages can create stress for a worker already struggling to pay the bills. Harassment or threats to penalize or fire the worker can cause fear and anxiety and give rise to mental health concerns. The worker may develop new health problems, and existing ones may be exacerbated.

Patients may be able to file an employment standards violation complaint with their provincial or territorial employment standards regulatory body. They may also have additional entitlements through civil litigation. It is important to be aware that complaints must be filed within a specified amount of time from when the alleged violation occurred. Patients who file a complaint may also give up the right to file a civil lawsuit if they file a complaint. It is best for patients to get legal advice about their options, where practicable, before proceeding with any complaint.

Table 5.1 provides a summary of key information about employment standards complaints across various jurisdictions in Canada, including which forum handles the complaints and how much time individuals have to file particular complaints.

Human Rights Legislation

Workers in Canada also have the right, under human rights legislation, not to be subject to workplace discrimination. Similar to employment standards legislation, each province and territory in Canada has its own human rights statute to protect workers from discrimination in the workplace. The *Canadian Human Rights Act* protects federally regulated workers from workplace discrimination. Human rights legislation usually applies to both employees and contractors.

However, the protections from discrimination are not without limit. Workers are protected from discrimination on the basis of specific grounds or characteristics that are listed in the human rights statute. For example, British Columbia's *Human Rights Code* states that a person must not refuse to employ or continue to employ someone,

Table 5.1. Forum and Limitation Periods for Employment Standards Complaints by Jurisdiction

Jurisdiction	Forum	Limitation period
Federal	Employment and Social Development Canada	*Unpaid wages*: within 6 months from the last day your employer was required to pay you[a] *Termination*: within 90 days from the date of your dismissal[b]
Alberta	Employment Standards Branch	*Termination*: within 6 months from the date of termination,[c] anytime up to 6 months after the date on which an averaging arrangement ceases to apply, or anytime up to 6 months after the end of the averaging period[d]
British Columbia	Employment Standards Branch	*Termination*: within 6 months from the last day of work[e] *Other*: within 6 months of the alleged contravention[f]
Manitoba	Employment Standards Branch	*Unpaid wages*: within 6 months from the last day your wages were payable[g] *Termination*: within 6 months from the date of the termination[h]
Ontario	Ministry of Labour, Immigration, Training and Skills Development	Claim must be filed within 2 years of the alleged *Employment Standards Act* violation[i]
Quebec	Commission des normes de l'équité de la santé et de la sécurité du travail	*Differential treatment based on hiring date*: within 12 months from the date on which the distinction became known[j] *Dismissal, suspension, transfer, reprisal, or discrimination*: within 45 days from the alleged violation if the violation falls under s. 122.[k] If the reprisal is based on the ground that the employee reached or passed the age at which they should retire, the claim must be made within 90 days[l] *Psychological harassment*: within 2 years of the last incident of the offending behaviour[m] *Dismissal without good and sufficient cause*: Employees with 2 uninterrupted years of service may make a claim within 45 days of dismissal.[n]
New Brunswick	Department of Post-Secondary Education, Training, and Labour	Complaint must be filed within 12 months after the alleged violation or denial.[o]
Newfoundland and Labrador	Labour Standards Division	*Termination*: within 6 months of the date the employee's contract is terminated[p] *Other*: Complaint must be made within 2 years of the date of the alleged violation.[q]

Jurisdiction	Forum	Limitation period
Northwest Territories	Department of Education, Culture and Employment	A complaint may be made at any time within 12 months after the date on which the subject matter of the complaint occurred.[r]
Nova Scotia	Labour Standards Division	Complaint must be made within 6 months from the date that the alleged violation took place.[s]
Nunavut	Labour Standards Compliance Office	Prosecution for an offence under the *Labour Standards Act* may not be commenced more than two years after the time when the subject matter of the prosecution arose.[t]
Prince Edward Island	Employment Standards Branch	Complaints respecting benefits or an employers' lack of pay transparency must be made within 12 months of the alleged violation.[u]
Saskatchewan	Employment Standards Branch	*Unpaid wages*: within 12 months of the last day that your wages were payable or 12 months of the last day on which payment of wages was to be made[v] *Other*: within 12 months after the date on which you knew or reasonably should have known about the alleged violation[w]
Yukon	Employment Standards Office	*Unpaid wages*: within 6 months from the last day wages were payable.[x] *Other*: within 6 months after the date on which the subject matter of the complaint arose[y]

[a] *Canada Labour Code*, RSC 1985, c L-2, s 251.01(2).

[b] *Canada Labour Code*, RSC 1985, c L-2, s 240(2).

[c] *Employment Standards Code*, RSA 2000, c E-9, s 82(2).

[d] *Employment Standards Code*, RSA 2000, c E-9, s 82(2.1).

[e] *Employment Standards Act*, RSBC 1996, c 113, s 74(3).

[f] *Employment Standards Act*, RSBC 1996, c 113, s 74(4).

[g] *Employment Standards Code*, CCSM c E110, s 87.

[h] *Employment Standards Code*, CCSM c E110, s 60(6).

[i] *Employment Standards Act*, 2000, SO 2000, c 41, s 96(3), s 114, s 139.

[j] *Act respecting labour standards*, CQLR c N-1.1, s 121.1.

[k] *Act respecting labour standards*, CQLR c N-1.1, s 123.

[l] *Act respecting labour standards*, CQLR c N-1.1, s 123.1.

[m] *Act respecting labour standards*, CQLR c N-1.1, s 123.7.

[n] *Act respecting labour standards*, CQLR c N-1.1, s 124.

[o] *Employment Standards Act*, SNB 1982, c E-7.2, s 61(1).

[p] *Labour Standards Act*, RSNL 1990, c L-2, s 62(3).

[q] *Labour Standards Act*, RSNL 1990, c L-2, s 62(3).

[r] *Employment Standards Act*, SNWT 2007, c 13, s 61(2).

[s] *Labour Standards Code*, RSNS 1989, c 246, ss 21(3D), s 81.

[t] Labour Standards Act, RSNWT 1988, c L-1, s 70.

[u] *Employment Standards Act*, RSPEI 1988, c E-6.2, ss 30(2–2.1).

[v] *Saskatchewan Employment Act*, SS 2013, c S-15.1, s 2–89(1).

[w] *Saskatchewan Employment Act*, SS 2013, c S-15.1, s 2–89(3).

[x] *Employment Standards Act*, RSY 2002, c 72, s 73(3)(a)

[y] *Employment Standards Act*, RSY 2002, c 72, s 73(3)(b).

or discriminate against them in relation to their job, because of that person's

> Indigenous identity, race, colour, ancestry, place of origin, political belief, religion, marital status, family status, physical or mental disability, sex, sexual orientation, gender identity or expression, or age of that person or because that person has been convicted of a criminal or summary conviction offence that is unrelated to the employment or to the intended employment of that person.[14]

The prohibited grounds of discrimination are similar in each jurisdiction in Canada, but not identical. For example, discrimination in employment on the basis of a worker's political belief is prohibited in most provinces and territories in Canada, but it is not a protected ground in the human rights statutes of Alberta, Saskatchewan, Ontario, and Nunavut.

If a protected ground is the reason, or even only one of the reasons, why a worker has been subject to adverse treatment in the workplace, then they may have a claim for workplace discrimination. One example of such discrimination includes the following:

> *Maya's case*: When Maya asks why she did not receive the promotion, her employer tells her they were worried she wouldn't be around for the next year. Maya has likely experienced discrimination in employment on the basis of her sex and her family status as a mother and expectant mother.

Finally, employers have a duty to accommodate workers who may have a specific need or barrier related to a characteristic protected by human rights legislation. Accommodation in the workplace may mean the employer changes aspects of the worker's workplace or working conditions, such as the schedule or number of hours they work, the provision of assistive tools and devices, the specific tasks they are required to perform, or other terms and conditions. Two examples follow:

> *Jasper's case:* Jasper's employer must accommodate his disability, which may include providing visual reading aids and devices, allowing him to take breaks throughout the day, and reducing the number of hours he works at a computer.

> *Khadeejah's case*: As an accommodation, the manager agrees to Khadeejah's suggestion that she wear a tight-fitting hijab with no loose ends that could get caught in machinery.

Employers are required to provide reasonable, but not perfect, accommodation to the point of undue hardship. Workers are entitled to reasonable accommodation, but not necessarily their preferred accommodation. A failure to accommodate a worker up to the point of undue hardship constitutes discrimination and may entitle the worker to damages and other types of compensation.

Patients may be able to file a human rights violation complaint with their provincial, territorial, or federal body responsible for regulating human rights (listed in Table 5.2). Depending on which province or territory they work in, unionized workers may or may not have the ability to instead file an independent human rights complaint on a labour grievance, and they should check with their union or their provincial or territorial human rights body. Patients who have experienced discrimination may also have additional entitlements through civil litigation. It is important to be aware that complaints must be filed within a specified amount of time from when the discrimination occurred. Patients who file a complaint may also give up the right to file a civil lawsuit. Where practicable, it is best for patients to get legal advice about their options before proceeding with any complaint.

Occupational Health and Safety Legislation

Workers have the right to be safe at work. Most workplaces in Canada are required to comply with their provincial or territorial occupational health and safety legislation. Federally regulated workplaces must comply with the health and safety requirements in the *Canada Labour Code*.

Occupational health and safety legislation usually applies to both employees and independent contractors, as well as employers, with some exceptions. The legislation generally covers the employer's and the worker's duties to ensure a safe workplace and addresses the handling of dangerous substances and the worker's right to refuse unsafe work. At the time of writing, all jurisdictions in Canada with the exception of Nova Scotia also require employers to have workplace harassment prevention policies and to take steps to address harassment complaints, such as an investigation. The employer, the overseeing board or Ministry, or both may be required to conduct a health and safety investigation in certain circumstances if they receive a complaint from a worker. Employers who receive a health and safety complaint or concern from a worker are not permitted to punish the worker for doing so, although in reality some employers do.

Workers who have a concern about their health or safety at work should speak to their workplace's health and safety representative

Table 5.2. Forum and Limitation Periods for Human Rights Claims in Employment by Jurisdiction

Jurisdiction	Forum	Limitation period
Federal	Canadian Human Rights Commission	Commission has the discretion to not deal with complaints based on acts or omissions that occurred more than 1 year before the claim.[a]
Alberta	Alberta Human Rights Commission	Within 1 year after the alleged violation of the *Alberta Human Rights Act*[b]
British Columbia	British Columbia Human Rights Tribunal	Within 1 year of the alleged contravention (or the last instance thereof)[c]
Manitoba	Manitoba Human Rights Commission	Within 1 year after the day of the alleged contravention or within 1 year after the day of the last alleged instance of the contravention[d]
New Brunswick	New Brunswick Human Rights Commission	Within 1 year of the alleged violation of the *Human Rights Act* or last instance thereof (if continuing)[e]
Newfoundland and Labrador	Newfoundland and Labrador Human Rights Commission	Within 12 months of the alleged contravention, or within 12 months of the last instance of the alleged contravention (if ongoing)[f]
Northwest Territories	Northwest Territories Human Rights Commission	Within 2 years after the alleged contravention of the *Human Rights Act* or last instance thereof (if continuous)[g]
Nova Scotia	Nova Scotia Human Rights Commission	Within 12 months of the action or conduct complained of, or within 12 months of the last instance of the action or conduct (if ongoing)[h]
Nunavut	Nunavut Human Rights Tribunal	Within 2 years after the alleged contravention of the *Human Rights Act* or last instance thereof (if continuous)[i]
Ontario	Ontario Human Rights Tribunal	Within 1 year after the incident to which the application relates or within 1 year after the last incident in a series[j]
Prince Edward Island	PEI Human Rights Commission	Within 1 year of the date that the alleged contravention of the *Human Rights Act* occurred[k]
Quebec	Commission des droits de la personne et des droits de la jeunesse	Commission has discretion to not deal with complaints based on acts or omissions that occurred more than 2 years before the claim[l]
Saskatchewan	Saskatchewan Human Rights Commission	Within 1 year after the complainant became aware, or should have been aware, of the alleged act of discrimination[m]

Jurisdiction	Forum	Limitation period
Yukon	Yukon Human Rights Commission	Within 18 months of the alleged breach or the last instance of a continuing contravention[n]

[a] *Canadian Human Rights Act*, RSC 1985, c H-5, s 41(1).
[b] *Alberta Human Rights Act*, RSA 2000, c A-25.5, s 20(2)(b).
[c] *Human Rights Code*, RSBC 1996, c 210, s 22(1–2).
[d] *Human Rights Code*, CCSM, c H175, s 23(1).
[e] *Human Rights Act*, RSNB 2011, c 171, ss 18(1–2).
[f] *Human Rights Act*, SNL 2010, c H-13.1, s 25(2).
[g] *Human Rights Act*, SNWT 2002, c 18, s 29(2)(a-b).
[h] *Human Rights Act*, RSNB 2011, c 171, s 29(2).
[i] *Human Rights Act*, SNu 2003, c 12, s 23(1–2).
[j] *Human Rights Code*, RSO 1990, c H.19, s 34(1).
[k] *Human Rights Act*, RSPEI 1988, c H-12, s 22(2).
[l] *Charter of Human Rights and Freedoms*, CQLR c C-12, s 77.
[m] *Saskatchewan Human Rights Code*, SS 1979, c S-24.2, s 29(5).
[n] *Human Rights Act*, SNWT 2002, c 18, s 29(2)(a).

or their union representative, if they have any. They may be able to file a complaint with the provincial, territorial, or federal ministry or board responsible for overseeing workplace health and safety. Table 5.3 includes some key information about where and how workers can do this.

Employment Insurance

Employment Insurance (EI) is a federal government program that provides temporary income support to workers who have stopped working. Eligible workers receive benefits in the amount of 55 per cent of their regular earnings, up to a maximum amount per week.[15] A number of different benefits are available through the program:

- *Regular benefits*: for workers who have lost their job through no fault of their own, and who are looking for and available for work. Workers who are fired for misconduct may not be eligible for this benefit. Workers who have quit their jobs may also not be eligible, unless they can prove they had just cause for leaving their job. Some examples of situations that could constitute just cause include discrimination, harassment, or unsafe working conditions.
- *Sickness benefits*: for workers who are unable to work because of illness, injury, or quarantine. To qualify for sickness benefits, workers need a medical certificate signed by their doctor or

Table 5.3. Forum and Limitation Periods for OHS Complaints by Jurisdiction

Jurisdiction	Forum	Information about filing complaints
Federal	Federal Public Sector Labour Relations and Employment Board	You must complain to your supervisor before exercising other recourse (unless it concerns ss 128, 129, or 132 of the *Canada Labour Code*).[a] *Reprisal*: If your employer punishes you for exercising your *Code* rights, you can complain to the board within 90 days of the date that you knew or ought to have known of the impugned conduct.[b]
Alberta	OHS Contact Centre	You should tell inform your supervisor or health and safety committee or representative about any OHS issues. You can also report to an OHS Contact Centre.[c] *Reprisal*: If you are disciplined for exercising your *OHSA* rights, you can file a complaint within 180 days from the date the action was taken against you.[d]
British Columbia	WorkSafeBC	If you become aware of unsafe or unhealthy conditions at work, you should report it to someone at your work or union or to WorkSafeBC. *Reprisal*: If your employer punishes you for exercising your OHS rights, you can file a complaint for unpaid wages within 60 days from the date the wages become payable, or for all other complaints within 1 year of the alleged prohibited action.[e]
Manitoba	Manitoba Workplace Safety and Health	Contact your supervisor or your workplace safety and health committee with any OHS concerns. If your concern is not resolved or is urgent, you can contact Manitoba Workplace Safety and Health. *Reprisal*: If your employer punishes you for exercising your OHS rights, you can file a complaint with a Safety and Health Officer within 6 months of the alleged punishment.[f]
Newfoundland and Labrador	Occupational Health and Safety Division (Service NL) Labour Relations Board	You should report OHS concerns to your supervisor, OHS committee, or WH&S designate. You can contact the Occupational Health and Safety Division if the concern continues. *Reprisal*: If your employer discriminates against you for exercising your OHS rights, you can file a complaint with the Labour Relations Board.[g]

Jurisdiction	Forum	Information about filing complaints
New Brunswick	WorkSafeNB	Report OHS concerns to your supervisor or joint health and safety committee. If the issue is not resolved, contact WorkSafeNB. *Reprisal*: If your employer discriminates against you (or threatens to) for exercising your OHS rights, you can file a complaint within 1 year of the conduct giving rise to the complaint.[h]
Northwest Territories	Workers Safety and Compensation Commission	You should report OHS concerns to your supervisor. If the concern persists, you can complain to your joint OHS committee or to the commission. *Reprisal*: If your employer discriminates against you for exercising your OHS rights, you can complain to the Supreme Court of the Northwest Territories.[i]
Nova Scotia	Safety Branch Department of Labour, Skills and Immigration	Contact your supervisor or joint health and safety committee with OHS concerns. You can also contact the Safety Branch to report health or safety issues. *Reprisal*: If your employer discriminates against you (or threatens to) for exercising your OHS rights, you can make a complaint within 30 days of the conduct giving rise to the complaint.[j]
Nunavut	Workers Safety and Compensation Commission	You should report OHS concerns to your supervisor. If the concern persists, you can complain to your joint OHS committee or to the Workers Safety and Compensation Commission. *Reprisal*: if your employer discriminates against you for exercising your OHS rights, you can complain to the Supreme Court of the Northwest Territories.[k]
Ontario	Ministry of Labour, Immigration, Training and Skills Development Ontario Labour Relations Board	You can file a complaint with the Ministry if the situation has not been corrected after you (a) speak to your employer and (b) consult your JHSC or health and safety representative. *Reprisal*: If you have been punished for exercising your *OHSA* rights, you can file a complaint with the Labour Relations Board.[l]
Prince Edward Island	Workers Compensation Board of PEI	You should report OHS concerns to your supervisor or joint OHS committee or representative. If the complaint is not resolved, you can contact WCB. *Reprisal*: If your employer discriminates against you for exercising your OHS rights, you can file a complaint by stating the nature of the complaint in writing to the WCB Director of OHS.[m]

(Continued)

Table 5.3. (Continued)

Jurisdiction	Forum	Information about filing complaints
Quebec	Commission des normes de l'équité de la santé et de la sécurité du travail	Contact your employer or health and safety committee with OHS complaints. You can also contact a confidential, on-call CNESST inspector to report a dangerous or risky occurrence. *Reprisal*: If you have been punished for exercising your OHS rights, you can file a claim with CNESST within 30 days of the events giving rise to the claim.[n]
Saskatchewan	Occupational Health and Safety Harassment and Discriminatory Prevention Unit	Contact your employer or Occupational Health Committee or representative for health and safety concerns. If the issue is not resolved, contact an OHO. *Reprisal*: If your employer discriminates against you for exercising your OHS rights, you can file a complaint with an OHO with the Harassment and Discriminatory Prevention Unit.[o]
Yukon	Workers' Safety and Compensation Board	You should report OHS concerns to your supervisor. If unresolved, you can report to your joint health and safety committee or health and safety representative. If still unresolved, you can complain to the WSCB. *Reprisal*: If you are punished for exercising your OHS rights, you can complain to the WSCB within 21 days of the conduct giving rise to the complaint.[p]

[a] *Canada Labour Code*, RSC 1985, c L-2, s 127.
[b] *Canada Labour Code*, RSC 1985, c L-2, ss 133, 147.
[c] *Occupational Health and Safety Act*, SA 2020, c O-2.2, s 5(1).
[d] *Occupational Health and Safety Act*, SA 2020, c O-2.2, ss 18–19.
[e] *Workers Compensation Act*, RSBC 2019, c 1, ss 48–49.
[f] *Workplace Safety and Health Act*, CCSM c W210, s 42.1(1).
[g] *Occupational Health and Safety Act*, RSNL 1990, c O-3, ss 49–51.
[h] *Occupational Health and Safety Act*, SNB 1983, c O-0.2, s 25.
[i] *Safety Act*, RSNWT 1988, c S-1, s 22.
[j] *Occupational Health and Safety Act*, SNS 1996, c 7, ss 45–46.
[k] *Safety Act*, RSNWT (Nu) 1988, c. S-1, s 22.
[l] *Occupational Health and Safety Act*, RSO 1990, c O.1, s 50.
[m] *Occupational Health and Safety Act*, RSPEI 1988, c O-1.01, ss 30–31.
[n] *Act respecting occupational health and safety*, CQLR c S-2.1, s 227.
[o] *Saskatchewan Employment Act*, SS 2013, c S-15.1, ss 3–35, 3–36.
[p] *Workers Safety and Compensation Act*, SY 2021, c 11, s 54.

OHS = occupational health and safety; *OHSA* = *Occupational Health and Safety Act*; OHO = occupational health office; JHSC = Joint Health and Safety Committee; CNESST = Commission des normes de l'équité de la santé et de la sécurité du travail; WCB = Workers Compensation Board; WH&S = Workers Health & Safety; WSCB = Workers' Safety and Compensation Board.

approved medical practitioner. The certificate should confirm (a) the date the doctor saw the patient, (b) that the worker is too sick to work, and (c) how long they need to be off work or when they can be expected to return to work. EI sickness benefits were recently significantly improved, so workers whose claim started on 18 December 2022 or later can now receive sickness benefits for up to 26 weeks. Workers whose claim began before that date can receive the benefits for up to 15 weeks. The duration of 26 weeks parallels many short-term disability insurance programs and is especially helpful for low-wage and precarious workers who do not have workplace benefits or insurance.

- *Maternity benefits*: for workers who are pregnant or who have recently had a baby.
- *Parental benefits*: for workers who are a parent to a newborn baby or a recently adopted child.
- *Compassionate care benefits*: for workers who need time off work to care for a person who is ill and who could die within the next six months.
- *Family caregiver benefit for children*: for workers who need time off work to care for a critically ill child.
- *Family caregiver benefit for adults*: for workers who need time off work to care for a critically ill adult.
- *Fishing benefits*: for self-employed fishers who are actively looking for work.

The EI program also offers a family supplement for low-income families. Families whose net family income is $25,921 or less, who have children, and in which at least one parent receives the Canada Child Benefit are considered low income. The family supplement may increase the EI recipient's benefit rate up to 80 per cent of their average insurable earnings.

Workers who have been fired or who are taking time off work should apply for EI right away. Delays in applying for the benefit may affect the ability to qualify for the benefit and could also result in lower benefit amounts. Workers who have been fired for cause (e.g., because of alleged misconduct) or who have voluntarily resigned from their job may be ineligible for EI, but there are important exceptions to these rules. As a result, these workers should still apply for EI in case they are found to fit within an applicable exception or are otherwise able to challenge the facts surrounding why their job came to an end.

EI is usually only available to workers who are employees. Most employees in Canada pay into the EI program through premiums that their employer takes out of their paycheques. However, workers who are self-employed or who are contractors do not pay premiums into the program and cannot receive EI unless they join a special EI program for the self-employed. Employees who have been misclassified as independent contractors are entitled to receive EI but may first have to prove that they are employees. Workers who are unsure about whether they are an employee or independent contractor can apply and request a determination of their status.

Access to EI is especially critical for low-wage and precarious workers, who are unlikely to have benefits and insurance, who are often denied termination and severance entitlements if they lose their job, and who are less likely to have savings or other sources of income to fall back on. However, low-wage and precarious workers, especially women, have historically been less likely to qualify for EI.[16(pp. 2–3)] This is because of onerous eligibility rules that disadvantage people who do part-time, temporary, and contract work. Even when these workers do qualify, the benefit amounts they receive are usually inadequate to support their basic living expenses. This means that many workers who pay into the EI system are unable to access it or meaningfully benefit from it. EI requires significant reforms to better support the workers in Canada most in need of it: low-wage and precarious workers.

Workers' Compensation

Workers' compensation is benefits for injuries or illness related to the work that a person does. Each province and territory in Canada has a workers' compensation board that pays these benefits to workers. There is also the Federal Workers' Compensation Service, which provides compensation to federally regulated workers.

Workers who have a work-related injury or illness may be entitled to a range of important benefits, such as loss of earnings, health care costs, travel costs to visit a doctor or attend therapy, retirement income that the worker could not get because of their injury, or compensation for permanent disability caused by work.

Workers' compensation is a no-fault system, meaning that workers who become injured or ill in relation to their work are entitled to the benefits, regardless of whose fault it was. The work does not have to be the only cause of the injury or illness, but it must typically be a significant cause.

Work-related injury or illness can occur in many different ways. Here we outline several examples, using Khadeejah's case to illustrate them:

- *Accident*: If Khadeejah trips over a cable while working at the factory, falls, and sustains a broken leg, this is a work-related injury that was caused by an accident.
- *Health problem that develops over time*: If Khadeejah experiences neck and shoulder strain and pain, this may be a symptom of a

longer-term health problem. It may not be apparent whether it
is related to Khadeejah's work because she did not experience
an accident or sudden onset of pain. Instead, the pain has been
ongoing for a long time. However, it may have been caused by
repetitive lifting and leaning while she works on the assembly line,
in which case it is a work-related injury.

- *Resurgence of a previous medical condition*: If Khadeejah had a
  previous medical condition that returns or becomes worse
  in relation to her work, this is also a work-related injury. For
  example, if she previously suffered a herniated disc in her lower
  back and experiences pain again because of repetitive lifting or
  straining at work, she may be entitled to workers' compensation
  benefits.
- *A work-related injury that leads to another injury*: If Khadeejah breaks
  her leg after tripping over a cable at work and then develops knee
  pain in her other leg as she heals because she is now forced to place
  more weight on it, the knee pain is also a work-related injury.
- *Mental health challenges*: Work-related injuries can be psychological
  as well as physical. For example, Khadeejah may develop
  depression because of significant pain from an injury at work, or
  she may develop posttraumatic stress disorder after witnessing a
  terrible accident at work.

A patient who may have a work-related injury or disease should report
it to their employer and workers' compensation board right away. The
passage of time can impede a worker's ability to prove that the injury
or illness is related to work.

It is crucial that health providers carefully document their patients'
symptoms and health issues. Health providers should ask what kind of
work the patient performs and be alert to the possibility of long-term
problems that may develop as a result of repetitive work and strain,
particularly for physical labourers. Although the patient may not need
workers' compensation at first, they may in the future, and health providers' documentation of the patient's condition over time could be key
to proving that the injury or disease is workplace related.

Finally, not all workplaces in Canada have workers' compensation
coverage. Whether a workplace or industry is covered will depend on
the workers' compensation legislation in the jurisdiction where the
worker works. For example, in Ontario employers in the agricultural,
manufacturing, and construction industries must have workers' compensation coverage. However, employers in certain industries, such as
banking, private daycares, and barbers and hair salons, are not required
to participate in the workers' compensation system. Employers in these

industries may apply for optional coverage, but most do not because it is an additional expense for them.

If a worker is not sure whether their workplace is covered by workers' compensation, they can ask their employer. However, some employers required to provide it may not (in violation of the law), so workers should also call their local workers' compensation board to confirm.

Migrant Workers

Migrant worker is a term that refers to workers without permanent resident immigration status in Canada. It can include workers with work permits, workers with study permits, or those who are undocumented. Migrant workers are employed in various sectors of the economy, including farm work, care work, and transportation work and in the food, retail, and construction industries. They typically fall within one of several federal programs:

- the Caregiver Program (formerly the Live-in Caregiver Program), largely made up of Filipina, Indonesian, and Latin American women;
- the Seasonal Agricultural Workers Program, largely made up of workers from Mexico and the Caribbean; or
- the Temporary Foreign Worker Program stream for low-wage positions (including people from countries in the Global South) in primary agriculture and other streams.[17(p. 2)]

More than 400,000 migrant workers have open work permits that entitle them to work for any employer.[18(p. 2)] Approximately 900,000 migrant workers have closed work permits, which restrict them to working only for a single employer and can lead to exploitation and abuse.[19(p. 2)]

The rules and laws that apply to migrant workers can be complex. Generally, even workers without a valid work permit or Social Insurance Number still have rights under employment standards, human rights, health and safety, and workers' compensation legislation. With some exceptions, this includes the right to entitlements such as the minimum wage and a safe workplace.

However, in spite of their rights, migrant workers are uniquely vulnerable and over-represented in precarious work.[20(p. 1)] Their lack of permanent resident status compounds their precarity by making them vulnerable to the risk of deportation if they speak out. As a result, they are consistently subject to abuse and exploitation in the workplace, including harassment, sexual harassment, unpaid or unfair wages, substandard living accommodations that pose health concerns, discrimination and other violations of their rights, having their passport and other legal documents taken away, and the threat of deportation if they attempt to report employer abuse or assert their rights.[21] They may lack documentation to access public health care and may not have private health insurance from their employer. Their geographic location, often rural, and lack of immigration status pose further barriers to equitable access to health care.[22(p. 6)] Many employers will discourage or prohibit migrant workers from taking time off work to seek health care, or else refuse to provide means of transportation to do so. Language barriers add a further level of precarity for migrant workers to understand or enforce their rights.

Later in this chapter we provide tips for working with patients who are migrant workers. However, we recognize that many migrant workers are unable to access health care at all and that much work remains to be done to ensure equitable and meaningful access to health care for all migrant workers.

Common Work-Related Issues and Challenges That May Arise in Clinical Encounters

Termination of Employment

One of the most common challenges many workers will experience in their lifetime is getting fired from their job. This event can cause enormous stress and other health problems, such as anxiety and depression. For many workers, the loss of a job and income has serious consequences: it can mean losing one's home; becoming unable to afford food, electricity, daycare, medication, or other basic needs; and being unable to care for one's family. Job loss can also lead to feelings of shame, humiliation, hurt, and loss of identity for the worker. In this context, it is important for workers to understand that they may be entitled to compensation for getting fired. Receiving adequate compensation from the employer, in accordance with the worker's legal entitlements, can reduce the financial strain and other challenges that result from the termination of employment.

In Canada, employers are entitled to fire non-unionized employees for almost any reason, as long as they provide sufficient notice to the employee.[23] This means advising the employee ahead of time about the date of their termination so that they have time to look for alternative work or paying them the equivalent amount of wages. Employers are usually required to pay their employees termination, severance pay, or both in accordance with employment standards legislation.[24] This usually means a week's worth of wages for each year that the employee worked for the employer, up to a maximum amount.

However, the employee may be entitled to additional compensation, commonly referred to as "common-law notice" or "reasonable notice of termination." This can be a significant amount, particularly when the employee is older and has worked for the employer for many years, making it difficult for them to become re-employed. For example, a 60-year-old individual who worked for a construction company for 18 years before they were fired may be entitled to wages equivalent to 12 to 18 months of pay as compensation.

Although some employers choose to provide common-law notice to employees they have fired, many do not – either deliberately or because they are unaware of legal obligations to do so. Workers will usually need the assistance of a lawyer to determine their entitlements and obtain them from the employer.

Finally, employees may be entitled to additional compensation if they have been subject to discrimination, harassment, or other poor treatment in the workplace.

Constructive Dismissal

Constructive dismissal is a specific type of termination of employment. It occurs when an employer unilaterally breaks the employment contract in a serious way or substantially changes the terms of an employee's job without the employee's consent. When this occurs, it is as though the employee has been fired, and they become entitled to termination pay and potentially common-law notice or other types of compensation.

Some common changes that may trigger a constructive dismissal include

- significantly reducing the employee's compensation;
- demoting the employee, reducing the employee's job responsibilities, or changing the employee's reporting relationships;
- requiring the employee to move to a different geographic location;
- requiring the employee to work in a poisoned work environment (i.e., work in an environment in which the employee faces ongoing harassment, discriminatory conduct, or improper employer discipline);
- refusing to address an employee's complaint of harassment or assault, including sexual harassment or assault; and
- failing to pay the employee or placing them on an unpaid leave.

Constructive dismissals can be complex. Some employees quit their jobs and later assert that a constructive dismissal occurred. However, an employee who quits and is later unable to prove that constructive dismissal occurred may not be able to receive any termination payments from their former employer. Wherever possible, it is important for patients to first consult a lawyer about whether they have a claim for constructive dismissal before taking further action.

Failure to Accommodate Disabilities

Discrimination in employment on the basis of disability is one of the most common complaints received by human rights tribunals in Canada. Workers with one or more disabilities often experience barriers to obtaining a job, keeping it, or performing their job duties. As we explained earlier, employers have a duty to accommodate workers with disabilities up to the point of undue hardship.

This includes a procedural duty to obtain all relevant information about the worker's disability and conduct an individualized assessment of their needs and accommodation measures. It also includes a substantive duty to provide reasonable accommodation measures or, if the employer cannot do so, it must justify that doing so would cause undue hardship to the employer.

The duty to accommodate is present at all stages of the working relationship, including when interviewing a worker (even if the worker ultimately does not get hired) and throughout the time the worker works for the employer up to the point of termination. For example, an employer who fails to accommodate a worker up to the point of undue hardship and then fires that worker on the basis that the worker allegedly cannot do the job has very likely discriminated against the worker.

Health providers should be aware that human rights legislation generally defines *disability* much more broadly than other schemes they may be familiar with, such as the Canada Pension Plan (CPP) disability benefit or provincial and territorial social or income assistance benefits. This generous approach to the definition of disability is intended to extend human rights protection to as many people as possible and give meaningful effect to human rights legislation. However, there are limits: human rights tribunals have found that the cold, flu, stress, and other conditions viewed as temporary or transitory do not constitute disabilities within the meaning of human rights legislation.

Workers who have experienced a failure to accommodate their disability may be entitled to compensation for their pain and suffering, lost wages, reinstatement to their job if they were fired in relation to their disability, and public interest remedies such as human rights training for the employer.

Harassment

Workplace harassment is a series of actions or comments that the perpetrator knows, or ought to know, are unwelcome. It includes actions or comments that demean, belittle, offend, or cause personal humiliation or embarrassment and acts of intimidation or threat. Generally, a series of actions or events is required to establish harassment, but in some cases a single serious occurrence can constitute harassment.

Workplace harassment is prohibited under human rights legislation if the harassment in question is related to the race, gender, disability, religion, or other protected characteristic of the worker. Harassment is generally not expressly prohibited under occupational health and safety legislation. However, as previously discussed, all jurisdictions with the exception of Nova Scotia require employers to have workplace harassment prevention policies and to address harassment complaints that may arise.

Harassment can occur within the workplace or at any event or location related to work, such as during travel to work; at employer-sponsored events, including social events; and at a conference where attendance is sponsored or sanctioned by the employer.

Some examples that can constitute harassment include

- yelling and swearing at a worker;
- unwelcome physical contact, such as touching, rubbing, patting, or slapping, which can constitute sexual harassment;
- making fun of a worker's religious garment;
- threatening the safety of the worker; and
- regular and inappropriate remarks about a worker's appearance.

Harassment is sometimes difficult to discern. Criticism and constructive feedback about work performance or management direction about work is usually not harassment, unless it is accompanied by offensive behaviour such as yelling and swearing. When harassment has occurred, workers may have options for a legal remedy under occupational health and safety legislation, human rights legislation, and workers' compensation or through civil litigation.

A note on workplace sexual harassment: Workplace sexual or gender-based harassment is a serious form of harassment that can include unwelcome physical contact, gestures, and actions, as well as unwelcome verbal conduct, such as insults, threats, suggestive comments, and propositions. Employers are responsible for providing a workplace that is free of sexual harassment and for taking action to prevent and address it where it occurs. Where it does occur, there can be serious repercussions for the mental and physical health of the person who experienced the harassment and cascading effects on their ability to work, support their family, and access income supports or other important aspects of their lives.

Workplace sexual harassment raises complex and overlapping issues of human rights, health, and criminal, tort, and health and safety laws that are beyond the scope of this chapter. However, we hope that future editions of this book will include discussion of sexual and gender-based harassment and violence (not only in the workplace but beyond it as well), how it affects patients' lives, and how health care workers can best support them. In the meantime, for further reading and resources, readers can consult the Ending Violence Association of Canada, Women's Legal Education and Action Fund, and the Sexual Harassment and Assault Resource Exchange (Ontario only).

Misclassification

As we discussed near the start of this chapter, some workers are employees, and others may be independent contractors. Some workers fall into a third, in-between category, dependent contractors.

The worker's classification is important because it determines their legal rights and entitlements. Employees are entitled to the protections of employment standards legislation, as well as other employment-related benefits such as EI, CPP, workers' compensation, and private health and dental insurance. Independent contractors generally are not. Dependent contractors may have some or all of these entitlements.

Many workers who are actually employees are misclassified as independent contractors or as self-employed and denied access to these important rights and protections. And misclassification is on the rise: many employers deliberately misclassify employees to avoid the costs and legal responsibilities associated with employment, such as health and safety requirements, paying the minimum wage, vacation and statutory holiday pay, EI and CPP premiums, and workplace safety insurance premiums and to avoid the right of employees to unionize and bargain collectively.

This problem has become prevalent in what is often called the "gig economy," especially when workers provide transportation and food delivery services through apps. However, misclassification can occur in any industry, such as cleaning, childcare, transportation, and trucking and even in industries that do commonly have independent contractors. The classification of the worker is individualized and depends on the worker's specific circumstances and working relationship with the employer.

The cost of misclassification to workers is steep: they are often "forced to absorb the cost of unpaid wages and to work longer hours or at multiple jobs."[25(p. 32)] This can contribute to poor physical and mental health for the worker.

It is important to note that just because an employer has told a worker that they are an independent contractor, and has even had the worker sign a contract stating they are a contractor, that does not necessarily mean that the worker is legally an independent contractor. The worker's legal status as an employee or independent contractor is not determined by these things alone. Rather, there are different legal tests, depending on the right or benefit the worker is seeking, that consider the degree of control the employer had over the worker to determine whether they were truly an employee or not. In reality, though, workers who have been told they are a contractor, or who have signed a contract to that effect, usually believe it – and believe they have no right to pursue legal action against the employer.

Misclassified workers do have legal options for redress and can end up reclaiming thousands of dollars in unpaid wages, EI, workers' compensation, and other entitlements, which can significantly improve their quality of life.

Health Interventions to Assist Patients with Work-Related Health Challenges

Identify the Issue

Some simple screening questions can assist with identifying whether the patient is experiencing work-related challenges that may be affecting their health:

- Are you currently working or looking for work? If yes, where and what do you do? If no, were you previously working? These simple questions can help to identify whether the patient lost their job. It can also invite further conversation about the nature of their work and any challenges they are experiencing, or have experienced, with it.
- Do you currently have difficulty paying for basic needs?[26] If yes, why? These questions can help identify whether the patient is

struggling financially and invite discussion about what may be causing it, such as unfair or unpaid wages, employment termination, or misclassification.
- Are you currently employed in a casual, short-term, or temporary position? Do you feel fearful that you could be fired if you raised employment concerns? Does your pay vary a lot from month to month?[27] These questions have been validated for screening for precarious employment, where a "yes" to two or more questions suggests a very high likelihood of precarious employment.

As discussed in chapter 1, an alternative to screening for health-harming legal needs related to work would be to take a case-finding approach. This approach would have the clinician inquire using the preceding lines of questioning for higher-risk populations.

Provide Appropriate Supporting Medical Documentation for Disability-Related Accommodation Requests

When a patient requests accommodation for their disability at work, they may need to provide supporting medical documentation. Requests for such documentation may come from the patient, their legal representative, or sometimes from the patient's employer. Health practitioners should prioritize these requests: the type and extent of accommodation that an employer provides will often hinge entirely on the medical documentation provided by the patient's treating health practitioner. The documentation can also become key evidence if the patient needs to litigate a human rights claim against their employer. Employees who do receive appropriate accommodation at work can experience significant improvements in work satisfaction and reduce or eliminate the worsening of work-related health problems. We therefore provide the following guidance and tips on how to best support a patient requesting accommodation:

- *Obtain the following medical information:*
  - Identify that the patient has one or more disabilities.
  - Identify the patient's functional limitations or needs in relation to the disability. For example, the functional limitations for a patient with multiple sclerosis may be no heavy lifting (above 35 pounds), no prolonged standing (more than 30 minutes), and frequent regular breaks (every 45 minutes). Health providers should ask the employer to provide a functional limitations form to fill out; however, be aware that not all employers will have one, and

the health provider may need to draft a letter describing those
limitations.
- Assess whether the patient can perform the essential duties of
their job, with or without accommodation. To make this assessment, health practitioners should first request a description of the
patient's job duties, confirm what the patient's essential job duties
are, or both.
- Determine the type of accommodations that may be needed to
allow the patient to fulfil the essential duties of the job. Although
it is generally up to the employer to propose a reasonable way to
accommodate the patient's functional limitations, in some cases
the health practitioner can provide suggestions.
- If the patient is on leave, provide regular updates about when the
patient can be expected to return to work.
- *Protect the patient's privacy*: As much as possible, health practitioners
should protect their patient's privacy and confidentiality
regarding the disability. In general, health practitioners providing
documentation to support an accommodation request do not need
to provide the patient's confidential medical information, such as
the cause of the disability, the diagnosis, or treatment, unless these
relate to the accommodation being sought or the person's needs are
complex, challenging, or unclear, and more information is needed.[28]
At the same time, a doctor's note that is vague and merely states,
for example, that the patient "feels depressed" or "stressed" will
likely not be enough to trigger the employer's duty to accommodate
the patient. Health providers should always confirm that the patient
has one or more disabilities and describe the patient's functional
limitations. If there is a question about whether the patient has a
disability, health providers may need to provide more information
(such as descriptions of symptoms) in addition to confirming that
the patient has a disability.
- *Be an expert, not an advocate (for purposes of legal settings)*: We
encourage health practitioners to be advocates for their patient's
health. But in the world of workplace-related challenges, courts and
tribunals will discount a medical opinion if they feel the medical
practitioner is not objective and impartial. Employers usually do not
have an automatic right to obtain an independent medical opinion
when assessing accommodation options and must usually rely
on the worker's treating health practitioner. However, if there is a
basis to find that the patient's treating health practitioner was not
objective, the employer may then have a right to an independent
medical opinion, which may or may not be harmful to the patient.

To maintain credibility and avoid this outcome, health practitioners should focus on answering the questions that have been asked of them. They should generally avoid suggesting the specific accommodations to be provided to the patient and focus on explaining the patient's functional limitations and needs.

Tips for Working with Patients Who Are Migrant Workers

Migrant workers experience unique challenges that impede their access to quality health care. We provide the following tips to help health providers overcome some of these barriers:

- *Confirm whether an injury or health problem is workplace-related*: Employers may try to threaten or trick migrant worker employees to keep them from telling their health provider that their injury or health problem is related to the workplace, to avoid higher worker's compensation premiums as well as workplace health and safety inspections. Health providers should be alert to this reality, particularly if the patient is reluctant to explain their health issue or if their story appears incomplete or does not make sense.
- *Ensure interpretation services are available*: Migrant workers often do not speak English or French well, which can significantly affect their ability to explain the nature of their health concerns and what may be causing them. Health providers should arrange for interpretation services before an appointment, which can include in-person or over-the-phone interpretation. Alternatively, the patient may be accompanied by a support person who can also interpret, but health providers should be cautious that the quality of such interpretation will vary and that the person interpreting should not be the patient's employer, as discussed next.
- *Be very cautious if the employer accompanies the patient to the medical appointment*: This can be a common occurrence, particularly for migrant workers in rural locations, who may have no means of transportation to an appointment other than their employer. Employers who accompany a patient to an appointment may downplay a patient's injury for their own interests, such as to avoid costs, liability, and recommendations that the patient not work or that their job duties be modified. These dangers are further compounded if the patient does not speak English or French and the employer is acting as interpreter. Wherever possible, insist on seeing the patient alone or with a support person of their choosing, and secure independent interpretation services if necessary.

- *Ask about potential health-affecting living and working conditions*: Migrant farm workers in particular often live in cramped, shared housing with deplorable conditions that contribute to illness. Domestic workers such as nannies who live with their employer may be forced to live in poor conditions. Farm workers may also be exposed to chemicals and pesticides that can affect their health. Often, they will not be aware of a potential connection between these conditions and their health and may not volunteer the information, so we encourage health providers to directly ask patients about their working and living conditions.

Provide Appropriate Referrals for Support

The health practitioner's role is to identify that the patient is experiencing work-related challenges that may have legal recourse. Their role is not to assess the patient's legal options or provide legal advice. To that end, health teams should make referrals for legal advice when practicable. Some resources that may assist patients can be found in Appendix 1.

Acknowledgment

The authors thank Marie Fiedler, a law student who assisted them in research and formatting this chapter.

NOTES

1 Leclerc A, Kaminski M, Lang T. Closing the gap in a generation: health equity through action on the social determinants of health: Commission on Social Determinants of Health final report. Rev Epidemiol Sante Publique. 2008;57(4):227–30. https://doi.org/10.1016/j.respe.2009.04.006.
2 Kivimäki M, Vahtera J, Virtanen M, et al. Temporary employment and risk of overall and cause-specific mortality. Am J Epidemiol. 2003;158(7):663–68. https://doi.org/10.1093/aje/kwg185.
3 Loopstra R, Tarasuk V. Severity of household food insecurity is sensitive to change in household income and employment status among low-income families. J Nutr. 2013;143(8):1316–23. https://doi.org/10.3945/jn.113.175414.
4 Benavides FG, Benach J, Muntaner C, et al. Associations between temporary employment and occupational injury: what are the mechanisms? Occup Environ Med. 2006;63(6):416–21. https://doi.org/10.1136/oem.2005.022301.
5 Ferrie JE. Is job insecurity harmful to health? J Royal Soc Med. 2001;94(2):71–6. https://doi.org/10.1177/014107680109400206.

6 Vives A, Amable M, Ferrer M, et al. Employment precariousness and poor mental health: evidence from Spain on a new social determinant of health. J Environ Public Health. 2013;2013: 978656. https://doi.org/10.1155/2013/978656.

7 Ferrie JE, Kivimäki M, Shipley MJ, et al. Job insecurity and incident coronary heart disease: the Whitehall II Prospective Cohort Study. Artherosclerosis. 2013;227(1):178–81. https://doi.org/10.1016/j.atherosclerosis.2012.12.027.Job.

8 Pinto AD, Hassen N, Craig-Neil A. Employment interventions in health settings: a systematic review and synthesis. Ann Fam Med. 2018;16(5):447–60. https://doi.org/10.1370/afm.2286.

9 Pinto AD. Building an advocacy network to address a key social determinant of health: Ontario's Decent Work and Health Network. Paper presented at the North American Primary Care Research Group 44th Annual Meeting; Colorado Springs, CO; 2016 Nov 12–16 .

10 *Employment Standards Act*, 2000, SO 2000, c 41, s 48(1).

11 Employment and Social Development Canada. Government of Canada will require employees in all federally regulated workplaces to be vaccinated against COVID-19 [Internet]. Cision; 2021 Dec. 7. Available from: https://www.newswire.ca/news-releases/government-of-canada -will-require-employees-in-all-federally-regulated-workplaces-to-be -vaccinated-against-covid-19-848302529.html.

12 Banks K. Employment standards complaint resolution, compliance and enforcement: a review of the literature on access and effectiveness [Internet]. Toronto: Queen's Printer for Ontario; 2016. Available from: https://cirhr.library.utoronto.ca/sites/default/public/research-projects /Banks-6B-ESA%20Enforcement.pdf.

13 Noack AM, Vosko LF. Precarious jobs in Ontario: Mapping dimensions of labour market insecurity by workers' social location and context [Internet]. Toronto: Law Commission of Ontario; 2011. Available from: https://www .lco-cdo.org/wp-content/uploads/2012/01/vulnerable-workers -call-for-papers-noack-vosko.pdf; Block S, Galabuzi G-E, Weiss A. The colour coded labour market by the numbers: a national household survey analysis [Internet]. Toronto: Wellesley Institute; 2014. Available from: https://www.wellesleyinstitute.com/wp-content/uploads/2014/09/The -Colour-Coded-Labour-Market-By-The-Numbers.pdf; Canadian Human Rights Commission. Report on the equality rights of Aboriginal people [Internet]. Ottawa: Canadian Human Rights Commission; 2013. Available from: https://www.chrc-ccdp.gc.ca/sites/default/files/publication-pdfs /equality_aboriginal_report_2.pdf ; Oxfam Canada, Canadian Centre for Policy Alternatives. Making women count: the unequal economics of women's work [Internet]. Toronto: Oxfam Canada; 2016. Available from: https://www.oxfam.ca/wp-content/uploads/2016/03/making-women -count-report-2016.pdf .

14 *Human Rights Code*, RSBC 1996, c 210, s 13.

15 For 2023, the maximum weekly benefit that a worker can receive from EI
is $650. See Government of Canada. EI regular benefits [Internet]. Ottawa:
Government of Canada; 2023 [last modified 2024 Oct 10]. Available from:
https://www.canada.ca/en/services/benefits/ei/ei-regular-benefit
/benefit-amount.html.

16 Acorn Canada, Masse. The Employment Insurance Act: a sexist law in
need of reform! [Internet]. Montreal: Le Masse; 2018. Available from:
https://lemasse.org/wp-content/uploads/2021/08/Feuillet_anglais
_F_web.pdf.

17 Migrant Rights Network. Underinsured: ending the exclusion of migrants
from EI [Internet]. Toronto: Migrant Rights Network; 2021. Available from:
https://migrantworkersalliance.org/wp-content/uploads/2021/04
/MRN-Submissions-to-HUMA-on-EI.pdf.

18 Migrant Rights Network. Underinsured: ending the exclusion of migrants
from EI [Internet]. Toronto: Migrant Rights Network; 2021. Available from:
https://migrantworkersalliance.org/wp-content/uploads/2021/04
/MRN-Submissions-to-HUMA-on-EI.pdf.

19 Migrant Rights Network. Underinsured: ending the exclusion of migrants
from EI [Internet]. Toronto: Migrant Rights Network; 2021. Available from:
https://migrantworkersalliance.org/wp-content/uploads/2021/04
/MRN-Submissions-to-HUMA-on-EI.pdf.

20 Migrant Rights Network. Underinsured: ending the exclusion of migrants
from EI [Internet]. Toronto: Migrant Rights Network; 2021. Available from:
https://migrantworkersalliance.org/wp-content/uploads/2021/04
/MRN-Submissions-to-HUMA-on-EI.pdf.

21 p. 2 of Migrant Rights Network. Underinsured: ending the exclusion
of migrants from EI [Internet]. Toronto: Migrant Rights Network; 2021.
Available from: https://migrantworkersalliance.org/wp-content
/uploads/2021/04/MRN-Submissions-to-HUMA-on-EI.pdf.; p. 5 of FCJ
Refugee Centre, Canadian Centre to End Human Trafficking. It happens
here: labour exploitation among migrant workers during the pandemic
[Internet]. Toronto: Canadian Centre to End Human Trafficking; 2023.
Available from: https://www.fcjrefugeecentre.org/wp-content
/uploads/2023/02/FCJ-CCTEHT-%E2%80%93-Labour-Trafficking
-Report-EN.pdf.

22 FCJ Refugee Centre, Canadian Centre to End Human Trafficking. It
happens here: labour exploitation among migrant workers during the
pandemic [Internet]. Toronto: Canadian Centre to End Human Trafficking;
2023. Available from: https://www.fcjrefugeecentre.org/wp-content
/uploads/2023/02/FCJ-CCTEHT-—-Labour-Trafficking-Report-EN.pdf.

23 However, employers are not entitled to fire employees for reasons
prohibited by the law. For example, employers are prohibited from firing

employees for a reason related to a ground protected by human rights legislation, such as the employee's disability, gender, or race, or as reprisal because the employee attempted to assert their legal rights, such as a harassment complaint or a complaint about unpaid wages. Where such terminations occur, the employee may be entitled to additional damages or to reinstatement to their job.

24 "Termination pay" may go by other names under different employment standards legislation, such as "wages in lieu of notice," "pay instead of notice," "payment in lieu of notice of termination," or other similar variations.

25 Workers' Action Centre. Working on the edge [Internet]. Toronto: Worker's Action Centre; 2007. Available from: https://workersactioncentre.org/wp-content/uploads/2016/07/WorkingOnTheEdge_eng.pdf.

26 Brcic V, Eberdt C, Kaczorowski J. 2011. Development of a tool to identify poverty in a family practice setting: a pilot study. Int J Fam Med. 2011;2011:812182. https://doi.org/10.1155/2011/812182; Pinto AD, Bondy M, Rucchetto A, et al. Screening for poverty and intervening in a primary care setting: an acceptability and feasibility study. Fam Pract. 2019;36(5):634–8. https://doi.org/10.1093/fampra/cmy129.

27 Bellicoso E, Bondy M, Hassen N, et al. Screening for precarious work in primary care: a validation study. Paper presented at North American Primary Care Research Group 47th Annual Meeting; Toronto, ON; 2019 Nov 16–20.

28 Ontario Human Rights Commission. 8. Duty to accommodate [Internet]. Toronto: Ontario Human Rights Commission [updated 2016 June 27]. Available from: https://www.ohrc.on.ca/en/policy-ableism-and-discrimination-based-disability/8-duty-accommodate.

Indigenous Legal Expert Reflection on Chapter 5

SARA MAINVILLE

I am a law partner at JFK Law LLP, working from our Toronto office. We serve many First Nations, Inuit, and Métis communities across Canada. My practice is all about nation-building, but we clearly understand and our lawyers are sensitive to intersectional issues, including the 2SLG-BTQIA++ community, of which I am a member, in addition to being a member of Couchiching First Nation.

Indigenous peoples face health issues that intersect with the workplace every single day. Sometimes they are not directly related, but the workplace may indirectly amplify an underlying health issue – or simply elucidate issues rooted in the social determinants of health.

I am keenly aware of the workplace health impacts that a First Nations community member may face on a day-to-day basis. For instance, micro-aggressions may not always rise, as Qureshi and Pinto described, to the definition of discrimination, but they can still lead to mental health challenges. Members of First Nations communities are either themselves employed precariously or are deeply involved in communities made up of precariously employed individuals. I know that this can contribute to or intersect with issues of poverty, systemic racism, intergenerational trauma, and discrimination on the basis of gender identity. Indigenous peoples often feel these social determinants of health more intensely, and multiple intersecting identities can exacerbate existing health issues or create new ones, inside or outside of the workplace.

I take seriously the need to advocate for safe workspaces everywhere, including my own.

We recently held an event in my current workplace that featured a presentation by Prairie Sky, a drag artist from my home community of Couchiching in Treaty 3. The presentation and discussion was rich and varied, spanning from the health issues faced by 2SLGBTQ+ people and how they intersect with precarious work and access to appropriate care, to ways of being a better ally and what community really means. Prairie Sky shared a story about Sunshine House, a community neighbourhood resource centre, that was expanding to deliver mobile harm reduction care. The team faced challenges in delivering this life-saving care because of legal hurdles for both the mobile care unit itself and for the health care professionals who sought to deliver health care services. As executive director of Sunshine House, Prairie Sky, also known as Levi Foy, was careful to ensure that their advocacy was centred on empowering clients as well as addressing the root causes of a health care crisis in the middle of the COVID-19 epidemic. It reminded me of the ways in which our systems are intertwined and the need for health care professionals to work closely with community, and sometimes with legal professionals, when individuals are facing legal challenges that have impacts on their health and well-being.

As it turned out, the story told by Prairie Sky to JFK Law was a story of allyship for the queer, Indigenous, and intersectional community, the local Member of Parliament, and other committed social organizations.

I like to think that my colleagues who participated in this discussion with Prairie Sky came away as savvier allies and more culturally competent individuals, even when their law practice is not centred on harm reduction. Ultimately, I hope that health care professionals might take something similar away from this discussion about community. Indigenous peoples face workplace health issues like anyone else, but the particular legacy of colonialism has had an impact on every single Indigenous person in a way that is unique to their communities. It is critical that health care professionals take a wide view of community when caring for Indigenous patients – understanding that each person will have a different background but is likely to carry intersecting identities that may be leading to or contributing to workplace health issues. I also hope that health care professionals will consider the ways in which members of seemingly different communities might come together to provide holistic care that always has the patient's health and well-being at the centre.

6 Income, Social Benefits, and Health

GARY BLOCH, ANU BAKSHI, AND LOUISE SIMBANDUMWE

Many people who live in poverty rely on social assistance or other income support programs for their survival. Social assistance programs are designed to be last-resort benefits for those who have exhausted all other options. Each province and territory has its own programs, each with different rules, eligibility criteria, and amounts paid. Some First Nations with self-government agreements have their own income assistance programs.

To effectively support people living in poverty to navigate income benefit programs, health providers must examine the deeply troubling narrative that reliance on social assistance is an individual personal failing. There are prevailing harmful concepts about who is deserving and undeserving of public income benefits.

Let's consider three common myths.

Myth 1: You Can Make Ends Meet Living on Social Assistance

Social assistance programs in Canada do not cover the actual cost of rent, food, medicine, transportation, clothing, Internet, and basic necessities. Each province's welfare rates are below the poverty line.[1] Take Halifax, for example: a single person receives only $8,232 per year. The official Halifax poverty line is $27,483.

Living on social assistance anywhere in Canada poses an extremely high risk of food insecurity. In Canada, about 70 per cent of households reliant on social assistance were food insecure in 2022.[2]

Myth 2: Welfare Fraud Is Rampant

Everyone has heard of fraud hotlines and welfare cheats and that the government needs to get tough on fraud. The fraud language dehumanizes patients seeking public benefits. In reality, welfare fraud is exaggerated. Few cases are actually prosecuted as fraud in criminal courts.[3]

Social assistance rules are complicated and have onerous reporting requirements. Accordingly, overpayments occur quite frequently in the social assistance context, often for innocent reasons.[4] An overpayment takes place when the government has provided an amount to a recipient in excess of their entitlement. If the government claims an overpayment has arisen, it can enforce collection of the overpaid amount against the recipient's future monthly entitlements. Sometimes, welfare caseworkers supply recipients with very little information about alleged overpayments and their calculation.[5] This makes it extremely difficult for a marginalized person to determine the accuracy of the overpayment and provide an informed response.

Myth 3: People on Social Assistance Just Don't Want to Work

Most people on social assistance are dealing with multiple barriers to leaving poverty, often including family, work, or health crises, and they need financial assistance to help them to survive. They seek social assistance as a last resort after depleting their emotional and financial resources because they lost their job, lost a family member, live with a disability, or are leaving a traumatic situation, such as violence. Many face some kind of adversity and need support to stabilize their lives.

Some people who receive social assistance do work. But the current rules mean that, even with employment income, working one's way out of poverty and off social assistance is difficult. For example, in Ontario, social assistance recipients keep only the first $200 of any income they earn in a month, and half of any income above that amount is deducted from their monthly entitlement.

Navigating Income Security

In this chapter, we aim to build the skills and knowledge health providers require to effectively support their patients to navigate income supports. We begin with an approach to screening for poverty and guiding patients to appropriate income benefit programs. We then turn to an exploration of the barriers to accessing income supports. We conclude with a discussion of common legal issues faced by health care providers and their patients in navigating income supports.

Cases, Part 1

Malalai, a 37-year-old woman, and her husband Ali (also your patient), are both new to the country and parents to two young children, also in your practice. Malalai begins to tell you of conflict in her relationship.

Rachel and Samuel come in with their three children, aged four, six, and nine years. The children are having difficulty concentrating in school, and their teachers wonder whether all of them might have problems with attention.

Jessica comes to see you in tears, not sure whether she will be fired from her job as she deals with an illness.

A Practical Approach to Health Office-Based Screening for and Intervention with Poverty

How to Screen for Poverty

The identification of income insecurity requires targeted approaches to screening in health offices. Health care providers cannot assume level of income without exploring the issue directly with patients. Any patient may be living with income insecurity, regardless of how they present, and the stresses of poverty play a large role in determining their risk of developing health conditions and their ability to limit morbidity and mortality from health conditions.

Canada has no universally accepted marker of poverty. Three commonly used poverty lines are the Market Basket Measure, the Low Income Cut-Off, and the Low Income Measure. Each uses a different methodology to determine the level of poverty. The latest calculations use Statistics Canada data from 2023 for the Market Basket Measure and data from 2022 for the Low Income Cut-Off and Low Income Measure.

- *Market Basket Measure*: a basket of goods and services representing a basic living standard for a family of four. In 2018, this was chosen as the official Government of Canada poverty line. It is calculated by province and size of community. For example, for a large city in British Columbia, it is $58,163; for a rural community in New Brunswick, it is $49,794.[6]
- *Low Income Cut-Off*: the income threshold below which a family spends 20 per cent more than average on necessities, such as food, shelter, and clothing. This is an absolute measure of poverty, meaning that it is not sensitive to income distribution in society. It is

adjusted by community size. For a family of four, in a large city it is $46,033, and in a rural community it is $30,112.[7]

- *Low Income Measure*: represents 50 per cent of the median adjusted household income. This is a relative measure of poverty, meaning that it is sensitive to income distribution in society. It is not adjusted by geography. For a family of four, it is $57,726.[8]

Health is not beholden to poverty lines, however. Evidence shows that income determines the prevalence of and morbidity from common health issues across the income spectrum.[9]

There are three approaches to income screening: simple screening, a guided social history, and a narrative story-based approach. These can be used alone or in combination and provide different context and information about individuals' and families' social situations.

1. *Simple income screening*: This approach uses one or a few questions to identify income insecurity among patients. The Clinical Tool on Poverty[10] proposes a single-question screen: "Do you ever have difficulty making ends meet at the end of the month?" This question was found to be 98 per cent sensitive and 40 per cent specific for people living below the Low Income Cut-Off.[11] Other simple screens have focused on identifying common markers of poverty, such as food security, access to transportation, and adequacy of housing.
2. *Social history*: A more complex directed approach to screening for social risks to health proposes a broader set of questions to gain a full understanding of patients' social situations and their impact on health. There is no one standard for a multi-domain social history, but an excellent Canadian guide with questions and resources is available.[12]
3. *Narrative approach*: There is a strong movement in primary care practice to encourage patients to tell their stories in their own words, with deep listening by health practitioners. Proponents of narrative medicine suggest that this approach allows patients to take control of their stories and represent themselves and their experiences authentically and that it encourages health providers to understand those experiences deeply, treating the stories like literature, to be considered and analysed. This approach takes time, but it may be the most transformative to the health care experience.[13]

Any screen for income security should be seen as a gateway to further conversation and to deeper understanding of the context in which patients' health is realized. A more complete understanding of the Canadian income security system will guide further targeted history taking for patients who are income insecure.

Malalai, Part 2

You ask Malalai to tell you more about her story. She tells you that she came to Canada as a visitor, and her husband Ali is a Canadian citizen. They have two young children together who are well settled in their school and community. Ali repeatedly promised to sponsor Malalai so that she could stay in Canada, but so far he has made no efforts to do so.

Malalai tells you that Ali's threats and violence are increasing. She is stressed. She is thinking about leaving the relationship for her safety and the well-being of her children. She is fearful and does not know how she can survive. Because her husband is a citizen, she is entitled to receive the Canada Child Benefit as long as they stay together. But if she leaves the abusive situation with her children, she will no longer be eligible. She also does not have status in Canada and may be at risk of removal.

Helping Patients Navigate the Income Security System

The system of income support programs is complex. Guiding patients towards income benefits that may alleviate their poverty is a major intervention to support low-income patients. Effective guidance requires a basic understanding of the structure of income support systems in Canada.

Income benefit programs can be categorized in several ways, for example, by the level of government or other entity that administers them, such as federal, provincial, or municipal government; private sector insurance; or extra-governmental non-profit entities. To aid navigation of these programs with patients in health care settings, we approach the organization of programs by demographic group and life stage.

We use a simple set of patient-oriented questions, modified from the Clinical Tool on Poverty, to frame an overview of the income security system in Canada.

HAVE YOU COMPLETED AND FILED YOUR INCOME TAX RETURNS?
The income tax system is the largest gateway to income security programs in Canada. Many programs, such as the Goods and Services Tax/Harmonized Sales Tax (GST/HST) tax credit and the Working Income Tax Benefit, and provincial grants, such as the Ontario Trillium Benefit, are automatically accessed through tax filing.

Tax-based credits are available retroactively, and there is significant benefit to people living at low income to file taxes for current and prior years. Tax-filing services for people living at low income, such as the SEED Access to Benefits program in Winnipeg, have garnered millions of dollars in income support in Canada.

Most tax credits for people living at low income are refundable, meaning they are paid out whether a person pays taxes or not. Some tax credits, however, are non-refundable, meaning that they pay out by increasing an individual's tax refund, which is only accessible if sufficient taxes have been paid to offset the credit. The Disability Tax Credit is non-refundable, but there is universal benefit to applying because approval allows access to other benefits, such as Registered Disability Savings Plans.

Most low- to lower-middle-income families experience a net increase in income from filing taxes, and this is especially pronounced for families with children.[14] Benefits are often payable for previous as well as current tax years. Everyone living on a low income, therefore, should be encouraged to file their taxes.

DO YOU HAVE CHILDREN OR ARE YOU YOUNGER THAN AGE 18?
Some of Canada's most generous income support programs are available to families with children. Most of these programs are accessible simply by returning the Canada Child Benefit (CCB) application when filing income taxes or to the Canada Revenue Agency at any other time.

Child benefits include federal and provincial programs that, for many families, raise incomes to or near the poverty line. Canadian governments have created a support system that essentially offers guaranteed annual incomes that raise the majority of at-risk children out of poverty.

Basic federal child benefits offer almost $7,000 per child per year, with additional supplements for younger children, children with disabilities, and children from provincial programs.

There are also specific programs, such as the Canada Education Savings Grant and the Canada Learning Bond, that can support children in low-income families with post-secondary education costs.

Rachel and Samuel, Part 2

You ask the family about their income. Both parents work part time for near-minimum wage. They earn less than $18,000 per year combined. They never have enough money to pay for groceries, and their children usually go to school without breakfast and often without a packed lunch.

> They have not filed taxes for many years because they did not feel they needed to pay taxes, they found the forms confusing, and they could not afford professional help. You refer them to a community income tax clinic where they file 10 years of tax returns. They qualify for more than $25,000 in child benefits for the current year,[15] and they also receive tens of thousands of dollars from eight years of back-paid child benefits. They come back a few months after their last visit to thank you profusely for your advice. They tell you that their children are doing much better in school, and they can now even afford a little time for relaxation and play with their family.

DO YOU RECEIVE SENIORS' BENEFITS?

Canada's first guaranteed annual income program is targeted people older than age 65. A combination of Old Age Security and the Guaranteed Income Supplement offered a maximum of $1,815 of monthly income for a single senior living on a low income in 2025.[16] Some provinces top this amount up further for seniors living at low income.

Contribution-based programs, including the Canada Pension Plan (CPP) and private pension plans, add significantly to the total available from government plans.

ARE YOU INDIGENOUS, AND DO YOU HAVE A STATUS CARD?

In addition to other income support programs, Indigenous people have access to specific income support programs, especially if they have Indian status. The Non-Insured Health Benefits program covers health-related services, including medical, dental, vision, mental health, rehabilitation, medical transportation, and prescription drugs.[17] Other specific programs offer tax credits, income benefits, and education and training supports. A listing of federal programs is available at https://www.canada.ca/en/services/benefits/audience/indigenous.html.

According to Jordan's Principle, named for Jordan River Anderson, a young Indigenous boy in Manitoba who died waiting for federal and provincial governments to agree on who would pay for his care, any Indigenous child must be provided with social supports available to other children in Canada. This legal requirement resulted from a ruling by the Canadian Human Rights Tribunal that "states that any public service ordinarily available to all other children must be made available to First Nations children without delay or denial."[18] A variety of supports and benefits can be accessed directly through a Jordan's Principle request at https://www.sac-isc.gc.ca/eng/1568396296543/1582657596387#sec1.

ARE YOU A NEW IMMIGRANT, A REFUGEE, OR WITHOUT LEGAL STATUS IN CANADA?
Income support programs are available to some classes of newcomers
to Canada. Eligibility may change with shifts in immigration status,
meaning some individuals receive benefits that are then cut off when
their status changes. The Resettlement Assistance Program supports
government-assisted and privately sponsored refugees. It provides
income supports similar to provincial social assistance programs,
which some newcomers are eligible for, and settlement services. The
Interim Federal Health Program provides health benefits for some
newcomers who do not have other health care coverage. Newcomers can qualify for some tax credits, including the CCB (available to a
permanent resident or citizen parent, although this limitation is currently being challenged in federal tax court on *Charter* grounds), the
GST/HST credit, and other federal and provincial credits by filing a
tax return.[19]

Many refugees hold significant debt because of the immigration process. The federal government offers loans to cover their transportation
to Canada, but they must be paid back with interest.

**ARE YOU RECEIVING SOCIAL ASSISTANCE? DO YOU RECEIVE EXTRA SUPPLEMENTS
AND BENEFITS?**
People living at low income may receive support through provincial
social assistance programs. These programs generally provide differing amounts of support for people with and without disabilities.
Some programs also offer separate funding to people with or without
housing.

Social assistance programs provide supplemental benefits. Some are
realized as additional income, such as for special dietary needs, medical
supplies, and transportation to health-related appointments. Other benefits are offered as ancillary, and often essential, services, such as dental
and prescription drug coverage. In some cases, individuals may be able
to receive ancillary benefits even if they do not qualify for income benefits, and in some provinces individuals may continue to receive these
benefits for a period of time after starting employment, even if they
earn too much money to qualify for income supports.

ARE YOU LIVING WITH A DISABILITY?
Support for people living with disabilities is offered through a complex array of federal, provincial, and private income support programs.
These programs can be categorized as asset tested, contribution based,
employment based, and tax based.

Asset-tested programs are available to individuals whose income and assets fall below a threshold. These include provincial social assistance disability support programs.

Contribution-based programs are available to those who have paid into government programs while employed. These include Employment Insurance sickness benefits and the CPP disability program.

Employment-based programs are available to those who are currently working. These include workers' compensation boards and private short- and long-term disability plans. Veterans of the Armed Forces and Royal Canadian Mounted Police are eligible for a separate disability pension.

Tax-based disability supports include the Disability Tax Credit, the related Registered Disability Savings Plans, and additional credits specifically for children with disabilities, such as the Child Disability Benefit and Assistance for Children with Severe Disabilities.

Jessica, Part 2

Jessica is a single mother of young children. You find out that she works part time in a salon washing hair. She earns minimum wage, but really survives on her cash tips. She is now dealing with a serious illness, and she is afraid that she will be fired from her job.

She likely does not have access to private disability insurance. She may not qualify for Canada Pension Plan disability or Employment Insurance sickness benefits because these are contributory income regimes, where eligibility is contingent on contributions to the plan or hours worked. Even if she is eligible, the amounts paid may not be sustainable because she worked part time for a low wage and earned unreported cash.

ARE YOU IN POST-SECONDARY SCHOOL AND RECEIVING GRANTS OR LOANS?
Low-income students may be eligible for grants to support tuition and living expenses and for student loans with interest relief. Students could receive up to $4,200 per year from the Canada Student Grant for the 2024–2025 school year. The loan amount available through the Canada Student Loan program is based on assessed financial need. Students may also be eligible to access loans and grants from provincial and territorial governments.[20]

ARE YOU IN TRANSITION, BETWEEN LIFE STAGES, OR INTO DISABILITY?

Some of the most challenging moments in supporting people through income support programs arise during times of transition, including from child to adult supports, from working-age to seniors' supports, and to disability-related supports.

As children transition to adult benefit programs, they lose access to multiple benefits. They may need to specifically apply for adult support programs and risk losing or seeing a gap in income if they are not approved in time for the transition.

When adults transition from provincial social assistance programs to seniors' benefits, they often gain income but lose essential ancillary benefits, such as dental and drug coverage. They also risk a period without income if they have not applied early enough for a seamless transition.

People applying for disability supports face some of the most challenging transitions because they need to obtain detailed assessments and attestations of the impact of their disabilities to access appropriate income support programs.

HOW MUCH DEBT DO YOU CARRY AND IN WHAT FORM?

Debt can pose a major barrier to exiting poverty. High-interest debts, such as to credit card companies or payday lending agencies, can be extremely difficult to pay back. Debt restructuring and consolidation can ease the burden of debt payments and offer a path to repayment. Non-profit debt counselling services offer free assistance with debt management to people living at low income.

Financial literacy education offers people living at low income the opportunity to learn essential financial management skills. These include budgeting, managing debt, understanding credit, and retirement planning. Programs are available, often for free, online and through community agencies.

Figure 6.1 provides a snapshot of various income support programs.

Barriers to Income Security in Canada

Income (In)Adequacy

Despite progress for certain groups, income supports for people living at low income still leave millions of people in Canada living in poverty. As illustrated by the Maytree Foundation's *Welfare in Canada* report, total welfare incomes (combining social assistance with other income benefit programs) fall well below the official poverty line for most individuals and families. Although targeted programs have raised income

Figure 6.1. Quick Guide to Navigating Income Supports

INCOME TAX	Have you filed your tax return?	• Most important gateway to tax credits, federal and provincial benefit programs
CHILDREN	Do you have children? Are you under 18?	• Federal and provincial supports, including Canada Child Benefit • Supports for post-secondary education (e.g., Canada Education Savings Grant)
SENIORS	Do you receive seniors' benefits?	• Minimum monthly income through Old Age Security and Guaranteed Income Supplement • Contribution-based programs (e.g., Canada Pension Plan)
INDIGENEITY	Are you Indigenous? Do you have a status card?	• Specific supports (e.g., Non-Insured Health Benefits Program) • Jordan's Principle guarantees Indigenous children equal social supports
IMMIGRATION STATUS	Are you a new immigrant, refugee, or without legal status?	• Some newcomers eligible for supports (e.g., Resettlement Assistance Program, provincial social assistance) • Eligibility may change with changes in immigration status
SOCIAL ASSISTANCE	Are you receiving social assistance?	• Provincial social assistance programs for low-income • Supplemental benefits (e.g., for special dietary needs) and ancillary services (e.g., dental and prescription drugs)
DISABILITY	Are you living with a disability?	• Asset-tested: provincial social assistance disability • Contribution-based: EI-Sickness, CPP-D • Employment-based: WCB, short- and long-term disability • Tax-based: Disability Tax Credit, child credits
EDUCATION	Are you in post-secondary school and receiving grants or loans?	• Grants for tuition and living expenses • Interest relief on loans
TRANSITIONS	Are you in a period of transition between life stages or into disability?	High-risk transitions: • Child to adult • Working age to seniors; social assistance to seniors benefits • Onto disability
INCOME: DEBT	How much debt do you carry and in what form?	• Restructure and consolidate debt, especially from high-interest lenders • Refer to debt counseling services and financial literacy education

EI-Sickness = Employment Insurance sickness benefits; CPP–D = Canada Pension Plan disability benefits; WCB = worker's compensation board.

Table 6.1. Highest and Lowest Adequacy of Welfare Incomes among Provinces (2023)

Benefit unit	Jurisdiction	Welfare income ($)	Official poverty line (MBM; $)	% of MBM
Unattached single considered employable				
Lowest	Nova Scotia	9,204	27,483	33
Highest	Quebec (Manpower Training; 12 mo)	26,368	24,212	109
Unattached single with a disability				
Lowest	Alberta (Calgary) – Barriers to Full Employment	12,820	28,954	44
Highest	Alberta (Calgary) – Assured Income for the Severely Handicapped	23,473	28,954	81
Single parent, one child				
Lowest	Nova Scotia	21,969	38,867	57
Highest	Prince Edward Island	32,294	37,552	86
Couple, two children				
Lowest	New Brunswick	30,395	51,082	60
Highest	Quebec (Manpower Training; 12 mo)	47,794	48,424	99

Source: Adapted from Laidley J, Tabbara M. Welfare in Canada, 2023 [Internet]. Toronto: Maytree; 2024. Available from: https://maytree.com/wp-content/uploads/Welfare_in _Canada_2023.pdf .

MBM = Market Basket Measure.

supports for certain groups and have lowered overall poverty rates significantly in the past few years, millions of Canadians remain unable to rely on income benefit programs to leave poverty. Table 6.1 provides a snapshot of social assistance (welfare) rates across Canada, and how they compare.

Targeted income support programs were developed for seniors in the 1990s. Through a combination of federal programs, such as Old Age Security, CPP, and the Guaranteed Income Supplement, and some provincial top-up programs, the rate of seniors' poverty was dramatically reduced to less than 10 per cent. Nonetheless, seniors remain disproportionately more likely to live near the poverty line than younger adults.

Children's poverty has been targeted through specific income benefit programs over the past decade. As a result, child poverty rates have dropped from more than 15 per cent to less than 10 per cent.[21] Children, however, remain disproportionately susceptible to the health and developmental impacts of growing up in poverty and should continue to be treated as a high-priority group for poverty elimination.

People living with disabilities are vastly over-represented among people living in poverty. In 2023, the federal government approved the Canada Disability Benefit, a specific targeted income benefit for people living with disabilities. Its initial roll-out date is June 2025, with a pay-out of $200 per eligible person per month. Eligibility criteria announced to date are restrictive and dependent on qualifying for the Disability Tax Credit. Under ongoing consultation, this program is expected to evolve significantly in the next few years.[22]

An examination of disaggregated statistics on poverty is required to truly understand the need for targeted programs for people living in poverty. These data demonstrate higher poverty rates for certain groups, including people who are racialized, Indigenous, newcomers, 2SLGBTQ+, unattached individuals, and women.[23] These data speak to the need to target income support programs in a more direct manner to those socially marginalized groups.

Access to Identification

Government-issued identification (ID) is critical to social and economic inclusion. Without the required identification, community members are denied access to essential government services, income support programs, employment, housing, banking, and other commercial services.[24] As detailed in Table 6.2, identification in Canada falls under both federal and provincial jurisdiction and is provided through different government agencies.

Lack of government-issued identification leaves financially vulnerable people unable to access essential income supports and services. The social and economic exclusion caused by this identification divide has far-reaching adverse impacts.[25] A study on access to identification for individuals living on low levels of income highlighted a number of barriers to obtaining or possessing required identification.[26] These barriers include the cost of identification, the lack of foundational ID required to obtain other pieces of government-issued ID, the challenges of receiving ID by mail or loss of ID because of precarious housing, and loss of ID because of incarceration. Immigrants and refugee claimants encounter language barriers as well as difficulties finding a guarantor who has known them for an extended period of time to vouch for their identity. The disproportionately high number of Indigenous community members who lack ID is attributable, in part, to the removal

Table 6.2. Identification in Canada: Jurisdictions and Services

Identification document	Jurisdiction	Services
Birth certificates[a]	Provincial	Often required to apply for other identification, such as SIN, driver's license, or passport, as well as services such as enrolling children in school
SIN[b]	Federal	Required to obtain employment, file taxes, and access banking and government services and benefits.
Driver's license or non-driver's photo identification[c]	Provincial	Often required to access banking
Health card[d]	Provincial	Required to receive health care coverage
Secure Certificate of Indian Status or status card[e]	Federal and First Nations	Required to access provincial and federal government services and programs available to individuals recognized as having status under the *Indian Act*.
Permanent resident card (PR card)[f]	Federal	Proof that an immigrant has permanent resident status. Often required to apply for other identification and government benefits.[g]

[a] Sarah. How to get a copy of a Canadian birth certificate [Internet]. InfoProcedures.com; 2024. Available from: https://www.infoprocedures.com/get-copy-canadian-birth-certificate/.

[b] Employment and Social Development Canada. Social insurance number: overview [Internet]. Ottawa: Government of Canada; 2024. Available from: https://www.canada.ca/en/employment-social-development/services/sin.html.

[c] Government of Canada. Driving in Canada [Internet]. Ottawa: Government of Canada; 2024. Available from: https://www.canada.ca/en/immigration-refugees-citizenship/services/new-immigrants/new-life-canada/driving.html#licences

[d] Government of Canada. Health cards [Internet]. Ottawa: Government of Canada; 2024. Available from: https://www.canada.ca/en/health-canada/services/health-cards.html

[e] Government of Canada. Indian status [Internet]. Ottawa: Government of Canada; 2024. Available from: https://www.sac-isc.gc.ca/eng/1100100032374/1572457769548

[f] Government of Canada. Get a permanent resident card [Internet]. Ottawa: Government of Canada; 2024 . Available from: https://www.canada.ca/en/immigration-refugees-citizenship/services/new-immigrants/pr-card.html.

[g] Government of Canada. Understand permanent resident status [Internet]. Ottawa: Government of Canada; 2023. Available from: https://www.canada.ca/en/immigration-refugees-citizenship/services/new-immigrants/pr-card/understand-pr-status.html.

SIN = social insurance number.

of Indigenous children from their families. Forced enrolment in residential schools and the Sixties and Millennial Scoops mean that many Indigenous community members are disconnected from their family histories and do not have ready access to the information required to fill out ID applications. Finally, the pandemic accelerated the shift towards service delivery through online and virtual channels by the government agencies responsible for the provision of ID. This resulted in reduced access to ID for individuals who do not have the required technology.

Community organizations address these barriers by introducing access to ID services and supports, such as covering the cost of ID, providing intensive in-person navigation, providing ID storage, allowing individuals to use a community organization as their mailing address, providing interpreters, and partnering with correctional facilities to obtain ID before release.

Jessica, Part 3

Jessica tries to start the process of applying for disability programs but realizes she cannot find any photo ID or proof of citizenship, both of which are required to apply. She worries she may have lost these in her last move from an apartment whose rent she could not afford.

A community organization in the nearest town helps her apply for a new birth certificate. Once she has that, she is able to obtain a copy of her driver's license and move ahead with disability program applications.

Barriers to Tax Filing

Many low-income patients do not file tax returns. Tax filing is a critical step in accessing poverty reduction income benefits, such as the CCB, Guaranteed Income Supplement, Old Age Security, Disability Tax Credit, and Canada Worker's Benefit. In 2016, an estimated 10–12 per cent of working-aged people did not file their personal income tax, resulting in $1.7 billion in unclaimed benefits.[27] In addition, many provincial programs require tax filing to verify income, such as provincial child benefits in Quebec and Manitoba, Ontario's income-tested drug program (Trillium), and British Columbia's housing subsidy and pharmacare programs.

Patients may face multiple barriers to tax filing, including the following:[28,29]

- lack of awareness of income benefits and how to file taxes;
- not knowing where to go for help;
- inability to afford tax help;
- difficulty finding and assembling the necessary documents;

- lack of confidence and fear of making mistakes and of government authorities;
- poor literacy and financial, digital, or language skills; and
- poor health, cognitive barriers, and other disability-related barriers

Volunteer tax clinics across the country support lower-income families in filing taxes and accessing benefits.[30]

Precarious Immigration Status

See chapter 7 of this text for a fulsome discussion of how immigration status affects various social determinants of health. Here we focus on the interplay between immigration status and income.

Many people with precarious immigration status work in essential services, which include cleaning offices, providing care and housekeeping in hospitals and nursing homes, working in grocery stores, or delivering meals. The Canadian immigration system provides many newcomers with temporary status to boost the labour supply.[31] Often, status is tied to a specific employer, and regularizing status is not within a person's own control, making them inherently vulnerable. Precarious-status migrants may experience precarious working conditions and job insecurity, marked by lower wages, lack of ability to control schedules, dangerous working conditions, and exploitative employers.

Pathways to permanent residence in Canada are limited, onerous, and delayed. Unexpected changes in employment and government policy can be confusing and problematic in regularizing status, even after living, working, and contributing to Canada for years.[32]

The majority of newcomers to Canada arrive with temporary student or tourist visas or work permits, or they submit a refugee claim.[33] If a visa or permit expires or a refugee claim is denied, another route to permanency may be initiated. Thus, individuals may fall in and out of recognized status for years, a situation that breeds frustration and hopelessness.[34,35]

Shifting status often affects a person's ability to engage with communities and receive services, such as income benefits.[36] Health providers must reject the dangerous narrative that those with precarious status are somehow undeserving of public benefits.

Individuals with precarious status may be afraid to access needed income benefits because doing so may have consequences for immigration pathways to permanency.[37] They are often fearful of revealing their precarious status to health providers.[38]

Access-without-fear initiatives attempt to provide services without immigration status information.[39] Service providers adopt a "don't ask, don't tell" policy with respect to immigration status. This means that service providers neither inquire into the individual's immigration status, nor notify the immigration authorities. Seven municipalities have enacted such policies since 2013: Toronto, Hamilton, Vancouver, Ajax, Montreal, Edmonton, and London.[40]

Provincial social assistance programs differ in eligibility on the basis of immigration status.[41] The CCB may not be available to children of parents without regularized immigration status, even if the children are Canadian citizens or permanent residents.

Migrant workers who contribute to the Canadian Pension Plan (CPP) may be able to receive income benefits upon retirement or when they can no longer work, even in their home country. However, migrant workers face multiple barriers to accessing these benefits from abroad.

Benefits navigation is particularly challenging for those with precarious status, and it often requires the services of a specialized financial services agency.[42]

Malalai, Part 3

Consider Malalai's complex needs: she may need help to address her immediate safety; she may need legal information regarding issues ranging from immigration to family law to income assistance; she may need assistance to make informed decisions about legal action and her legal rights; and she needs to find legal help to help her navigate a Canadian legal system that is foreign to her.

Racialization and Intersectionality

Poverty is racialized in Canada. In 2022, the overall poverty rate was 9.9 per cent, but for racialized persons, it was 13 per cent.[43] In 2022, 16.4 per cent of immigrants who had been in Canada for four years or less were living in poverty, and 17.5 per cent of Indigenous people living off reserve were living in poverty.[44]

Often, patients who need income support the most face the greatest intersectional barriers in accessing benefits as a result of systemic and institutional discrimination. Many of those facing intersecting barriers have difficulty applying for, receiving, and maintaining benefits, including Indigenous communities, individuals living with disabilities, individuals with precarious housing, and newcomers, including refugees, seniors, and youth.[45] Barriers include poor literacy, digital, or language skills; distrust of government; difficulty filing tax returns; complex multi-step application processes; lack of identification documents; limited access to financial services, such as a bank account; lack of knowledge about benefits; and geographical location.

Jessica, Part 4

Think about the overlapping and multiple barriers Jessica may face. For example, being a female sole-caregiver wage earner affects how much money she earns and her ability to work. Her employment is precarious and low wage.

Failing to consider the impact of intersectionality on Jessica provides an incomplete understanding of poverty and the barriers to income support. For example, in 2022, the overall poverty rate was 9.9 per cent, but for female sole-caregiver families, it was 23.8 per cent. Data from 2020 show that 30.2 per cent of female sole-caregiver families living with disabilities lived in poverty.

Sources: Employment and Social Development Canada. A time for urgent action: The 2024 report of the National Advisory Council on Poverty [Internet]. Ottawa: Employment and Social Development Canada; 2024. Available from: https:// www.canada.ca/content/dam/esdc-edsc/documents/programs/poverty -reduction/national-advisory-council/reports/2024-annual/4877-NACP_2024 -Report-EN-Final.pdf; National Advisory Council on Poverty. Poverty in Canada and update on progress. In: Understanding systems: the 2021 report of the National Advisory Council on Poverty [Internet]. Ottawa: Employment and Social Development Canada; 2021. p. 16–37. Available from: https://www.canada.ca/en /employment-social-development/programs/poverty-reduction/national-advisory -council/reports/2021-annual.html.

Indigeneity (Impacts of Colonization)

Colonialism has systematically dispossessed Indigenous peoples of their lands, independence, and traditional economies. Indigenous peoples in Canada experience significant health disparities, such as a higher incidence of chronic conditions and higher prevalence of related risk factors.[46] The legacy of colonialism, racism, and social exclusion have far-reaching effects on health inequities.[47]

Social assistance programs have historically played a role in the attempt to assimilate Indigenous peoples. Since 1964, Canada has enabled Indigenous Services Canada (ISC) to adopt provincial rates and eligibility criteria in the administration of income assistance to First Nations people. ISC's Income Assistance Program is also a program of last resort. There is no single delivery model for income assistance because individual First Nations communities or organizations manage program delivery.

A recent report, *Income Supports and Indigenous Peoples in B.C.*, identifies a multitude of barriers for Indigenous income support recipients, including systemic racism and some government workers' deeply disrespectful attitudes to those accessing government services.[48] Racist experiences perpetuate mistrust of government and may prevent Indigenous families from receiving much-needed income supports. For example, only 79 per cent of eligible First Nations families accessed the CCB in 2017, compared with 97 per cent of the general population.[49]

Indigenous persons with disabilities face additional barriers to accessing income benefits, including lack of access to health practitioners willing to complete medical forms, lack of coordination between federal and provincial governments, and lack of understanding of the severe trauma rooted in colonial assimilation policies passed through the generations.

Disability

In 2022, more than 1.5 million people living with disabilities were living below the poverty line.[50] From 2013 to 2022, the poverty rate among people living with a disability was on average twice as high as the poverty rate for people without disabilities.[51] This over-representation of poverty points to the systemic barriers faced by people living with disabilities when they try to obtain adequate income and access income supports.

People living with disabilities often experience intersecting barriers to accessing support and to avoiding poverty. These intersectional experiences of marginalization often result in increased rates of poverty, as illustrated in Table 6.3.

People with disabilities face particular barriers to accessing income support programs, including highly complex application processes, requirements for medical documentation of disability and its impact on function, and hard-to-understand eligibility criteria and assessment processes. These processes often require a relationship with a health provider who has a deep knowledge of an individual's disability. The

Table 6.3. Poverty Rates among Persons with Disabilities with Marginalized Identities (2019)

Characteristics	Persons with disabilities (%)	Persons without disabilities (%)
Overall	13.5	9.0
Singles (0–64 years old)	42.8	29.2
Female sole-caregiver families	30.2	24.9
Indigenous (off-reserve)	24.0	13.5
Immigrants (10–19 years since landed)	18.6	12.0

Source: Adapted from National Advisory Council on Poverty. Poverty in Canada and update on progress. In: Understanding systems: the 2021 report of the National Advisory Council on Poverty [Internet]. Ottawa: Employment and Social Development Canada; 2021. p. 16–37. Available from: https://www.canada.ca/en/employment-social -development/programs/poverty-reduction/national-advisory-council/reports/2021-annual .html#h2.4.

application process can be dehumanizing and frustrating for applicants and their professional and personal supports.[52]

Digital Divide

Accessing government benefits requires multiple digital steps, technology access, and digital literacy. The basic digital steps – downloading benefit information and forms, filling out online applications, printing or sending forms to health practitioners, gathering online supporting documents, and attaching all required documents to an application – are onerous. Those who need benefits the most are the least likely to have access to stable and affordable Internet, quality computers or laptops, smartphones, adequate cellular data, and digital skills and literacy.

Digital inequalities are significantly correlated with demographic and socio-economic factors. Indigenous and rural and remote communities, low-income individuals, older adults, people with disabilities, youth, and newcomers are less likely to have an Internet connection with sufficient speed.[53] As a result of intersectional barriers, many low-income patients have limited digital access and poor digital skills that are intensified by language barriers and disability-related impairments.

Patients may need help downloading forms and filling out and submitting online documents, and they may not be able to read large electronic documents on their smartphones. Referrals to social services agencies that provide in-person one-to-one services and public libraries with Internet access may be appropriate.

Rural and Remote

From the moment they think about applying for income assistance, rural and remote patients face barriers in accessing income assistance compared with their urban counterparts. They may not be able to find a local health practitioner or community agency to aid them in completing applications and medical forms. In some remote and rural areas, Internet and digital services are limited.

Most rural and northern communities do not have public transit systems. Without public transit, residents face the extra burden associated with the high costs of arranging private transportation and increased travel time. Travel time may influence which services individuals seek. It may be difficult to collect documents from multiple parties in different locations to complete benefits applications.

In particular, disability benefits are often denied because of the lack of sufficient medical documentation, including efforts to obtain treatment, referrals to treatment, or ongoing treatment by specialists. Providing sufficient evidence is difficult in a rural environment because there is a scarcity of medical professionals. Specialist consultation and ongoing specialist involvement may be impossible. When completing medical forms or letters for disability applications in the rural context, health practitioners may want to note rural systemic barriers to income support, such as the lack of a local health practitioner, driver's license, treatment, and specialists, as well as long wait lists and financial barriers (e.g., paying for gas and other travel costs).

In small communities, low-income people living on income assistance may face a backlash or long-standing stigma. Certain individuals or families may be branded as "on welfare" and morally inferior in the wider small community.

Debt Trap

Many low-income earners take out payday and high-interest alternative lender loans because they do not have enough money to make ends meet from month to month. The average term for a payday loan in Ontario is 10 days.[54] Low-income earners face a greater risk of being trapped in a cycle of high-cost debt repayment because of precarious employment and a lack of access to mainstream financial institutions. The departure of banks from financially distressed neighbourhoods exacerbates the vulnerability of these households to high-cost lenders.[55] Examples of high-cost lenders include pawn loans, rent-to-own financing, cheque cashing, and sub-prime auto loans. There are also firms that specialize in providing advance loans for individuals who are entitled to tax refunds or provide payday advances on government benefits such as Employment Insurance, the CCB, and Old Age Security.

Interest and fees charged on payday and alternative loans are typically well in excess of 30 per cent per year. A review of high-cost financial services in Alberta found interest rates of 46.9 per cent for an instalment loan, 60.0 per cent for a pawn loan, and a median annual percentage rate of 70.8 per cent for rent-to-own financing.[56]

Immigration loans are a financial burden on resettled refugee families. Many families cannot afford to pay their own travel costs. As a result of immigration loans, many refugee families start their new life in Canada with debt of up to $10,000. They do not have enough money to cover even their basic needs, let alone debt repayment. Defaulting on immigration loans can also undermine efforts to sponsor other family members. Owing the government money may be a source of stress and a deterrent to tax filing and applying for benefits.

Rachel and Samuel, Part 3

Rachel returns to your office in tears. She says that, once again, she is unable to afford groceries this month. She reveals that, over years of living in deep poverty, she and Samuel took out a number of loans to help pay for their rent and essential needs in the hardest months. Their debt is on credit cards and from payday loan agencies. They are paying 20–60 per cent annual interest on these debts, and they can barely keep up with minimum interest payments, let alone pay down the capital.

You refer them to a financial counselling agency that helps them consolidate their debt into a bank loan at 6 per cent interest. Without exorbitant interest payments, they are able to put a monthly payment schedule in place that will allow them to fully pay off their debts in two years without compromising their ability to afford food and shelter.

Benefit Program Interactions and Reviews

Income programs have complex rules that keep people trapped in poverty. These rules and inadequate benefit levels make it difficult to save money, earn a living wage, and receive other income support benefits. Each provincial social assistance program has its own rules and eligibility criteria that perpetuate institutional poverty, including asset tests, earning exemptions, clawback rates, and overpayment recovery.

Asset tests calculate the amount of cash or cashlike assets a household must stay below to qualify and remain eligible for benefits. For example, to be eligible for New Brunswick's Transitional Assistance, an individual applicant cannot have assets that exceed $1,000.[57] This stringent asset limit means recipients do not have the savings necessary for an emergency, leaving them vulnerable to precarious housing, food insecurity, and predatory lenders.

Earning exemptions relate to the amount of income recipients can earn without altering their income support payment. Once they earn more than the exemption, a recipient's income assistance is reduced. For example, if an individual Saskatchewan Income Support program recipient works part time, making $1,000, only the first $325 of net earnings from wages is exempt; support is reduced dollar for dollar after that.[58] As a result, it is difficult for recipients to work their way out of poverty because when they do work, they often work in low-wage precarious employment, and the income earned is deducted. Very few can work to financial independence in a single leap.

The clawback rate is the percentage by which income support programs reduce their benefits to account for other income the recipient receives via earnings; other benefits, such as insurance benefits or CPP disability benefits; gifts; inheritance; and so forth. In some cases, a recipient's income assistance benefit may be clawed back dollar for dollar on each dollar earned through other sources. This deduction is called a 100 per cent clawback rate.

An overpayment occurs when a recipient receives an amount over what they are entitled to under the income support program. Overpayments can be triggered in many ways, such as through unreported income or assets, changes in family relationships, the receipt of a lump sum applicable to earlier months, administrative errors, and communication issues. Income support administrators can recover overpayments from recipients through court proceedings, a referral to the Canada Revenue Agency, and deductions from the recipient's ongoing assistance. As a result of an overpayment, the government may reduce a recipient's inadequate social assistance payment every month, plummeting them deeper into poverty.

The social assistance system is administratively burdensome and police-like because of these complex rules. Recipients must be responsive to requests for information. If they do not respond, miss an appointment, or do not provide updated medical forms, administrators may suspend or cancel benefits. To stay eligible for benefits, recipients give up their privacy about their finances, family, children, living arrangements, relationships, and medical information.

Income Security Navigation Skills for Health Providers

The evidence linking poverty and poor health outcomes points to a responsibility for health providers to address poverty as a health issue. Income security interventions should be integrated into routine health interactions and the day-to-day functioning of health care teams. There are two roles for health providers in addressing income security: to guide patients to income benefits and to support patients' applications for income benefit programs.

Helping patients navigate income benefits requires some knowledge of income security systems and skills in guiding patients in navigating them. Health providers should, at minimum, have a general appreciation for the categories of income security programs outlined in "Helping Patients Navigate the Income Security System." The ability to ask simple questions to direct patients to high-yield programs can serve as a powerful intervention. Health providers may choose, through research and education, to develop a deeper knowledge of income security programs, especially those their patient population is most likely to benefit from.

Effectively supporting patients' applications for income benefit programs depends on adequate knowledge of those programs and skills in conducting relevant assessments and conveying information through application forms and other communications. A few core principles and approaches guide effective intervention:

- Prioritize completing income security applications as a core health intervention: achieving income security is as important as other health interventions and should be engaged in with urgency and priority.
- Health providers' role in income security applications is to provide information, not to determine eligibility: Health providers are asked to conduct careful assessments of health and functional status and to communicate those assessments to income security programs. That information is then analysed by adjudicators trained in the particularities of that program. Income security programs have different criteria for eligibility, including different definitions of disability. Health providers rarely have an adequate understanding of those criteria or definitions to enable them to contemplate eligibility.
- Be an ally; lower barriers to income security application processes: Access to income benefits is essential to improving health, and health providers have a responsibility to support and facilitate their

patients' access to those benefits. Providers should avoid posing barriers, including charging low-income patients more than they can afford to complete forms, taking excessive time to complete forms, making patients feel uncomfortable by complaining about forms, and failing to complete forms for patients who do not follow office rules, such as attending or arriving on time for scheduled appointments.

We now elaborate on the core components of income security program navigation for health providers.

Health Providers' Role and Disability Benefits

Health providers are central to a patient's ability to access disability income benefits. For some patients, the difference in income can be substantial. For example, under Ontario's social assistance system, as of July 2024, a single person received only $733 per month from Ontario Works, compared with $1,368 if they were a person living with a disability and qualified for the Ontario Disability Support Program (ODSP). It is important to note that access to ODSP includes access to Extended Health Benefits such as prescription drugs, dental care, physiotherapy, transportation to health appointments, and medical supplies.

HEALTH PROVIDERS' ROLE

Sometimes health providers are unaware of how much power they wield and do not prioritize spending the time to provide an opinion. Others are reluctant gatekeepers, unilaterally determining a patient's access to benefits. Both approaches are problematic. In the end, the health provider's role is to provide detailed and accurate information about the patient's health status. Patients face increased stress when health providers delay providing information.

For some disability benefit program applications, health providers are asked to provide an opinion on a patient's health status and disability. Generally, treating health providers are "participant experts" who form opinions based on observing and participating in the patient's care and treatment.[59] Opinions may be found in the clinical notes and records, completed forms, referral notes, and letters. They must be "fair, objective and non-partisan" and confined to the provider's area of expertise.[60] The most effective health providers keep their evidence simple and straightforward. They understand the purpose of providing their opinion and basic legal concepts. An overview of key information on major disability income support programs is provided in Table 6.4.

Table 6.4. Legal Resources for Major Disability Income Support Programs

Resource	Web page
Canada Child Benefit	
Forms and overview	https://www.canada.ca/en/revenue-agency/services/child-family-benefits/canada-child-benefit-overview.html
Info sheet	https://connectingottawa.com/wp-content/uploads/2022/05/CCB-Infosheet_May-17_2022.pdf
How to apply	https://www.canada.ca/en/revenue-agency/services/child-family-benefits/canada-child-benefit-overview/canada-child-benefit-apply.html
	https://stepstojustice.ca/questions/income-assistance/how-do-i-apply-child-tax-benefits/
How to appeal	https://stepstojustice.ca/questions/income-assistance/can-i-appeal-decision-about-child-tax-benefits/
Disability Tax Credit	
Forms and overview	https://www.canada.ca/en/revenue-agency/services/tax/individuals/segments/tax-credits-deductions-persons-disabilities/disability-tax-credit.html
Toolkit	https://disabilityalliancebc.org/dtc-app/
Tip sheet	http://disabilityalliancebc.org/wp-content/uploads/2018/03/HS14.pdf
Practitioner's Guide to the Disability Tax Credit	https://disabilityalliancebc.org/publications/rdsp-dtc/
Webinar for practitioners	https://www.youtube.com/watch?v=7CpsQ8KO70Q
How to dispute	https://disability.benefitswayfinder.org/resource/if-your-dtc-application-is-denied
Seniors	
Low-income and seniors retirement info	https://openpolicyontario.s3.amazonaws.com/uploads/2024/07/Low-Income_Maximizing-GIS_-Determining-OAS-and-GIS-English-booklet_JULY-2024.pdf
Forms and overview – CPP retirement	https://www.canada.ca/en/services/benefits/publicpensions/cpp.html
Forms and overview – OAS	https://www.canada.ca/en/services/benefits/publicpensions/cpp/old-age-security/apply.html
OAS Toolkit	https://www.canada.ca/en/employment-social-development/programs/old-age-security/reports/oas-toolkit.html
Reconsideration and Appeals – OAS	https://stepstojustice.ca/questions/income-assistance/can-i-appeal-oas-decision/
OAS and GIS appeals	https://www.sst-tss.gc.ca/en/your-appeal/oasgis-general-division-your-reasons-appealing
Self-help legal guides to challenge OAS-CPP decisions	https://clasbc.net/wp-content/uploads/2019/06/Challenging Decision-CPP-OAS.pdf
How to appeal CPP decisions	https://stepstojustice.ca/questions/income-assistance/can-i-appeal-decision-about-my-cpp-retirement-pension/

(Continued)

Table 6.4. (Continued)

Resource	Web page
CPP-D	
Forms and overview	https://www.canada.ca/en/services/benefits/publicpensions/cpp/cpp-disability-benefit.html
Toolkit	https://www.canada.ca/en/employment-social-development/programs/pension-plan-disability-benefits/reports/toolkit.html
CPP-D self-help appeals	https://stepstojustice.ca/guided-pathways/guided-pathway-for-cpp-d-denials/
How to appeal	https://sst-tss.gc.ca/en/your-appeal/cpp-disability-general-division-your-reasons-appealing

CPP-D = Canada Pension Plan disability benefit; OAS = Old Age Security.

STANDARD OF PROOF

The standard of proof is the level of certainty necessary to prove a case. Generally, when health providers give an opinion, the standard of proof required is a balance of probabilities. In other words, the health provider should be 50 per cent plus one, or more likely than not, certain of their opinion. Medical certainty is not required. The opinion should be realistic.

Putting this into context, consider the employment question on the medical report for a CPP disability application.[61]

Canada Pension Plan Disability
From a strictly medical standpoint, do you expect your patient to return to any type of work in the future?

Standard of Proof Reframing
From a strictly medical standpoint, is it more likely than not that your patient will return to any type of work in the future?

LEGAL TESTS VARY

Each income benefit system has a different legal test. When providing an opinion, health providers should review the requirements of the test they need to apply when answering the questions posed.

For example, to qualify for the CPP disability benefit, a patient is disabled if they have a "severe and prolonged mental or physical disability." A disability is severe if the person is "incapable regularly of pursuing any substantially gainful occupation" and is prolonged if "likely to be long continued and of indefinite duration or is likely to result in death."[62] This may sound complicated, but courts apply a real-world

Table 6.5. Legal Definitions of Disability

Program	Definition of disability
EI–Sickness	At least 40% reduction in work hours due to illness
Short-term disability (insurer)	Substantially unable to perform important duties of own occupation/regular job
Ontario Disability Support Program	Substantial restrictions (work, social, self-care) for 1 year or more[a]
Long-term disability (Insurer)	Substantially unable to perform the tasks of any employment for which they are suited by way of education, training, and experience[b]
Canada Pension Plan disability	Severe and prolonged mental or physical disability – regularly incapable of pursuing any substantially gainful occupation
Disability Tax Credit[c]	Impairment in physical or mental functions that is severe and prolonged, resulting in a marked restriction in the person's ability to perform a basic activity of daily living all, or substantially all, of the time[d]

[a] Section 4(1), *Ontario Disability Support Program Act*, 1997, S.O. 1997, c 25, Sch B.
[b] Usually, for the first 24 months for private long-term disability, the legal test is the own occupation, and then after 24 months, the legal test changes to the any occupation legal test.
[c] Qualifying for the Disability Tax Credit is a gateway to other benefits, such as Registered Disability Savings Plan, Child Disability Benefit, and Canada Caregiver Credit.
[d] Section 118.3 and 118.4 of the *Income Tax Act*, RSC, 1985, c 1 (5th Supp.).

EI = Employment Insurance

approach to the application of the severity requirement, such that the applicant's age, skill level, life experience, past work, digital skills, education, and language proficiency should be taken into account when deciding whether the claimant is able to find "substantially gainful occupation."[63]

A health provider unfamiliar with the real-world approach applied to the disability definition may discourage a patient from applying for this benefit or leave out important details of the impairment when completing the forms.

Table 6.5 presents examples of different legal definitions of disability.

CHARTING

Health providers are well versed in their obligations to chart a patient's health care journey. However, some do not consider how easily, and often unintentionally, notations shift a patient's ability to access benefits. Medical records are legal documents. Adjudicators and insurers comb through medical records to determine whether patients should be granted disability benefits. They check for notations about diagnosis, prognosis, consistency of complaints, treatment recommendations, and specialists' referrals and commentary.

Stigmatizing and critical language in medical records has "the potential to exacerbate racial and ethnic health care disparities."[64] Health providers must consider the potential for implicit clinician bias in the clinical setting that may be communicated in charting. Out-of-context, offhand, missing, or imprecise commentary can fuel disability benefit denials.

There are some simple things that health providers can do when charting to avoid unintentionally creating problems:

- Clearly note the diagnosis or working diagnosis.
- Consistently detail all impairments, not just chief impairments. Ask patients about their worst days. If impairments are chronic, keep a running list.
- Describe stress tolerance, energy levels, or endurance, if appropriate.
- Detail medication, side effects, and challenges. Instead of just noting "off meds" or "non-compliant with medication," include the reason why. If appropriate, document the reason, such as "cannot afford medication," "patient has difficulty understanding/accepting condition," "poor literacy/ability to follow through," or "medical distrust."
- Make appropriate specialist referrals or note challenges with referrals, such as long wait lists, lack of resources or transportation, or difficulties communicating with patients because of precarious housing.
- Avoid irrelevant, incomplete, non-essential notations, such as vacations or embarrassing details about family or work disputes. Comments such as "went out of country for a funeral," "on a vacation," or "missed specialist appointment" can disentitle your patient to income support benefits or trigger an investigation. Furthermore, some adjudicators inappropriately assume, without knowing the full context, that if a patient travels or misses an appointment that their impairment is not serious.
- Avoid noting legal proceedings and solicitor–client advice. A "lawyer-said" notation can be extremely prejudicial to your patient. Solicitor–client advice should never appear in charts.

LETTERS

Health providers receive many requests for letters. Sometimes, primary care health providers hesitate to write letters because they assume that their opinion is less compelling than a specialist's opinion. This

Table 6.6. Words to Use to Communicate the Standard of Proof

Write this	Not this
Probably	May
Likely	Possibility
Will	Perhaps
More likely than not	Can, could
On a balance of probabilities	A chance that

assumption is incorrect.[65] Health providers' opinions are valuable because they observe patients on multiple occasions over an extended period of time, providing holistic patient assessments.

Health providers should use objective and impartial language, even when they feel strongly that their patient is entitled to benefits. Avoid words such as *advocate*, *believe*, *medical certainty*, and *obviously* and absolutes such as *never*, *always*, and *cannot*. If the adjudicator perceives the health provider as a passionate advocate, they may discount the opinion as not credible.

Consider the following example:

- *Before*: I strongly believe that Jessica cannot do any housekeeping work!
- *After*: Jessica has limitations with standing and walking for prolonged periods, repetitive bending, weight bearing, kneeling, and crouching. She fatigues quickly and has poor stamina. Her pain levels increase with poor sleep and stress. She has substantial difficulty carrying out housekeeping duties that will likely continue into the future.

COMMUNICATING THE STANDARD OF PROOF

Generally, when health providers present an opinion, the standard of proof required is on a balance of probabilities. Medical certainty is not required. Table 6.6 presents some words commonly used to communicate the standard of proof, and Figure 6.2 provides some broader tips for letter-writing for practitioners.

FORMS

Disability benefit programs require health providers to complete forms for patients to apply for benefits. For the patient, a great deal rides on how thoroughly the health provider completes these forms. A missing

Figure 6.2. Letter-Writing Tips for Practitioners

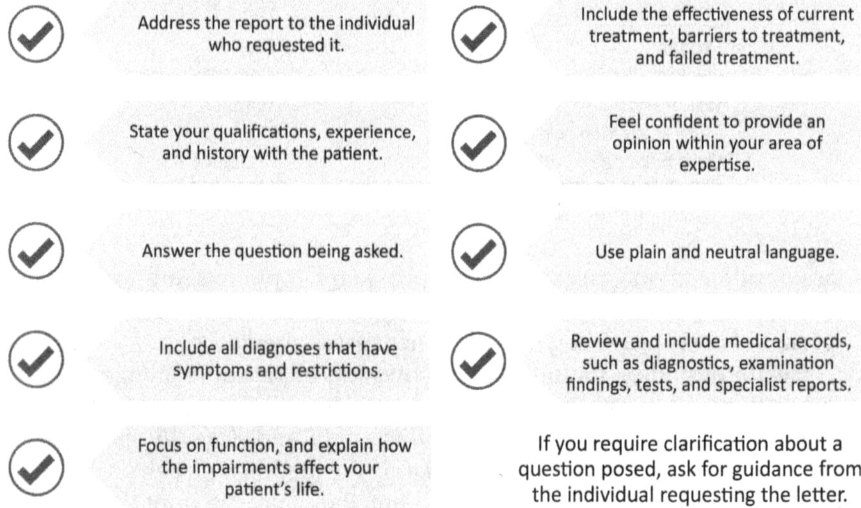

impairment, misplaced checkmark, or delayed medical form can have severe unintended consequences for a patient's entitlement to income support.

No matter how routine the form may seem, health providers should take the time to fully review and assess their patient's condition before completing it to ensure the information is accurate and complete. Patients are often denied benefits because medical forms were filled out quickly, without complete and accurate information.

Functional limitations and restrictions should be detailed, including physical, cognitive, or mental. Prognosis sections should be filled out to a realistic, more-likely-than-not standard. Generally, treatment details should mention prior, current, and future recommendations, including any barriers associated with the recommendations.

Health providers should screen for patients who have difficulty completing their portions of the application forms. Some patients face significant barriers in filling out forms, such as poor literacy, digital, and language skills; a reluctance to disclose information to the government; confusion with the complex application process; and feeling overwhelmed by scheduling appointments and gathering documents. For a person living with a disability, the application process can be stressful, dehumanizing, and draining.[66]

APPEALS

Some patients may feel discouraged after receiving a disability benefit denial. In some situations, denied applications are common, and this does not mean that the patient will not eventually qualify for the benefit.

When income benefits are denied, changed, or stopped, the patient may have the right to request a review of the decision. Health providers should direct patients to review the denial letter. If the patient does not have the denial letter, the patient should contact the decision maker to request the denial in writing.

Health providers should also warn patients that they may face a short deadline to challenge a benefit denial and make appropriate referrals. For example, in Ontario, patients have 30 days from the date they received an ODSP denial to request an internal review of the denial, unless granted an extension.[67] Health providers should encourage the patient to move quickly to seek legal advice to ensure that this first deadline and additional deadlines during the appeal process are not missed.

EMPOWERMENT AND ADVOCACY

The process of navigating and applying for income and disability support programs can be profoundly counter-therapeutic for patients. Dealing with complex systems that are designed to identify ineligible applicants rather than welcome eligible applicants often leaves patients feeling distressed and dehumanized, sometimes reigniting experiences of trauma and marginalization. Health providers can counter these experiences through active attempts to empower and advocate for patients.

A sense of empowerment begins with patients feeling that health providers understand and empathize with their stories. Patients should be encouraged to express the impact of their disabilities in writing (with assistance, if necessary), and these accounts should be considered in developing health provider opinions. Patients can be explicitly involved throughout the application process when health providers share drafts of written opinions and forms, discuss detailed functional assessments in collaboration with patients, and double check information directly with patients.

Empowerment is enhanced when patients feel their health providers are acting as their advocates. Health providers should develop knowledge of income support programs and applications and appeals processes, enabling them to serve as confident guides to patients. This role need not infringe on health providers' ability to provide objective accounts of the impact of disability. It makes it clear to patients, however, that the health provider is ably applying their expertise to the therapeutic process of income security system navigation.

Jessica, Part 4

With your support and careful description of her situation and provision of collateral health information, Jessica is able to apply for a combination of federal and provincial disability support programs. Unfortunately, her application for the provincial social assistance disability program is denied. You explain the appeals process, give her a copy of her application, and help her set up an appointment with a local legal aid clinic. You reassure her that you will provide further information to support her appeal, with the guidance of her legal advisor. You make a note to call her in two weeks to check on her progress.

Luckily, her appeal is accepted in the first stage, on internal review by the provincial adjudication unit, and her benefits are delivered the following month. Although she is not living above the poverty line, she is able to afford rent and has access to coverage for medications, transportation to health appointments and medical supplies, and a minimal degree of financial security.

Building Supports for Income Interventions

Although income interventions may be undertaken by individual health providers supporting their patients, capacity for these interventions can be multiplied through targeted program development and partnerships. A 2021 evidence-based overview of the literature detailed a wide range of interventions for social risks to health being explored by health providers and their teams, in partnership with their communities.[68] Health teams can reorient and direct resources towards income interventions. Community organizations with expertise in income interventions support patients with both basic interventions and navigating complex income support situations. Legal aid clinics, where available, are essential for patients who require support with complex challenges and income program appeals.

Growing Your Health Team

To implement income security interventions, teams can leverage internal resources, build new team positions, or create programs for patients through partnerships with external agencies.

Existing health team resources can be used effectively to enhance income security interventions for patients. Every health team has a different structure and has been built around a different set of priorities. Refocusing on income interventions may be possible within available resources. Some team members, such as social workers, may already have significant expertise in this area. Other team members, such as nurses, physicians, or dieticians (who are often the first to identify poverty through food insecurity) can develop expertise to support income interventions.

Internal team experts can further enhance team capacity through the development of assessment and management algorithms and provider- and patient-oriented resource packages. Algorithmic approaches to income security interventions can be tailored to local team and community resources and can enable a team approach to addressing income security needs. Handouts targeting high-prevalence income security interventions or listing community or other supports increase intervention efficiency and offer direct intervention tools to patients. These handouts have been developed in some jurisdictions, including the excellent Get Your Benefits booklet in Manitoba that is available in an editable format to enable it to be tailored to local resources and needs.[69] As income security interventions are prioritized, teams can continually assess capacity and target resources appropriately.

New team positions can be developed to enable income security interventions. The St. Michael's Hospital Academic Family Health Team in Toronto created a position for an income security health promoter in 2013.[70] Two permanent full-time income security health promoters are presently funded through core Ontario Ministry of Health funding. Similar positions have been created in other jurisdictions in Ontario and in other provinces. The Downtown/Point Douglas MyHealthTeams program in Winnipeg offers interdisciplinary care providers, including income security specialists, to solo and small group primary care practices. Although these specialists support multiple health providers, they are considered internal to each team, including charting in and communicating directly through patient electronic health records.[71]

Health teams can expand their capacity through partnerships with community agencies. Direct relationships may enable facilitated referrals, for example for assessment of complex income security situations or more comprehensive case management support for patients with multiple social needs. Community agencies can be encouraged to provide direct services at health clinics, including time-limited services such as low-income tax filing support.[72] Medical–financial partnerships, including Welfare Rights Advice services in the United Kingdom, have a long history of providing co-located services with health teams.[73,74] Medical–legal, or health justice, partnerships, offer on-site legal services to low-income patients, with direct health team referral pathways, using government or private funding.[75] The South Georgian Bay Ontario Health Team partnered with 211 Ontario to offer phone-based social needs assessments and community resource connections to socially marginalized patients.[76]

Community Organizations

There are community organizations across Canada who support income security and financial wellness for Canadians living on low levels of income through the provision of a range of financial empowerment interventions. Figure 6.3 illustrates five pillars of financial empowerment. The program interventions associated with these pillars include financial literacy workshops, financial coaching and counselling, access to identification, tax filing, benefits navigation, access to bank accounts, access to credit, matched saving programs, and consumer protection advocacy.

Prosper Canada is the national champion of financial empowerment in Canada and has worked with local and regional partners to develop these interventions It should be noted that community demand for these services and supports often outstrips the program delivery capacity of these organizations. Several organizations provide train-the-trainer and capacity-building services to support service delivery through other avenues, including the health care system. Prosper Canada has worked with cross-sectoral partners to develop an online tool, the Benefits Wayfinder, and its companion, the Disability Benefits Compass, to help quickly identify income benefits that Canadians may be eligible for. Support staff, volunteers, or community members can use this tool to identify government benefits available to an individual. Prosper Canada may also be able to help health care practitioners identify financial empowerment agencies in their communities who can provide financial empowerment supports to community members, capacity-building training to other service providers, or both. These supports can be found at https://prospercanada.org/.

Community organizations and other institutions (including health care centres) are able to host free income tax clinics with training and support from the Canada Revenue Agency. Health care centres can also partner with community agencies to provide access to tax filing through drop-off taxes and virtual tax filing services. Free tax clinics are provided through the Community Volunteer Income Tax Program (CVITP), and information about how to host a clinic through CVITP or

Figure 6.3. Five Pillars of Financial Empowerment

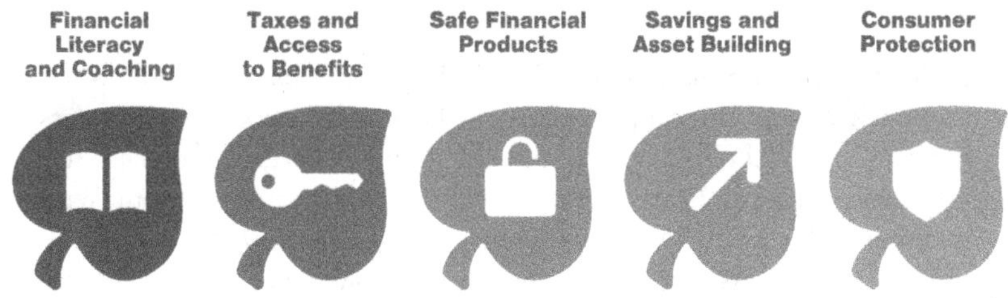

the location of free tax clinics in different communities is available at https://www.canada.ca/en/revenue-agency/services/tax/individuals /community-volunteer-income-tax-program.html.

Non-profit credit counselling organizations across Canada provide guidance and information to Canadians to help them manage their finances. Services offered include credit counselling to provide community members with the information and tools to manage their debts. Credit Counselling Canada operates an accreditation program for their member organizations. Information about certified non-profit credit counselling organizations can be found at https://creditcounselling canada.ca/.

The Financial Consumer Agency of Canada is responsible for protecting the rights and interests of consumers with respect to financial products and services. Their mandate includes the provision of financial literacy education. Financial literacy materials can be found at https:// www.canada.ca/en/financial-consumer-agency.html.

Legal Aid Clinics and Legal Professionals

Law can be a powerful tool to boost a patient's income so that they do not have to choose between food, rent, Internet, or medicine. Income benefit denials are disputed through the courts, tribunals, or both. Health practitioners can identify legal needs, foster awareness of legal rights, and support patients in accessing legal services. Generally, income security legal professionals require the medical documents that form part of the application process and the benefit denial letter. Legal intervention is a slow process – practitioners may receive a medical report request months after a legal referral.

Legal aid and community legal clinics can help to appeal the suspension and denial of income benefits. Online legal resources also provide legal information about benefits and appeal routes.

> **Malalai, Part 4**
>
> Malalai's complex situation necessitates a team-based, multifaceted approach to support. You engage your team social worker, who refers her to a legal aid clinic with a specialization in domestic violence. You also use your local 2-1-1 service to help her find a support group with members who speak her first language. She slowly builds a foundation of legal protections and social supports that enable her to feel less anxious and ready to enrol in a vocational program with a goal of entering the workforce in 18 months.

Conclusion

Health providers are well positioned to support their patients who live at low income as they improve their financial security and navigate income support programs. Intervention begins with identification of people living at low income and the particular income, financial literacy, and community supports they may benefit from. Health providers' skill in supporting patients is driven by knowledge of income security program eligibility criteria and applications and appeals processes.

Patients face multiple barriers to income security program access, often worsened by intersectional identities of social marginalization. Health providers are well positioned to identify those barriers and assist patients in reducing their impact directly or by accessing community and legal supports. The impact of health providers' involvement in income security applications and appeals is enhanced through knowledge-driven approaches to charting and letter writing that enable clear and effective communication of patients' situations to income support programs.

The evidence points to a dramatic potential impact from improving patients' income security. Health providers who develop individual and team knowledge, skills, and resources to facilitate patients' access to income benefits are building a powerful foundation for improved and maintained health and wellness.

Acknowledgment

The authors thank Marie Fiedler, a law student who assisted them in research and formatting this chapter.

NOTES

1 Laidley J, Tabbara M. Welfare in Canada, 2023 [Internet]. Toronto: Maytree; 2024. Available from: https://maytree.com/welfare-in-canada/.
2 Tarasuk V, Li T, Fafard St-Germain AA. Household food insecurity in Canada, 2022 [Internet]. Toronto: PROOF; 2023. Available from: https://proof.utoronto.ca/resource/household-food-insecurity-in-canada-2022/.
3 Mosher J, Hermer J. Welfare fraud: the construction of social assistance as crime [Internet]. In Mosher J, Brockman J, editors. Constructing crime. Berlin: De Gruyter; 2010. p. 17–52. Available from: https://digitalcommons.osgoode.yorku.ca/scholarly_works/494.
4 *Surdivall v. Ontario (Disability Support Program)*, 2014 ONCA 240 (CanLII), at para 35. See paras 39–40 for other examples.
5 See, for example, *2011-07297 (Re)*, 2021 ONSBT 2550 (CanLII). The director failed to provide any documents justifying the $20,000 alleged overpayment and the cancellation of income benefits. The director did not attend the hearing.
6 Statistics Canada. Market Basket Measure (MBM) thresholds for the reference family by market basket measure region, component and base year [Internet]. Ottawa: Statistics Canada; 2024. Available from: https://www150.statcan.gc.ca/t1/tbl1/en/tv.action?pid=1110006601.
7 Statistics Canada. Low Income Cut-Offs (LICOs) before and after tax by community size and family size, in current dollars [Internet]. Ottawa: Statistics Canada; 2024. Available from: https://www150.statcan.gc.ca/t1/tbl1/en/tv.action?pid=1110024101.
8 Statistics Canada. Low Income Measure (LIM) thresholds by income source and household size [Internet]. Ottawa: Statistics Canada; 2024. Available from: https://www150.statcan.gc.ca/t1/tbl1/en/tv.action?pid=1110023201.
9 An excellent overview of the evidence linking income and health can be found in Raphael D, Bryant T, Mikkonen J, et al. Income and income distribution in social determinants of health. In: Raphael D, Bryant T, Mikkonen J, et al. The Canadian facts. Oshawa: Ontario Tech University Faculty of Health Sciences and Toronto: York University School of Health Policy and Management; 2020.
10 Centre for Effective Practice. Poverty [Internet]. Toronto: The Centre; 2016. Available from: https://cep.health/clinical-products/poverty-a-clinical-tool-for-primary-care-providers/.
11 Brcic V, Eberdt C, Kaczorowski J. Development of a tool to identify poverty in a family practice setting: a pilot study. Int J Family Med. 2011; 2011:812182. https://doi.org/10.1155/2011/812182.
12 Centre for Effective Practice. A social history tool using the IF-IT-HELPS mnemonic [Internet]. Toronto: The Centre; n.d. Available from: https://cep.health/download-file/1542915867.061284-96/.

13 Samuel S. This doctor is taking aim at our broken medical system, one story at a time. Vox [Internet]; 2020. Available from: https://www.vox.com/the-highlight/2020/2/27/21152916/rita-charon-narrative-medicine-health-care.

14 Government of Canada. Child and family benefits calculator [Internet]. Ottawa: Government of Canada; 2024 [cited 2022 Sep 13]. https://www.canada.ca/en/revenue-agency/services/child-family-benefits/child-family-benefits-calculator.html.

15 Canada Revenue Agency. Child and family benefits calculator [Internet]. Ottawa: Government of Canada; 2021 [cited 2022 November 22]. Available from: https://www.canada.ca/en/revenue-agency/services/child-family-benefits/child-family-benefits-calculator.html.

16 Government of Canada. Old Age Security amounts [Internet]. Ottawa: Government of Canada; 2025. Available from: https://www.canada.ca/en/services/benefits/publicpensions/cpp/old-age-security/payments.html.

17 Government of Canada. About the Non-Insured Health Benefits program [Internet]. Ottawa: Government of Canada; 2024. Available from: https://www.sac-isc.gc.ca/eng/1576790320164/1576790364553.

18 Assembly of First Nations. Jordan's Principle Summit [Internet]. Winnipeg (MB): The Assembly; 2018. Available from: https://www.afn.ca/policy-sectors/social-secretariat/jordans-principle/#:~:text=Jordan's%20 Principle%20is%20a%20child,children%20without%20delay%20or%20 denial.

19 Government of Canada. Benefits, credits, and taxes for newcomers [Internet]. Ottawa: Government of Canada; 2024. Available from: https://www.canada.ca/en/revenue-agency/services/tax/international-non-residents/individuals-leaving-entering-canada-non-residents/newcomers-canada-immigrants.html#benefitsCreditsEligibility.

20 Government of Canada. National Student Loans Service Centre (NSLSC): how to apply [Internet]. Ottawa: Government of Canada; 2025. Available from: https://www.csnpe-nslsc.canada.ca/en/how-to-apply.

21 Employment and Social Development Canada. Canada's poverty reduction strategy – an update [Internet]. Ottawa: Employment and Social Development Canada; 2022. Available from: https://www.canada.ca/en/employment-social-development/programs/results/poverty-reduction.html.

22 Government of Canada. Canada Disability Benefit Regulations. Canada Gazette, Part 1 [Internet]. 2024;158(26). Available from: https://www.gazette.gc.ca/rp-pr/p1/2024/2024-06-29/html/reg2-eng.html.

23 Employment and Social Development Canada. "Understanding systems: The 2021 report of the National Advisory Council on Poverty." Ottawa: Government of Canada: 2021. Available from: https://www.canada.ca/content/dam/esdc-edsc/documents/programs/poverty-reduction

/national-advisory-council/reports/2021-annual/advisory-council
-poverty-2021-annual(new).pdf.

24 Smirl E. Access to identification for low-income Manitobans [Internet].
Winnipeg: Canadian Centre for Policy Alternatives; 2017. Available from:
https://policyalternatives.ca/sites/default/files/uploads/publications
/Manitoba%20Office/2017/10/Access_to_ID_Low_income_Manitobans.pdf.

25 Swire P, Butts CQ. The ID divide: addressing the challenges of identification
and authentication in American society [Internet]. Washington (DC):
American Constitution Society for Law and Policy; 2008. Available from:
https://www.acslaw.org/wp-content/uploads/2018/07/Swire-Butts
-Issue-Brief.pdf.

26 Smirl E. Access to identification for low-income Manitobans [Internet].
Winnipeg: Canadian Centre for Policy Alternatives; 2017. Available from:
https://policyalternatives.ca/sites/default/files/uploads/publications
/Manitoba%20Office/2017/10/Access_to_ID_Low_income_Manitobans
.pdf.

27 Robson J, Schwartz S. Who doesn't file a tax return? A portrait of non-
filers. Can Public Policy. 2020; 46(3):323–39. https://doi.org/10.3138
/cpp.2019-063.

28 Bajwa U. Income tax filing and benefits take-up: challenges and
opportunities for Canadians living on low income [Internet]. Toronto:
Prosper Canada; 2019. Available from: https://prospercanada.org
/CMSPages/GetFile.aspx?guid=b0a3599b-1b10-4580-bd2f-9887f5165edb;
Canada Revenue Agency. Ethnography of vulnerable newcomers'
experiences with taxes and benefits. Ottawa: Canada Revenue Agency;
2019. Available from: https://www.canada.ca/content/dam/cra-arc
/corp-info/aboutcra/ncmrsfnl2019-en.pdf.

29 Office of the Auditor General of Canada. Access to benefits for hard-to-
reach populations [Internet]. Ottawa: Office of the Auditor General of
Canada; 2022. Available from: https://www.oag-bvg.gc.ca/internet/English
/parl_oag_202205_01_e_44033.html.

30 Canada Revenue Agency. Free tax clinics [Internet]. Ottawa: Government
of Canada; 2019 [cited 2020 June 23]. Available from: https://www.canada
.ca/en/revenue-agency/services/tax/individuals/community-volunteer
-income-tax-program.html.

31 Immigration, Refugees and Citizenship Canada. IRCC Minister Transition
Binder 2019: Temporary Workers [Internet]. Ottawa: Government of
Canada; 2020 [last modified 2020 June 11;. Available from: https://www
.canada.ca/en/immigration-refugees-citizenship/corporate/transparency
/transition-binders/minister-2019/workers.htm.

32 See, for example, *Rimando v. Canada (Citizenship and Immigration)*, 2022 FC
254 (CanLII).

33 For example, in 2019 Canada admitted 1,211,870 newcomers, yet only 28 per cent were automatically permitted to stay permanently (Yalnizyan A. Permanently temporary: the problem with Canada's immigration policy. *Open Democracy*, 2021 Feb 26. Available from: https://www.opendemocracy.net/en/pandemic-border/permanently-temporary-the-problem-with-canadas-immigration-policy/).

34 Goldring L, Berinstein C, Bernhard JK. Institutionalizing precarious migratory status in Canada. Citiz Stud. 2009;13(3):239–65. https://doi.org/10.1080/13621020902850643. Precarious migrants may include refugee claimants, refused refugee claimants, temporary foreign workers, victims and survivors of human trafficking, undocumented, people who have entered Canada by way of law but no longer have valid immigration status and people involved in sponsorship breakdown.

35 There is a backlog of more than 1.8 million immigration applications as of 1 February 2022. Work permit extension applications take 133 days. Dayal P. Ongoing immigration delays leave nearly a million waiting to become citizens and permanent residents [Internet]. *CBC News*, 11 March 2022,. Available from: https://www.cbc.ca/news/canada/saskatoon/immigration-delays-canada-1.6390170.

36 Goldring L, Berinstein C, Bernhard JK. Institutionalizing precarious migratory status in Canada. Citiz Stud. 2009;13(3):239–65. https://doi.org/10.1080/13621020902850643.

37 Community Legal Education Ontario (CLEO). Status, eligibility, and immigration consequences chart [Internet]. Toronto: CLEO Connect; 2022. Available from: https://cleoconnect.ca/wp-content/uploads/2022/01/Status-Eligibility-and-Immigration-Consequences-Chart.pdf.

38 Campbell RM, Klei AG, Hodges BD, et al. A comparison of health access between permanent residents, undocumented immigrants and refugee claimants in Toronto, Canada. J Immigr Minor Health. 2014;16(1):165–76, https://doi.org/10.1007/s10903-012-9740-1.

39 Hamilton K, Johnston K. Fast facts: our city's undocumented. Winnipeg: Canadian Centre for Policy Alternatives; 2018. Available from: https://www.policyalternatives.ca/news-research/fast-facts-our-citys-undocumented/.

40 Paquet M, et al. Sanctuary cities and Covid-19: the case of Canada [Internet]. In: Triandafyllidou A, editor. Migration and pandemics. Cham: Springer; 2022. p. 85–102. Available from:https://link.springer.com/chapter/10.1007/978-3-030-81210-2_5.

41 A person must also meet all other eligibility requirements of each program to receive benefits.

42 Canada Revenue Agency. Ethnography of vulnerable newcomers' experiences with taxes and benefits [Internet]. Ottawa: Canada Revenue

Agency; 2019. Available from: https://www.canada.ca/content/dam
/cra-arc/corp-info/aboutcra/ncmrsfnl2019-en.pdf.

43 Employment and Social Development Canada. A time for urgent action:
The 2024 report of the National Advisory Council on Poverty [Internet].
Ottawa: Employment and Social Development Canada; 2024. Available
from: https://www.canada.ca/content/dam/esdc-edsc/documents
/programs/poverty-reduction/national-advisory-council/reports/2024
-annual/4877-NACP_2024-Report-EN-Final.pdf.

44 Employment and Social Development Canada. A time for urgent action:
The 2024 report of the National Advisory Council on Poverty [Internet].
Ottawa: Employment and Social Development Canada; 2024. Available
from: https://www.canada.ca/content/dam/esdc-edsc/documents
/programs/poverty-reduction/national-advisory-council/reports/2024
-annual/4877-NACP_2024-Report-EN-Final.pdf.

45 Office of the Auditor General of Canada. Access to benefits for hard-to-
reach populations [Internet]. Ottawa: Office of the Auditor General of
Canada; 2022. Available from: https://www.oag-bvg.gc.ca/internet
/English/parl_oag_202205_01_e_44033.html.

46 Kim PJ. Social determinants of health inequities in Indigenous Canadians
through a life course approach to colonialism and the residential school
system. Health Equity. 2019; 3(1):378–81. https://doi.org/10.1089
/heq.2019.0041.

47 Reading C, Wien F. Health inequalities and social determinants of
Aboriginal Peoples' health [Internet]. Prince George (BC): National
Collaborating Centre for Aboriginal Health; 2009. Available from: https://
www.nccih.ca/495/Health_inequalities_and_the_social_determinants_of
_Aboriginal_peoples_health_.nccih?id=46.

48 Kessler A, Quinless, J. Income supports and Indigenous peoples in B.C.: an
analysis of gaps and barriers. Victoria: First Nation Leadership Council of
BC and Ministry of Social Development and Poverty Reduction. Available
from: https://www2.gov.bc.ca/assets/gov/british-columbians-our
-governments/initiatives-plans-strategies/poverty-reduction-strategy
/indigenous-income-support.pdf.

49 AFOA Canada and Prosper Canada. Increasing Indigenous benefit take-
up in Canada [Internet]. Toronto: Prosper Canada; 2018. Available from:
https://www.prospercanada.org/getattachment/f4add5df-0edb-4883
-b804-60661f500c56/Increasing-Indigenous-benefit-take-up-in-Canada.aspx.

50 Statistics Canada. Poverty and low-income statistics by disability
[Internet]. Ottawa: Statistics Canada; 2025. Available from: https://www
150.statcan.gc.ca/t1/tbl1/en/tv.action?pid=1110009001.

51 Campaign 2000. 2024 disability report: Canada earns an F on addressing
disability poverty [Internet]. Toronto: Campaign 2000; 2024. Available

from: https://campaign2000.ca/2024-disability-report-canada-earns-an
-f-on-addressing-disability-poverty/.

52 Prosper Canada. Roadblocks and resilience: insights from the Access to
Benefits for Persons with Disabilities Project. Toronto: Prosper Canada; 2021.

53 Canadian Radio-television and Telecommunications Commission.
Communications monitoring report 2020 [Internet]. Ottawa: The
Commission; 2020. Available from: https:/crtc. gc.ca/pubs/cmr2020-en
.pdf; Davidson J, Schimmele C. Evolving internet use among Canadian
seniors [Internet]. Ottawa: Statistics Canada; 2019. Available from: https://
www150.statcan.gc.ca/n1/pub/11f0019m/11f0019m2019015-eng
.htm; Bizier C, Contreras R, Walpole A. Canadian Survey on Disability,
2012 [Internet]. Ottawa: Statistics Canada; 2016. Available from: https:
/www150. statcan.gc.ca/n1/pub/89-654-x/89-654-x2016001-eng.htm;
Statistics Canada. Canadian Internet Use Survey, 2020 [Internet]. Ottawa:
Statistics Canada; 2021. Available from: https:/www150.statcan.gc.ca
/n1/daily-quotidien/210622/dq210622b-eng.htm.

54 Dijkema B. Banking on the margins: the changing face of payday lending
in Canada [Internet]. Hamilton (ON): Cardus; 2019.

55 Buckland J, Guenther B, Boichev G, et al. "There are no banks here":
financial & insurance exclusion in Winnipeg's North End [Internet].
Winnipeg: Winnipeg Inner-city Research Alliance; 2005. Available from:
http://hdl.handle.net/10680/373.

56 Momentum. Summary brief: high-cost alternative financial services.
Calgary: Momentum; 2017. Available from: https://learninghub
.prospercanada.org/knowledge/summary-brief-high-cost-alternative
-financial-services/.

57 Laidley J, Tabbara M-D. Welfare in Canada, 2023 [Internet]. Toronto:
Maytree; 2024. Available from: https://maytree.com/welfare-in-canada.

58 Laidley J, Tabbara M-D. Welfare in Canada, 2023 [Internet]. Toronto:
Maytree; 2024. Available from: https://maytree.com/welfare-in-canada.

59 *Westerhof v. Gee Estate*, 2015 ONCA 206, paras. 60–62.

60 *Westerhof v. Gee Estate*, 2015 ONCA 206, paras. 60–64; *St. Marthe v.
O'Connor*, 2021 ONCA 790 (CanLII).

61 Government of Canada. Canada Pension Plan disability benefits [Internet].
Ottawa: Government of Canada, [last modified 2022 June 9]. Available
from: https://www.canada.ca/en/services/benefits/publicpensions
/cpp/cpp-disability-benefit/apply.html#h2.02.

62 *Canada Pension Plan*, RSC 1985, c C-8, sections 42(2)(*a*)(i) and (ii).

63 *Villani v. Canada (Attorney General)*, 2001 FCA 248, *Villani* at paras. 31, 32, and 38.

64 Sun M, Oliwa T, Peek MEE, et al. Negative patient descriptors:
documenting racial bias in the electronic health record. Health Aff. 2022;
41(2):203–11. https://doi.org/10.1377/hlthaff.2021.01423.

65 This resource from Ontario's Income Security Advocacy Centre sets out that
    mental health care too often falls to primary health care providers because
    of the paucity of specialist resources, long wait times, and prohibitive costs.
    This report rebuts the often-held presumption that if an individual is not
    under the care of a psychiatrist, then they must not be very ill: Sunderji N,
    Powles K, Tau M, et al. Understanding the complexity of treatment of mental
    illness and addictions in Ontario [Internet]. Toronto: University of Toronto,
    Departments of Psychiatry and Family & Community Medicine; 2020.
    Available from: https://incomesecurity.org/wp-content/uploads/2020/04
    /Understanding-the-complexity-of-treatment-of-mental-illness-and-addictions
    -in-Ontario-w-2-headers-updated-May-2018-_2.pdf.

66 Prosper Canada. Common steps to get disability benefits [Internet]. Toronto:
    Prosper Canada; 2021. Available from: https://prospercanada.org
    /CMSPages/GetFile.aspx?guid=402aae78-3848-42dc-9d88-18baecbcaa7e.

67 O Reg 222/98 (General) at s 58 (1) and s. 58 (3).

68 Bloch G, Rozmovits L. Implementing social interventions in primary care.
    CMAJ. 2021 Dec;193(44):E1696–701.

69 Health Sciences Center Winnipeg, Manitoba College of Family Physicians.
    It's a fact: better income can lead to better health: get your benefits.
    Winnipeg: University of Manitoba; 2022 [cited 2022 June 28]. Available
    from: https://static1.squarespace.com/static/5fcec5785ecf630459448ae0
    /t/6583602cace7e901cd1b4727/1703108653478/getyourbenefits2022en.pdf.

70 Jones MK, Bloch G, Pinto AD. A novel income security intervention to
    address poverty in a primary care setting: a retrospective chart review.
    BMJ Open. 2017;7:e014270.

71 L'Esperance S. Exploring income security offered through primary care: a
    mixed-methods process [thesis]. Winnipeg: University of Manitoba; 2019
    [cited 2021 Jan 28]. Available from: hdl.handle.net/1993/34500.

72 Black S, Sisco S, Williams T, et al. Return on investment from co-locating tax
    assistance for low-income persons at clinical sites. JAMA. 2020;323(11):1093–5.

73 Adams J, White M, Moffatt S, et al. A systematic review of the health, social
    and financial impacts of welfare rights advice delivered in healthcare
    settings. BMC Public Health. 2006 Mar 29;6:81.

74 Bell ON, Hole MK, Johnson K, et al. Medical-financial partnerships: cross-
    sector collaborations between medical and financial services to improve
    health. Acad Pediatr. 2020; 20(2):166–74.

75 Sandel M, Hansen M, Kahn R, et al. Medical-legal partnerships:
    transforming primary care by addressing the legal needs of vulnerable
    populations. Health Affairs. 2010;29(9):1697–705.

76 South Georgian Bay Ontario Health Team. Closed loop referrals: patients
    impacted by the social determinants of health. Wasaga Beach (ON): The
    Team; 2021.

Indigenous Legal Expert Reflection on Chapter 6

DOUGLAS VARRETTE

I have worked as a legal clinic lawyer for the past seven years. I am also a member of the Algonquins of Ontario, and more specifically a part of the Mattawa/North Bay Algonquin community. I spent many years working exclusively with Indigenous clients in Toronto and helped many with disability-related appeals.

In my work I have learned of the importance of social determinants of health or non-medical factors that influence health outcomes. It is also important to understand that Indigenous Peoples do not have equitable access to health services compared with the general Canadian population.

There are many reasons for this. One is geography, because many Indigenous people live in rural communities and on reserve. Much like education and justice, more remote communities lack access. There are also issues with the availability of health care services created by jurisdictional complexities. One need only to look at the case of Jordan River Anderson, discussed in more detail in chapter 11 (p. 385) to understand the way in which different levels of government prevent equitable access to health care services.

In addition, perceptions and distrust of the government and health care systems affect the willingness to seek services. There is a long history of discrimination and abuse against Indigenous peoples in the Canadian health care system. One example was the death of Brian Sinclair in a Winnipeg, Manitoba, hospital in 2008 and the manner in which health care providers ignored him for 34 hours before his passing, as discussed in more detail in chapter 3 (p. 13). To some Indigenous people, the Canadian health care system does not reflect traditional beliefs and knowledge and has been used as a system of oppression in the past, and even recently.

These significant factors and social determinants can be lost when the government adjudicates health, such as through provincial disability support programs. The determination of whether someone is a person with a disability is made within a colonial, rules-based model. The process does not take the particular barriers facing Indigenous people into account.

- First, many health care providers are under the mistaken belief that they are completing the disability determination application to be reviewed by another person of similar expertise. However, in many jurisdictions, such as Ontario, the medical information provided in the determination package is reviewed by unknown government officials who do not have medical qualifications. Instead, there are policy guides and manuals written by unknown persons, to be used by unknown government staff, to determine whether the applicant meets a legal test of disability.
- Second, although there is often no explicit requirement for documentary medical evidence, applications are often rejected when no medical records are attached. If medical providers do not provide a copy of helpful, relevant medical records as part of the initial application package – with their patient's consent, of course – it then becomes the patient's responsibility to seek their own records, review and determine what is helpful and relevant to their case, and file the records as evidence. This is often at the applicant's own cost.
- Third, if (and often when) the applicant is denied and an appeal is filed, they are now in a legal, administrative system that places the full burden to prove their case on them. They are expected to be able to provide detailed information about their medical history and respond to questions to which often only their doctor will know the answer. If the application has any errors or missing information, then it is the applicant who is responsible. If they are not receiving the medical treatments that the unknown government staff deems appropriate, it is up to the applicant to explain why.

    For example, many of my Indigenous clients would not want to take strong painkillers and opioids for personal reasons. Instead, they would try and manage pain using traditional methods or different kinds of medication that are not opioid based. Without more explanation, this sometimes leads disability adjudicators to wrongly presume that the impairment must not be substantial.

Those in the health and justice systems can often lack cultural competency and an understanding of how discrimination affects Indigenous patients and their access to and experience with the health care system.

This forces Indigenous patients to educate health care providers and government officials about the history of colonialization and the way in which discrimination affects Indigenous people to this day. Indigenous people must endure the trauma of having to educate others and re-experience the discrimination. They must justify their treatment decisions to government officials in a legal, administrative system.

How to Better Assist Indigenous Patients to Access Benefits to Which They Are Entitled

- To better assist Indigenous people, health care providers need to ensure that the forms and applications they are completing provide all available information about all conditions, as well as the degree of impairment and restriction. This includes attaching relevant and helpful medical records to support the application and reduce the administrative barriers on patients having to collect this information afterwards.

  It is important to discuss the applications, and potential evidence, with patients so that there are no misunderstandings or missing information from the beginning. Be sure to include any specialist reports or clinical notes, with your patient's consent, that are helpful and relevant as evidence of the symptoms, restrictions, and the degree of impact caused by the medical conditions.

  Often the mere existence of a symptom is not enough; instead, the focus is on the degree of impact created by the symptoms or impairments. If there is little information about the manner in which the condition affects the person, then the scope of adjudication in the entire process is limited. There can be a presumption by government officials that all important information is provided in the first instance, and information that comes later is often given less weight.

- Be mindful of the disconnect between medical knowledge and terminology and terminology in the legal and administrative systems. For instance, the term *conservative* means different things depending on the context, and it is helpful for health care providers to understand that they are often not completing these forms for people with similar training and knowledge. A doctor may think that strong painkillers are an effective treatment, rather than a more intrusive surgery treatment. This doesn't mean that the doctor considers the impairments to be mild or trivial, but the term *conservative* is often seen in the legal, administrative system as being mild or minimal.

- It would be helpful for Indigenous patients if health care providers included information about particular treatment choices and treatment plans. If an Indigenous patient wants to avoid certain medications or cannot undergo certain treatments because of a lack of access to particular health care services, then it is important to include this information. This is why it is advisable to meet with the patient when completing the application to ensure all helpful and relevant information is included. It is very helpful for government officials to understand the particular barriers facing Indigenous people in the health care system and to provide context for and an understanding of why certain treatment plans are made and how the lack of equitable access to health care may exacerbate their patient's health conditions. This can also take some burden off the Indigenous patient having to re-traumatize themselves later in the process by having to educate officials and justify their choices.

7 Immigration Status and Health

MICHAELA BEDER, DILAN BRAR, RITIKA GOEL, VANESSA REDDITT,
JENNIFER STONE, DIANA GALLEGO (ADVISOR), AND
LUIS ALBERTO MATA (ADVISOR)

Immigration status is a foundational social determinant of health
(SDOH) because the state ties access to various political, social, and
economic rights to it.[1] Primary care providers are often the first point
of contact for many who have been marginalized by social structures.
They are therefore well placed to see how complex intersecting systems
of exclusion, and the policies that uphold them, manifest in the experiences of their migrant patients.

Harsha Walia notes in her book *Border and Rule* that "classifications
such as 'migrant' or 'refugee' do not represent unified social groups
so much as they symbolize *state-regulated* relations of governance and
difference."[2(p. 2)] Governments, including Canada's, create complex categories predicated on a national imperialist–neo-colonialist–capitalist
demand for cheap labour and control. As Walia goes on to say, "We are
told that immigration policy is about law and order, not racial exclusion in an allegedly post-racial society. But there is no objective fact of
migrant illegality; as Catherine Dauvergne maintains, 'Illegal migration
is a product of migration law. Without legal prohibition, there is no
illegality.'"[3(p. 3)] Similar state controls have been enacted for centuries
on Indigenous Peoples in Canada, leading to many points of solidarity
between migrants to this land and its original peoples.

Being aware of the impact and relevance of a patient's immigration status to their health is paramount because immigration status is often tied
to access to income support benefits, employment, health care, housing,
education, and the right to vote and the right to mobility. Understanding these impacts, as well as potential ways to support and intervene,
allow primary care providers to better serve their communities.

This chapter lays out concepts around health and immigration status
in four parts. First, we survey the categories of immigration status and
comment on how each type of status affects access to other SDOHs.

In so doing, we call on all health care providers to be attentive to immigration status and to better understand the complexities of how immigration status affects and intersects with one's identities and experiences. Second, we provide practical tools for primary care providers to create health care spaces that support migrants. Third, we provide practical tips for providing medical documentation to support migrants. Finally, we end the chapter with a summary of important moments when the health community in Canada has added its unique perspective to advance positive systemic change for migrants. We hope this chapter encourages the reader to effectively serve and act in solidarity with migrants, with the ultimate goal of a healthier and more just society.

Case Scenarios

- *Carlos*: You are working at a family medicine office. The front desk clerk asks whether you can see someone who does not have a health card. Carlos is a 51-year-old man who has come in for a severe flare of a work-related injury to his lower back. You learn that he has not had any health care in a few decades because he is an undocumented migrant. He works in the construction industry under the table. During the visit, he mentions that he is also worried about blood in his stool and weight loss over the past 10 months. He has avoided seeking care because he was worried about medical bills and the risk of a health care provider calling immigration authorities.
- *Maria*: You are working in an emergency department (ED). Maria, a 29-year-old woman, presents for care at 28 weeks pregnant because of vaginal bleeding. As you build trust with her during your assessment, she hesitantly explains that her pregnancy is the result of a sexual assault. However, she does not want to report this to the police because she has fallen out of status and fears it will lead to her deportation. She did not seek health care because she cannot afford to pay. She is worried about how she will be able to support a child.
- *Elias*: You are working at a walk-in clinic. Elias, a 43-year-old man, seeks care because he heard from a friend that your clinic would accept patients with Interim Federal Health Program (IFHP) coverage. He says a previous doctor's office turned him away because they did not recognize his document. He is a refugee claimant and has been having debilitating flashbacks, making it hard for him to find work.

Immigration Categories and How They Affect Social Determinants of Health

Consider the real-life case of Lilia Ordinario Joaquin. She came to Canada as a live-in caregiver, and her first employer treated her very poorly. She had to wait months for her new work permit to be issued to work with a new employer, during which time she fell out of status. With no choice, to feed her family, Lilia had to work under the table. Despite this being a situation created by the government, she was deemed inadmissible to Canada for working without authorization and ordered to be deported. The Canada Border Services Agency (CBSA) halted her deportation only when the *Toronto Star* newspaper ran a cover story about her after a petition and support from a local legal clinic.[4]

Understanding Immigration Status Categories and Pathways

There are many ways in which one might enter Canada and move through various forms of immigration status. These streams and classifications are set out in the *Immigration and Refugee Protection Act (IRPA)*,[5] and the rules that govern obtaining and maintaining Canadian citizenship are set out in the *Citizenship Act*.[6] Three main immigration streams exist under *IRPA* and its accompanying regulations: (a) economic immigration (which includes students and temporary workers), (b) family class sponsorship, and (c) refugee (which includes humanitarian considerations). There is a wide spectrum of access and precarity based on immigration status; the most precarious are those who have no immigration status (i.e., those who are non-status), followed by those with a temporary status (i.e., visitors, temporary foreign workers, international students, refugee claimants), permanent resident status, and, finally, the most secure, citizenship status. Canada considers anyone who does not have permanent residency (PR) or citizenship to be a foreign national.

Figure 7.1 is a visual of common pathways to PR status and then to citizenship. Once PR status is obtained, there can still be barriers along the path to citizenship, whereas those with temporary status can lose their status and become undocumented because of various issues, such as a failed refugee claim, relationship breakdown with a spouse or employer, or a medical issue. For some, loss of immigration status can mean deportation to unsafe situations they had fled. If an individual becomes undocumented, depending on the pathway of arrival and their eligibility, they may be able to regain status through some limited mechanisms, such as a pre-removal risk assessment, an application for

Figure 7.1. Visual of Pathways (and Pitfalls) to Citizenship

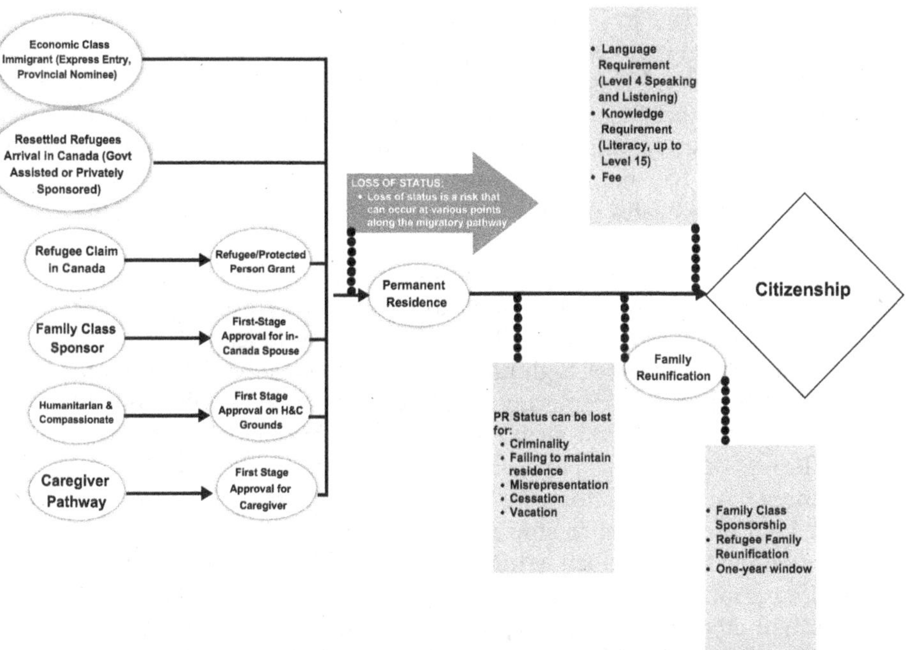

Note: Recognized refugees in Canada do not have to wait to get PR status to start the process of including their overseas spouse and children for PR status; this should be initiated together and is discussed further in the text.

PR = permanent residency; Govt = government; H&C = humanitarian and compassionate.

PR on humanitarian and compassionate (H&C) grounds, or an inland spousal sponsorship if they are in a relationship. These pathways, however, are rife with barriers, as is much of the broader immigration and refugee system. Outside of this picture are temporary foreign workers (i.e., agricultural and service sector workers), who at the time of writing do not have a pathway to PR status. Individuals can also arrive in Canada without status and may or may not be eligible for or pursue these pathways, depending on their situation.

UNDOCUMENTED AND PEOPLE WITHOUT STATUS

There are estimates that upwards of 500,000 people without status live in Canada, although the real number is not known; it is obviously not captured in census data.[7] As described throughout this chapter, we do know that in many cases, it is unfair rules that create a lack of status or so-called "illegality."[8]

People can arrive in Canada without status (by "irregular entry") or can lose status in various ways. People without status in Canada live in fear of deportation.[9] There is a constant inherent risk for those who are undocumented because any authority, such as police, Children's Aid Societies, or even health care providers, could contact CBSA, leading to deportation. This has been known to happen in health care settings in violation of a health provider's duty of confidentiality and requirements to keep information private.[10]

Individuals can arrive without status, or they can fall out of status by overstaying a visa or remaining in Canada after a refugee or PR application or appeal is denied. If an individual has fallen out of status, state interaction becomes high risk because it carries the risk of immigration detention and deportation. If detained, some people are held in immigration detention facilities, and others are held in provincial jails through agreements between CBSA, Corrections Canada, and the provinces.[11] Advocacy efforts are underway to call on all provinces and the federal government to stop using provincial jails as immigration detention facilities,[12] which is further discussed later in the chapter in the "Immigration Status and the Criminal Justice System" section. Once an individual or family is detained in an immigration detention facility, it can be very difficult for them to find and retain legal counsel. Often immigration detention facilities are far from larger cities where migrant communities and supports exist and where immigration and refugee lawyers[13] work. In addition, immigration detention can be indefinite.

Humanitarian and Compassionate Application

Note that people without status can apply for permanent residence from within Canada on humanitarian and compassionate grounds. This application, which costs $1,210 to make (in addition to legal fees that may range from $2,500 to $5,000 if there is no legal aid), requires putting forward evidence of both establishment in Canada and hardship if the person would have to leave to apply for permanent residence from outside of Canada. For further information about what this type of application entails, see the "Medical Documentation to Support an Application for Permanent Residence on Humanitarian and Compassionate Grounds" section.

TEMPORARY STATUS HOLDERS

Temporary status, which can be lost, includes visitors, students, temporary foreign workers, and refugee claimants.

Refugee Claimants

Refugee claimants are individuals who arrive in Canada and then make a refugee claim that the Immigration and Refugee Board (IRB) of Canada assesses on the basis of evidence provided by the individual. A refugee is defined, based on the 1951 United Nations *Convention Relating to the Status of Refugees*,[14] as someone having a well-founded fear of persecution on the basis of race, religion, political opinion, nationality, or membership in a particular social group (such as, but not limited to, victims of gender-based violence). Resettled refugees are deemed to meet the UN *Convention* definition outside of the country and then brought to Canada either as government-assisted or privately sponsored refugees and granted PR on arrival.

Refugee claimants can be in Canada for a long time with this precarious and temporary status while they await the outcome of their refugee claim and any subsequent appeals they may pursue. If accepted, they must pay $635 to apply for permanent resident status, as well as additional fees to reunite with their overseas spouse or common-law partner, children, or both; these fees can be a barrier for many. There have also been many critiques of the refugee claims system because of the extremely variable decisions of different adjudicators at the IRB.[15] Figure 7.2 illustrates the complexity of the refugee claim system in Canada.

Temporary Foreign Workers

Canada's Temporary Foreign Workers Program allows Canadian employers to hire foreign nationals for temporary work; it is widely criticized for its exploitation of low-income migrant workers.[16] As Walia notes in her book *Border and Rule*, temporary migration programs tie immigration status to employment: "This turns migrant workers into a state-sanctioned pool of unfree, indentured labourers. The state differentiates these workers as *migrant* labourers, whose labour power is first captured by the border and then manipulated and exploited by the employer."[17(p. 7)] Furthermore, "Migrant worker programs are carceral regimes, where many workers have their identification confiscated, are held captive in their place of employment, and are traded between employers like goods."[18(p. 7)]

One large category of temporary foreign workers is the Seasonal Agricultural Worker Program (SAWP), predominantly men from Latin

Figure 7.2. Refugee Claim Process in Canada

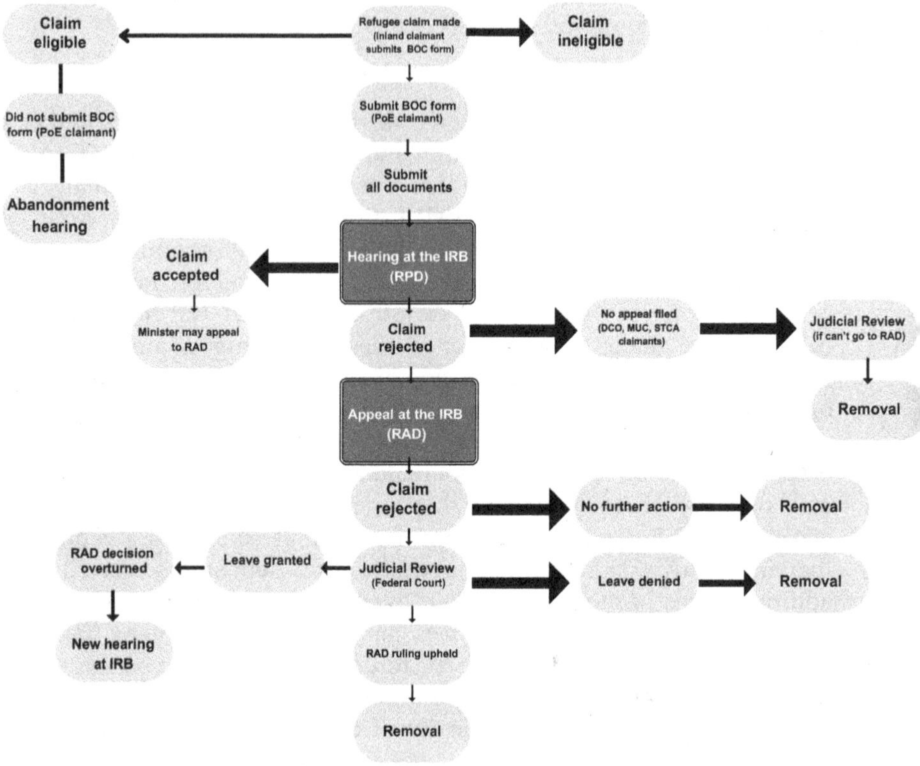

Claim eligible

Refugee claim made (Inland claimant submits BOC form)

Claim ineligible

Did not submit BOC form (PoE claimant)

Submit BOC form (PoE claimant)

Abandonment hearing

Submit all documents

Claim accepted

Hearing at the IRB (RPD)

Minister may appeal to RAD

Claim rejected

No appeal filed (DCO, MUC, STCA claimants)

Judicial Review (if can't go to RAD)

Removal

Appeal at the IRB (RAD)

Claim rejected

No further action

Removal

RAD decision overturned

Leave granted

Judicial Review (Federal Court)

Leave denied

Removal

New hearing at IRB

RAD ruling upheld

Removal

Source: Adapted from FCJ Refugee Centre.

BOC = basis of claim; PoE = port of entry; IRB = Immigration and Refugee Board; RPD = Refugee Protection Division; RAD = Refugee Appeal Division; DCO = designated country of origin; MUC = manifestly unfounded claim; STCA = Safe Third Country Agreement.

America and the Caribbean, who are allowed to come to Canada for eight months of the year and required to work 240 hours within any six-week period.[19] In the late 2000s, Southern Ontario saw a number of concerted raids of migrant farm workers by CBSA looking to arrest and detain undocumented individuals.[20]

SAWP workers notoriously live in extremely close quarters.[21] Farm-workers' rights are limited; although they are generally covered by provincial Employment Standards laws, enforcement of these rights is poor. Poor safety equipment and lack of training are well documented[22]; this was especially true during the COVID-19 pandemic when uncontrolled

Figure 7.3. Canada Immigration Levels (2017–21)

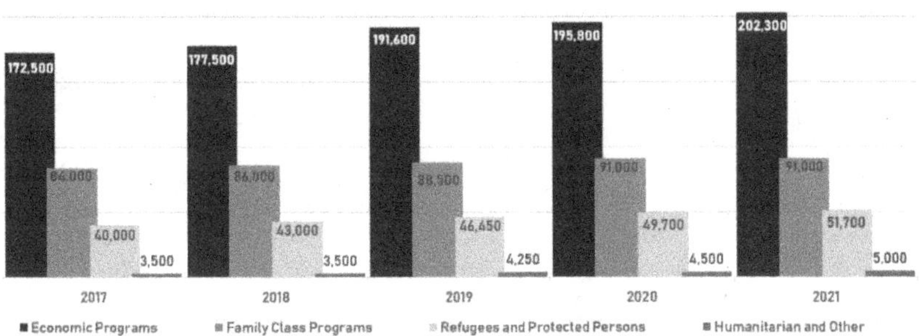

Source: Smith S, Katem E. Canada extends immigration targets into 2021 with prominent roles for express entry, PNPs [Internet]. CIC News, 2022 June 29. Available from: https://www.cicnews.com/2018/11/canada-extends-immigration-targets-into-2021 -with-prominent-roles-for-express-entry-pnps-1111368.html#gs.6f6n2k.

outbreaks among SAWP workers led to many preventable deaths.[23] SAWP workers live on the farms that employ them, and many cases have been documented of workers being medically repatriated if they become sick or injured.[24] As noted in a 2014 study, in 2001–2011, there were 787 repatriations among migrant farm workers in Ontario.[25] As a result, many farm workers are afraid to disclose that they have health needs because their employer will sometimes hold on to their health card. Furthermore, language and transportation barriers often leave them reliant on employers to be able to seek care.

Another large category includes the Home Child Care and Home Support Worker pilot programs (which have replaced the Live-In Caregiver program and which will, as of this writing, soon be replaced with a new Home Care Worker Immigration pilot). These programs predominantly bring women from the Philippines, who leave behind their own families to live in Canada and care for others' families for two years before they can access a path to permanent status and their own family reunification, which can take much longer. Home caregivers generally live with their employers, creating conditions ripe for exploitation, which have been widely documented.[26]

See chapter 5 of this text for a further discussion of rights under law (and lack thereof) for migrant workers.

Figures 7.3 and 7.4 illustrate the significant increase in temporary foreign workers (included under "Economic Programs") in Canada in recent years, demonstrating an increasing "permanence of the temporary." Having a larger share of temporary workers allows the state to simultaneously access labour while denying state membership rights.

Figure 7.4. Permanent and Temporary Economic Newcomers in Canada (2000–20)

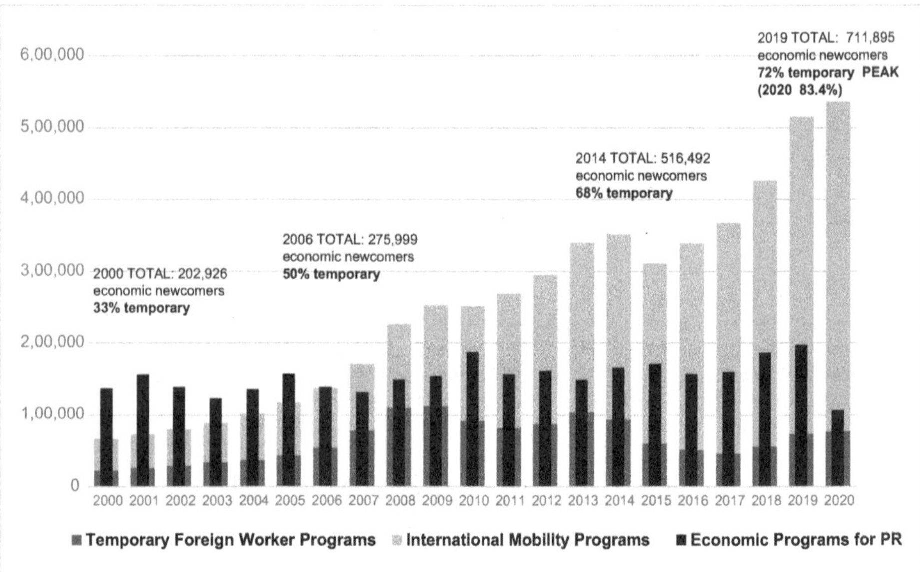

Source: @ArmineYalnizyan based on Immigration, Refugees and Citizenship Canada Open Data Portal Statistics.

PERMANENT RESIDENTS

There are various pathways to PR status in Canada. The largest pathway is through economic immigration streams, where individuals can be accepted into Canada on the basis of their level of education, professional skills, training or experience, and financial assets. These "high-skilled" immigrants must meet a certain level of points to be invited to apply[27] and are often seen as the "desirable" immigrants that Canada has chosen for its economic success. Immediate family members (i.e., spouses or common-law partners and children) of those who are granted PR status through economic streams are also granted permanent residence.

This category is juxtaposed with the so-called "low-skilled" categories, which are mostly temporary, with a long and barrier-filled pathway to permanent residence if they have a pathway at all. This structural contrast became particularly stark during the COVID-19 pandemic, when it was the latter category of workers that kept essential services going.[28]

Eligibility for Permanent Residence

Permanent residents also include Government-Assisted Refugees (GARs) or Privately Sponsored Refugees (PSRs), who are UN *Convention* refugees or protected persons resettled to Canada and granted PR status on arrival. Permanent residents who were once refugees (either from an in-land claim or a refugee resettlement process) can have both their refugee status and their PR status revoked if it is later established that they returned to their country of origin, misrepresented a material part of their refugee claim,[29] or obtained a serious criminal conviction.

Only permanent residents and citizens can sponsor family members. Family members who can be sponsored include spouses, dependent children, and parents or grandparents (the latter two only if higher financial eligibility criteria are met). Family members can be deemed inadmissible on security, criminality, or medical grounds. An exception to this is that spouses and children do not have to meet medical admissibility requirements related to excessive demand on health and social services.[30] The family sponsorship process can take several years and be inaccessible to many because of the prohibitive financial requirements to undertake it (see Table 7.1).[31]

Accepted refugees in Canada can include their spouse or common-law partner and dependent children for concurrent processing for PR status. This is not, per se, a family sponsorship, and so sponsorship undertaking rules do not apply. This is simply a process that recognizes that refugees are entitled to certain rights under the *Convention*, including the right to family reunification. This is why special rules apply to refugees. However, extremely long wait times for refugee family reunification reflect inadequate allocation of government resources for this stream.[32]

Generally, permanent residents or citizens who are on social assistance cannot sponsor a family member to join them in Canada. An exception is those who are on provincial or federal disability supports. Permanent residents who were sponsored by a family member can apply for social assistance, but if a sponsorship undertaking to financially support the sponsored person is still in force, the sponsor will be required to pay the province back, with almost no exceptions.[33] An individual who previously sponsored someone who then went on social assistance will not be able to sponsor anyone else until that debt is paid off.

Admissibility for Permanent Residence

Anyone seeking PR in Canada must be admissible. That is, they cannot have a medical condition posing an "excessive demand" on Canada's social and health care system (note that this criterion is waived for refugees and their dependents, protected persons, and family-sponsored dependent children, spouses, and common-law partners). They cannot have misrepresented themselves on another application within recent years. They cannot have any criminal convictions in Canada or reasonable grounds to believe they have engaged in criminal activity overseas. They must establish that they will be able to support themselves without relying on social assistance.

Later, we consider the impact of the *Immigration and Refugee Protection Act*'s inadmissibility provisions further to criminal convictions.

In chapter 10 of this text, on legal issues facing people with HIV, you will find a fulsome discussion of the excessive demand provision related to medical inadmissibility, who is exempt, and strategies to overcome such a finding.

The reader may note a disconnect between this chapter and others that delve into human rights law and various human rights codes that prohibit illegal discrimination. Mental health disabilities are often cast as injuries in the immigration context, which relies heavily on H&C discretion, as opposed to being seen as a protected identity. In a case called *Hilewitz v Canada (Minister of Citizenship and Immigration)*,[34] the court found that a finding of "excessive demand" could be overturned when the immigrating family had the means to pay privately for the needs of their child with a disability. The ongoing case of Nell Toussaint, who passed away in January 2023 after decades of fighting for the rights of non-status persons to life-saving medical care, is, at the time of writing, still before the Ontario Superior Court of Justice.[35] As of December 2024, several groups have been granted intervener status, and the litigation continues to proceed.[36] These cases illustrate, as Catherine Dauvergne writes, that the *Charter of Rights and Freedoms* has indeed failed non-citizens in Canada.[37]

Table 7.1 illustrates how long permanent residents or citizens who want to sponsor family must agree to be financially responsible for them. This exemplifies how immigrants must pay their own way or beg for discretion; this is not a rights-based area of law.

CITIZENS

Citizenship is said to have a positive impact on several key SDOHs, including, but not limited to, increased earning power and civic participation.[38] Only citizens can vote. Those who have PR status can eventually apply for citizenship after meeting certain criteria. For individuals who arrived in Canada as refugees, only obtaining Canadian citizenship will permit travel back to their home country without the risk of losing their refugee and PR status.

Permanent residents who want to become Canadian citizens must meet a number of specific requirements, including being physically

Table 7.1. Length of Financial Responsibility Undertaking for Sponsored Individuals

Sponsored individual	Duration of responsibility (as of March 2025)
Spouse, common-law partner, or conjugal partner	3 years
Dependent child (biological or adopted) or child younger than age 22 years to be adopted in Canada	10 years or age 25 (whichever comes first)
Dependent child aged 22 years or older	3 years
Parents or grandparents	20 years

present in the country long enough. Applicants must also have filed their taxes and have no recent convictions or criminal charges pending.

The citizenship application requires a $630 fee and, for applicants aged 15–54 years, up-front proof of proficiency in English or French.[39] These are barriers for more vulnerable migrants to accessing citizenship. Applicants aged 18–54 years must demonstrate adequate knowledge of Canada through a citizenship test.[40] Research has shown that family class–sponsored immigrants, refugees, and women are disproportionately affected by these barriers.[41,42]

***

The following section outlines SDOHs as they relate to different immigration statuses.

Immigration Status and Access to Health Care and Health Insurance

In Canada, access to health insurance is based on immigration status.[43] Health insurance plans (e.g., the Medical Services Plan in British Columbia, Ontario Health Insurance Plan in Ontario) are administered by the provinces and provide coverage for medically necessary and insured care services to those who are eligible. Helping patients with precarious status navigate the health care system is one of the biggest challenges for a health care provider. Many health care administrative staff and practitioners do not know where to begin serving someone who does not present with a provincial health insurance card. The patient may be uninsured or have alternate insurance, such as IFHP. As such, individuals may be asked to pay out of pocket upfront or told that they will receive a bill for services, both of which are a major deterrent to care.

INTERIM FEDERAL HEALTH PROGRAM

The IFHP provides comprehensive health insurance for refugee claimants while they go through the claims and appeals process. However, many providers are unfamiliar with IFHP, and patients may be turned away from care despite having coverage, as in the case of Elias in the case examples for this chapter.[44] IFHP provides basic coverage, comparable with health care coverage under provincial or territorial insurance plans. This includes hospital care, physician and nurse practitioner services, and laboratory and diagnostic services, as well as supplemental coverage similar to the coverage provided to recipients of provincial or territorial social assistance, such as prescription medications, psychotherapy, basic dental and vision care, physiotherapy, medical devices, home care, and other supplementary benefits.[45] Unfortunately, many patients are often unaware of the services available via IFHP or that coverage is linked to their refugee identity or IFHP document. GARs and PSRs receive provincial or territorial health insurance for basic coverage on arrival, and they can use IFHP for supplemental services (generally available for their first year of resettlement in Canada), whereas refugee claimants rely on IFHP coverage for all medical care. Although IFHP provides for comprehensive health care coverage, in practice, refugee claimants often face barriers to care because many health care providers are not registered to bill IFHP (administered through Medavie Blue Cross), and many health facilities do not accept the IFHP document and coverage (because of either a lack of familiarity or a decision to not accept it).

Key Tips for Facilitating Access to Health Care for Refugees and Claimants with Interim Federal Health Program Coverage

- Sign up as an Interim Federal Health Program (IFHP) provider (a quick and easy process) with Medavie Blue Cross and encourage others to sign up, too: https://www.medaviebc.ca/en/health-professionals/register.
- Ensure that administrative staff in your workplace are familiar with IFHP and the associated documents so your facility can provide barrier-free care if a patient arrives: https://ifhp.medaviebc.ca/.
- Ensure that patients know that IFHP provides coverage for medical services similar to provincial health care, as well as supplementary services (medications, some dental and vision care, physiotherapy, psychotherapy, assistive devices, etc.).
- Check the easily searchable IFHP cross-country provider database when referring to a specialist or recommending a service provider

(dentist, physiotherapist, optometrist, psychologist, and many more): https://ifhp.medaviebc.ca/en/providers-search.
- Certain services and devices require prior approval or referral (e.g., psychotherapy services require physician referral); this can be easily determined on the IFHP provider portal through the Benefits Grid.
- Always send a copy of the IFHP document with any referral.
- Remind the patient to always show their IFHP document for any appointments or investigations (bloodwork, imaging), as they would a health card.
- If a refugee claim is denied, but the patient is working on an appeal, IFHP coverage is valid through this process until the claim is accepted or the date of deportation.
- If there are questions or concerns about a patient's coverage, use the Medavie Blue Cross Provider Portal or phone to confirm a patient's coverage status. Alternatively, because the underlying refugee claimant status entitling someone to IFHP could have changed, email IRCC.IFHP-PFSI.IRCC@cic.gc.ca to verify whether there is still IFHP coverage.
- IFHP coverage expires 90 days after the decision date if a refugee claim is accepted; it is important to remind patients to apply for provincial health coverage during this time.

UNINSURED

People who are uninsured face significant marginalization and may not even make it past the door into clinic rooms. Hospital-based clinics and EDs often charge uninsured people an upfront registration fee in the hundreds of dollars for any visit, effectively turning people away right at the front desk. Many primary care clinics may even have standardized policies where they charge uninsured patients out of pocket for the visit, and there is no regulation of what these fees may be.[46]

Given that uninsured individuals often avoid health care for fear of debt, denial, or deportation, they may present at walk-in clinics or EDs with urgent issues because of lack of access to a regular primary care provider, as in the case of Carlos.[47] A review of ED visits for uninsured individuals in Ontario from 2002/03 to 2010/11 found that uninsured people disproportionately presented for obstetrical issues, injuries, and mental health conditions.[48] In large cities, advocates are often aware of the hospitals that are more likely to see patients without charging them upfront, although patients will usually still receive a bill after their care. After an ED visit or hospitalization, uninsured patients and their advocates often have to negotiate payment plans with hospital finance departments because bills can be prohibitively expensive.

The provincial variability in eligibility for health care related to immigration status leads to significant gaps in care and provider confusion. In Ontario, Community Health Centres have been provided limited funding that allows them to serve uninsured people for their primary care needs, as well as to refer them for specialist consultations and investigations. As well, many clinics that are designed or funded to serve marginalized communities (such as clinics for people experiencing homelessness) may not ask for insurance, thereby providing another avenue for uninsured individuals to seek services. In Ontario, midwives accept patients regardless of insurance status and provide excellent care for those with low-risk pregnancies. In Alberta, uninsured persons can get midwifery care, although there is a billing cap per midwife.[49]

Table 7.2 summarizes entitlements to health care by different type of immigration status.

Key Tips for Facilitating Access to Health Care for Uninsured People

- If you work in an emergency department setting, clarify administrative processes and policies to ensure uninsured people are not being denied care.
- If you work in a primary care or walk-in setting, determine whether your province has billing codes for uninsured care (as in Ontario during the COVID-19 pandemic).
- Consider providing pro bono care or connecting clients to pro bono care or clinics with funding for uninsured patients (e.g., Community Health Centres or homeless health services in some provinces).
- For pregnancy-related care, midwifery services may be available in your province, regardless of health insurance.
- Support patients to negotiate a payment plan with hospital finance departments, and provide assistance with this process.

Table 7.2. Immigration Status and Access to Health Care and Health Insurance

People without status	Study permit holders	Refugee claimants	Work permit holders, including special programs for temporary foreign workers	Permanent residents	Citizens
No access to provincial health insurance Individuals must pay out of pocket or rely on limited care from non-profit or volunteer organizations. During the COVID-19 pandemic, some provinces brought in temporary coverage for medical care.	May have private insurance through their educational institution, although not all do.	Have access to IFHP. Accepted refugee claimants can apply for provincial health insurance.	Eligible for OHIP if they are under the Caregiver or the Seasonal Agricultural Workers Programs. This may vary by province. With a valid work permit and proof of working full time for 6 months, work permit holders can be eligible for provincial health insurance in Ontario. Barriers remain when coverage is linked to work permits; loss of employment can lead to loss of insurance, increasing risk of employer exploitation.	Have provincial health coverage, but wait time depends on province (0–3 months). GARs and PSRs receive provincial health insurance upon arrival and are eligible for IFHP supplementary coverage for the first year (and longer in some cases).	Eligible for provincial health coverage as long as they meet residency requirements.

IFHP = Interim Federal Health Program; OHIP = Ontario Health Insurance Plan; GARs = Government-Assisted Refugees; PSRs = Privately Sponsored Refugees

Immigration Status and Personal Safety

People with precarious immigration status face an increased risk of violence, with a fear of reaching out for support because abusive partners or employers may threaten to call immigration authorities. This threat is exacerbated by mandatory charging policies, in which both the aggressor and the victim could face charges.[50]

In particular, migrant women and gender-diverse individuals who experience intimate partner violence face many intersecting barriers to accessing supports and disclosing abuse.[51,52,53] Challenges specifically related to immigration status include fear of deportation, particularly for those with precarious immigration status; negative experiences with authority figures, including police; fear of losing children; discrimination and racism; lack of familiarity with rights and local laws; social isolation; stigma related to abuse; language barriers; lack of culturally appropriate services; economic dependence on a partner; limited access to financial supports based on immigration status; and inadequate and difficult-to-access services, including legal supports and shelter.[54] They may also be more vulnerable to exploitative relationships, including abusive work relationships or spousal sponsorship arrangements, human trafficking, and financial dependence.

Although some municipalities, such as Toronto, have "don't ask, don't tell" policies,[55] which should limit the circumstances under which municipal services are allowed to ask for or report a person's immigration status to CBSA, police services do not see themselves as covered by these policies, unfortunately.[56] A No One Is Illegal (NOII) report titled "Often Asking, Always Telling" showed that Toronto Police Services were found to be frequently checking immigration status: of 3,278 calls made to CBSA by the Toronto police from 4 November 2014 to 28 June 2015, 83 per cent were listed as status checks (checking on the immigration status of an individual when there is no immigration warrant, a practice that is also highly linked to racial profiling).[57,58]

It is important for health care providers to be sensitive to these circumstances and to use a trauma-informed and person-centred approach, following the individual's lead on what they would like to share and identifying what supports they would like, which may evolve over time. As with other forms of trauma, it is not necessary to know the details of abuse to provide trauma-informed care and support. Building connections with community organizations that offer culturally and linguistically appropriate services sensitive to the needs of migrants can help to facilitate warm referrals to these supports. In Maria's case, you may explore with her what support she is interested in and help her to connect with appropriate organizations.

Key Tips for Supporting Safety for Migrants

- Be aware of the ways in which immigration status can affect an individual's interactions with and access to various systems and services.
- Use a trauma-informed approach and recognize that many migrants have experienced trauma (i.e., are fleeing state or interpersonal violence or living in fear or limbo while awaiting status decisions, have had experiences of immigration detention and criminalization and inappropriate conduct from employers). These experiences will influence their interactions with you and their concern about interactions with other authorities and institutions.
- Be aware that calls to police or to Children's Aid Services may result in a person without status being reported to immigration authorities; consider this risk along with your professional obligations to report.
- Demonstrate an understanding of these structural challenges and experiences for migrants to create a trusting patient–provider relationship in which patients can feel more comfortable to disclose.
- When working with precarious-status individuals, clearly notify them that you respect confidentiality and do not share information with immigration authorities.

Table 7.3 summarizes personal safety vulnerabilities tied to different types of immigration status.

Immigration Status and Access to Education

The educational system is structured in a way that poses challenges for people without immigration status, both adults and children. Access to federal government–funded English or French as an Additional Language classes is limited by immigration status,[59] with funding available only for permanent residents and accepted refugees. Provincially funded programs also have restrictions. For example, in Ontario,[60] undocumented individuals do not qualify. Having a handout sheet with local language learning resources and eligibility criteria can be valuable for your patients.

Children who are undocumented, or who have undocumented parents, also face challenges in access to education, and there have been

Table 7.3. Immigration Status and Its Impacts on Safety

People without status	Study permit holders	Refugee claimants	Work permit holders, including special programs for temporary foreign workers	Permanent residents	Citizens
May be at risk of abuse and exploitation and at risk of deportation if they come into contact with the criminal justice system or other state entities (e.g., traffic police, child protection).	Share the same concerns as people without status because of precarity of status.	Share many of the same concerns as people without status because of precarity of status.	Vulnerable to abuse and exploitation from employer because status is directly tied to employment.	Vulnerabilities due to immigration status decrease as individuals move closer to citizenship, such as being able to move jobs freely without work permits and qualifying for the Canada Child Tax Benefit, removing the need to rely on abusive partners. Permanent resident status may be lost for certain criminal convictions or by failing to meet residency obligations, so some structural vulnerabilities remain.	Citizenship is the most secure form of status

cases[61] of immigration enforcement coming to schools to detain children of parents who do not have status.[62]

In Ontario, section 21(1)(a) of the *Education Act*[63] provides for the compulsory attendance of minor children in school.[64] Furthermore, section 49.1 notes that "a person who is otherwise entitled to be admitted to a school and who is less than eighteen years of age shall not be refused admission because the person or the person's parent or guardian is unlawfully in Canada." However, in practice, upholding the right to access education has required advocacy. Too often, primary and secondary schools charge exorbitant fees for children without status to attend, failing to understand that they are not in fact here on study permits.

Many community groups, including NOII,[65] were instrumental in getting the Toronto District School Board to pass its own "don't ask, don't tell" policy in 2007. Implementation of the policy has been challenging, as mentioned earlier. Even when migrant students have access to education, challenges remain in ensuring that students have sufficient settlement supports and access to social workers, linguistic supports, and housing and financial supports.

For post-secondary students, access to education is dependent on financial means; scholarships and bursaries are not available to people without at least permanent resident status, with rare exceptions.[66] In addition, undocumented youth and refugee claimants are charged international student fees,[67] which are many times more expensive than fees for local residents. Across the country, only accepted refugees,[68] permanent residents, and citizens are allowed to apply for provincial student loans.

Tables 7.4 and 7.5 summarize entitlements to education based on type of immigration status.

Key Tips for Supporting Access to Education for Migrants

- Be aware that access to education is highly variable on the basis of immigration status.
- Provide handout sheets with local language learning resources, including eligibility criteria, to your patients.
- Advocate for families when children are denied access to education or face barriers in accessing school-based supports (e.g., social workers, linguistic supports).

Table 7.4. Immigration Status and Access to Primary and Secondary Public Schooling

People without status	Study permit holders	Refugee claimants	Work permit holders, including special programs for temporary foreign workers	Permanent residents	Citizens
As mentioned in the text, all children have a right to attend school, but fees may apply. Required documentation varies, and it is best to check what is required at https://www.canada.ca /en/immigration-refugees -citizenship/services /study-canada/study -permit/prepare/minor -children.html.	If the parent is a study permit holder, the child does not need a study permit; however, it is recommended that they get one. They must provide their passport or be listed on their parent's passport.	No study permit is required. Will need a determination-of- eligibility letter from IRCC, as well as their passport or being listed on their parent's passport, to not be charged fees.	If the parent is a work permit holder, the child does not need a study permit; however, it is recommended that they get one. They must provide their passport or be listed on their parent's passport.	No study permit is required.	No study permit is required.

IRCC = Immigration, Refugees, and Citizenship Canada.

Table 7.5. Immigration Status and Access to Post-Secondary Schooling

People without status	Study permit holders	Refugee claimants	Work permit holders including special programs for temporary foreign workers	Permanent residents	Citizens
A study permit is required for any course of study longer than 6 months. Foreign nationals may take courses shorter than 6 months if the course will be completed during their authorized period of stay. Do not have access to federal or provincial student loan programs.	A study permit is required for courses longer than 6 months, just as with any other foreign national. Do not have access to federal or provincial student loan programs.	A study permit is required, even for courses shorter than 6 months, but they are exempt from application fees. If a temporary resident makes a refugee claim, they do not lose their existing status, so they may attend courses shorter than 6 months without a study permit as long as the courses are completed within their period of authorized stay. Protected persons are eligible for student loans in every province.	A study permit is required for courses longer than 6 months, just as with any other foreign national. Do not have access to federal or provincial student loan programs.	Do not need a study permit to study in Canada. Can apply for federal or provincial student loans in every province.	Do not need a study permit to study in Canada. Can apply for federal or provincial student loans in every province.

Immigration Status and Access to Employment Insurance, Other Income Support, and Housing

In Canada, many undocumented workers find employment in the construction and housekeeping industries, and there is a secondary economy that exploits such workers, who too often become victims of labour trafficking practices.[69] Lack of access to safe stable work makes it more likely that precarious-status or undocumented people will live in poverty or experience housing instability.

Entitlement to provincial social assistance for people without PR or citizenship can be challenging to obtain. There are many barriers to applying, including, at times, inaccurate information provided by misinformed social assistance office staff.

Refugee claimants are entitled to access social assistance. In Ontario, anyone who has applied for permanent residence is entitled to social assistance, whereas people without status, including visitors, are not. It is important to note that anyone can apply for provincial social assistance and get a decision letter, which may then be challenged, and there have been cases of individuals without status receiving social assistance. Having a connection to your local community legal clinic or legal services provider can be key to helping your patients navigate income supports.

Migrants without status face significant financial insecurity and generally do not have access to social assistance or Employment Insurance if they are working without authorization. Exceptions include individuals who cannot be deported for reasons beyond their control. This includes, but is not limited to, those from countries under a moratorium on deportation because of the security situation in their country of origin.[70]

Migrants often face discrimination in access to housing, compounding issues of housing unaffordability.[71] For example, in the City of Toronto, individuals cannot apply for subsidized housing unless they are permanent residents, citizens, or refugee claimants or can prove that they have an application for permanent residence in process.[72]

Key Tips for Supporting Access to Income and Employment Based on Immigration Status

- Be aware of the different ways in which immigration status affects access to income and employment.
- Form relationships with local community legal clinics and legal services.

- Refer patients without status to community legal clinics for a consultation to see whether their status can be regularized (i.e., whether they can file a refugee claim or a humanitarian and compassionate application).
- Know that refugee claimants, accepted refugees, and anyone with a permanent resident application in process may be eligible for social assistance if they can show financial need.
- Offer to complete provincial or federal disability benefit applications (e.g., Ontario Disability Support Program in Ontario, federal Disability Tax Credit) for migrants if they are eligible.
- Screen for abuse in the workplace; connect patients who are working in unsafe settings to legal services or community-based supports.

Given that income is a key social determinant of health, Table 7.6 summarizes the stark variations in entitlements to income and employment supports on the basis of immigration status.

Immigration Status and the Criminal Justice System

In addition to the structural racism inherent in policing and the criminal justice system, which results in the disproportionate incarceration of Black, Indigenous, and other racialized people, non-citizens face additional vulnerability when interacting with the criminal justice system.[73] PR status may be refused or lost for reasons including security grounds, human or international rights violations, serious criminality, and organized criminality. People with precarious status who have been charged or incarcerated, including people with mental illness, are at risk of loss of status. As a primary care provider, connecting such patients to immigration legal supports, along with their criminal lawyer, is essential to ensure they are receiving the best advice.

Despite international standards to the contrary,[74] in Canada, migrants are too often detained in immigration detention, including to ascertain their identity.[75(paras 12, 14)] When provincial immigration detention facilities are full, or when individuals are experiencing severe mental health needs such as suicidal ideation, they may be sent to provincial prisons and mixed with the general prison population.[76] These practices are devastating to migrants' mental health.[77] Although Canadian law

Table 7.6. Access to Income and Employment Supports Based on Immigration Status

People without status	Study permit holders	Refugee claimants	Work permit holders, including special programs for temporary foreign workers	Permanent residents	Citizens
Unable to access employment or income support without a work permit because they are generally not eligible to work in Canada. Non-status parents of Canadian-born children do not have access to the Canada Child Tax Benefit, but this is being challenged in federal court	Precarious immigration status can be a barrier to stable employment with decent wage and benefits. Even in situations in which they can work, if employment is precarious or temporary, they may not be eligible for Employment Insurance if they do not meet the required 420 hours of insurable employment. Work permits and temporary social insurance numbers must be renewed regularly.	Eligible for social assistance if financial need can be proven. Eligible for work permits. Eligible for Employment Insurance benefits if they meet eligibility criteria and are unable to work for specific reasons (i.e., they did not quit).	Eligible for some Employment Insurance benefits if they are in Canada, meet eligibility criteria, and are unable to work for specific reasons (i.e., they did not quit) Delays in obtaining permits may cause loss of status. Even though those with "implied status" are permitted to continue working while awaiting permit renewal, employers often do not understand this and will be unwilling to hire someone whose papers have expired. Not eligible for other social assistance programs	Resettlement Assistance Program provides funding for basic living needs to GARs in the first year of resettlement. PSRs are supported in their first year by private sponsor groups. GARs and PSRs are eligible for provincial social assistance after the first year. The Canada Child Tax Benefit is available to citizens and permanent or temporary residents of 18 months or more.	No systemic barriers stem from citizenship status.

GAR = Government-Assisted Refugees; PSR = Privately Sponsored Refugees requires detention reviews within 48 hours, 7 days, and then 30 days thereafter,[78] a 2018 external review of the Immigration Division of the IRB found serious concerns about procedural fairness, leading to lengthy incarceration and multiple human rights breaches.[79]

In Canada, the number of children in detention has decreased, from 232 in fiscal year 2014/15 to 118 in fiscal year 2018/19.[80] However, the number of children held in Quebec has sharply increased, and it remains unclear how many children are separated from their detained parents across the country because CBSA is no longer collecting or publishing these data.[81]

Furthermore, shamefully, at least 16 migrants have died in immigration detention in Canada since 2000.[82] After years of advocacy, the federal government finally announced an independent review body for the CBSA.[83] After extensive community advocacy, British Columbia became the first province to end immigration detention in its jails, and other provinces are following suit.[84]

"Crimmigration" law (as it is known colloquially to immigration and criminal lawyers) is a complex area of law, and helping your patient access competent legal advice is key. Your patient's criminal lawyer should be competent in understanding the immigration consequences of criminal pleas and sentencing. Immigration lawyers must also understand how inadmissibility provisions work. The impact of a criminal conviction can be life-altering for non-citizens.[85]

Key Tips for Supporting Justice Based on Immigration Status

- Be aware of the ways in which migrants are affected by the criminal justice system on the basis of their immigration status.
- Assist patients who are facing legal challenges to connect with legal resources for both criminal and immigration representation.
- Connect with legal supports to determine how you may be able to provide medical documentation to assist migrants in accessing justice.

Being convicted a crime has varying consequences depending on immigration status, as summarized in Table 7.7.

Table 7.7. Criminal Justice Based on Immigration Status

People without status	Study permit holders	Refugee claimants	Work permit holders, including special programs for temporary foreign workers	Permanent residents	Citizens
May be found inadmissible for criminality if they apply for PR status. This may be followed by a removal order (deportation). Criminal inadmissibility may be a barrier to entering Canada in the future, requiring an immigrant to prove rehabilitation or a record suspension or obtain a valid temporary resident permit.	Same as for people without status	In some instances, may be inadmissible for PR status but maintain *Convention* refugee status, resulting in an indefinite need to apply for work permits. This results in discriminatory treatment in accessing services, such as health and housing.	Same as for people without status.	Can lose PR status and face deportation if they become inadmissible for criminality because they are convicted of a serious offence. There will also be no right to appeal if the sentence is a detention of 6 months or longer.	Can interact with the criminal justice system without fear of immigration consequences.

PR = permanent residency.

Creating Health Care Spaces That Support Migrants

Creating a welcoming and safe clinical space, from the initial booking, to office entrance, to clinical encounter, is essential to provide care to people with precarious immigration status who may have experienced trauma, either before coming to Canada or since arrival, and who may be facing intersecting marginalizations related to racism, homophobia, poverty, and other factors. A trauma-informed care approach[86] that takes into consideration the client's and their family's lived experience; fosters autonomy and collaboration; and is attentive to cultural, historical, and gender issues will provide staff with the tools to ensure physical and psychological safety.

Best institutional practices enshrine their commitment to the care of people with precarious status through policies and procedures. These practices outline and communicate to clients (in multiple languages)

- that patient information will be kept confidential; specifically, that staff will not provide information if CBSA or police call;
- that front desk staff ask for a health card and other personal information in a non-stigmatizing manner;
- how to support patients in navigating care with other health partners, such as hospital-based inpatient care or outpatient specialist consultation; and
- an attentiveness to anti-racism, including office signs that show that the clinic is a welcoming space. Examples can include "we do not communicate with immigration authorities," "Racism is not tolerated here," and "You do not need a health card to receive care here."

Training for all members of the clinical team, including front desk staff, is key to ensuring that everyone has the knowledge and skills to provide care to people with precarious status. Clients seeking care may fear the "the Three Ds" – debt, denial of care, or deportation. For any demographic information collected by the clinic, care must be taken to not share personal information with immigration authorities or police, and the manner of collection should provide reassurance to people without status and prioritize confidentiality. Front desk staff may need to ask for certain demographic information, such as a provincial health card or IFHP document, and training is essential so that any questions are asked in a way that reassures clients that information will not be shared with police or border or immigration services.

Access to interpretation services is a vital component to enable care.[87,88] Interpretation may be provided virtually, such as via telephone, or in person by a trained interpreter. Some people may strongly wish for family members to interpret; if a patient requests this, it is important to always confirm whether this is truly their choice. For more complex or sensitive matters, it is particularly important to get a professional interpreter to ensure client comfort and confidentiality. General guidelines for working with interpreters include starting with introductions, speaking in short sentences, allowing time for answers, and booking a longer appointment time.[89]

In supporting migrant health and well-being, it is essential to also consider structural and SDOHs. In addition to helping patients navigate the health care system, health care providers may be an initial point of contact for newcomers and can help connect individuals with valuable social and community resources.

Health care providers can build relationships with trusted local settlement agencies and community organizations that serve migrants, including those with precarious immigration status, and they can facilitate referrals to these organizations to help individuals access critical social supports. One national resource is the 211 resource hub – a comprehensive countrywide service that provides a service directory database of community and government services. It can be accessed by phone (calling 211, with interpretation available in more than 150 languages) and online. This resource is available to health care providers, patients, and community members.[90]

Key Tips for Creating Safer Health Care Spaces for Migrants

- Use signage and posters to signal safety in the care space.
- Create institutional policies to ensure safe access to care for migrants:
  - Confidentiality – information is not shared with immigration enforcement or police.
  - Identification or health card requested in a safe and non-stigmatizing manner.
- Ensure training for all staff, including front desk, regarding access to care for migrants.
- Ensure training for all clinical staff in how to meet the needs that migrants present with (e.g., the various social determinants of health presented earlier and tips on documentation presented later).

- Ensure systematic access to interpretation services for all patients with a language barrier.
- Connect patients with community supports, including for immigration needs, settlement, income supports, and so forth.

Providing Medical Documentation to Support Migrants

There can be many reasons why advocates will ask their clients to obtain medical documentation to support a refugee or other immigration-related application, including to outline physical and mental health impacts of torture, psychological impacts of precarious status, the importance of family reunification, diagnoses, and required treatments.

Obtaining consent to communicate with an individual's legal counsel is an important first step in providing this support. Legal counsel can clarify the nature of medical documentation needed and information on the individual's immigration status and background. When individuals do not have legal counsel, it is critical to help them connect with legal aid supports. One way to do this is to reach out to your provincial legal aid office.

General Documentation Tips for Immigration Reports

- When possible, talk to the lawyer or legal counsel in advance of writing the report. Note that your communication regarding their request may not be privileged.
- Focus on an objective account of reported symptoms, examination findings, and treatment plans and recommendations.
- Use neutral, professional language.
- Avoid commenting on the patient's credibility.
- Avoid a lengthy summary of the patient's history.
- Avoid statements that may be perceived as overt advocacy for the patient.
- Medical and mental health report structure should include the following:
  - introduction, including
    - writer's background and credentials and
    - duration of clinician–patient relationship and frequency of visits;

- description of symptoms at multiple visits, if possible;
- description of exam findings, including mental status exam;
- consideration of head injuries and cognitive impairments;
- known past medical history and medications;
- summary of diagnosis and findings and treatment plan;
- if applicable, how medical conditions may affect the individual's ability to testify; and
- if applicable, how medical conditions require accommodations (include examples).

Next, we outline several scenarios in which medical documentation can be helpful and tips on how to approach them.

Medical Documentation to Support a Refugee Claim

If a refugee claimant connects with you as a health care provider, the best thing you can do is ensure they are connected with reputable legal counsel in your community. Refugee claimants are 275 per cent more likely to be granted refugee protection when represented by a lawyer than when unrepresented.[91] Access to counsel has been shown to affect fairness and efficiency in the refugee system in many ways.[92]

Generally, key medical documentation for refugee claims has relied on psychiatric or psychological reports. If a client has a counsellor, psychologist, or psychiatrist or has had a psychiatric ED visit or hospital admission, a mental health report can be valuable. However, claimants may increasingly turn to primary care providers for medical documentation, including for mental health, to support their claim because specialist reports can be costly and access is limited. A resource from Ontario's Income Security Advocacy Centre sets out that mental health care too often falls to primary health care providers and rebuts the often-held presumption that if an individual is not under the care of a psychiatrist, then they must not be very ill.[93]

Primary care providers can provide supportive documentation detailing physical injuries and scars, mental health and cognitive conditions (particularly as they pertain to a person's ability to testify), recommended treatment, and required supports.

This medical evidence can substantiate that persecution took place, a key legal test in a refugee claim. The "Ready for my Refugee Hearing" guide[94] for refugee claimants is a helpful resource for physicians who are asked to provide documentation to support their patients' claims.

Other Resources for Preparing Refugee Claim Reports

- Cleveland J, Rousseau C, Guzder J. Cultural consultation for refugees [Internet]. In: Kirmay LJ, editors. Cultural consultation: encountering the other in mental health care. New York: Springer; 2014. p. 245–68. Available from: https://multiculturalmentalhealth.ca/wp-content /uploads/2019/07/Cleveland_2014_Refugees.pdf.

Refugee claim process:

- Steps to Justice. Refugee rights in Ontario [Internet]. Toronto: Steps to Justice; n.d. Available from: https://refugee.cleo.on.ca/en/refugee -protection-hearing.
- For claimants: Steps to Justice. Refugee law [Internet]. Toronto: Steps to Justice; n.d. Available from: https://refugeehearing.cleo.on.ca/.

Medical Documentation to Support Accommodations at a Hearing

Lawyers may request documentation to obtain human rights accommodation at the hearing.

Medical documentation can be used to support what is called a "vulnerable person application" at the IRB regarding a need for special accommodations. In such cases, a medical opinion can be key to establish that

- a person's vulnerability may affect memory, behaviour, and their ability to recount relevant events;
- the vulnerable person may be suffering from symptoms that have an impact on the consistency and coherence of their testimony;
- a person who fears persons in a position of authority may associate those involved in the hearing process with the authorities they fear; and
- a vulnerable person may be reluctant or unable to talk about their experiences.[95]

The IRB has broad discretion to tailor the hearing according to the particular needs of a vulnerable person, and a medical letter can advocate for the accommodations needed. This can look like

- allowing the vulnerable person to provide evidence by videoconference or other means;
- allowing a support person to participate in a hearing;
- creating a more informal setting for a hearing;
- varying the order of questioning so that the claimant can go first;
- excluding non-parties from the hearing room;
- providing a panel and interpreter of a particular gender;
- explaining IRB processes to the vulnerable person; and
- allowing any other procedural accommodations that may be reasonable in the circumstances.[96]

Medical Documentation to Support Expediting Family Reunification

At the time of writing, refugee claimants in Canada wait about two years for their hearing.[97] If accepted, they can then initiate the process to reunite with their spouse or common-law partner and children who remain overseas as part of their PR application. Often family members were left behind in the same situation of persecution that forced the accepted refugee to flee. However, the Canadian government has devoted too few resources to process dependent-of-refugee applications in a timely way. The last published processing time for this category of applicants was 39 months.[98] This protracted family separation under very stressful conditions has a profound impact on individuals' mental health.[99,100]

Health care providers can support individuals in this situation by providing a detailed letter setting out the mental and physical health impacts of prolonged family separation on their patient. This kind of medical opinion can be used by patients or their advocates or lawyers to push for expedited family reunification processing or early-entry Temporary Resident Permits.[101]

Medical Documentation to Support an Application for Permanent Residence on Humanitarian and Compassionate Grounds

If an individual is in Canada but is inadmissible (i.e., their refugee claim has been denied or they would not meet the definition of a refugee), they may instead apply for permanent residence on H&C grounds, known as an H&C application.

These applications are highly dependent on the individual facts and context of the applicant. If you are asked to contribute a medical support letter for an H&C, we strongly suggest you connect with the advocate or lawyer so that you can provide on-point medical documentation.

IRCC has produced guidelines on what H&C decision-makers must consider. This is generally framed as compelling factors, often referred to as "unusual, undeserved and disproportionate hardship" the individual would suffer if the exemption were not granted. Specifically, Inland Protection Manual IP-5[102] states at s. 5.11,

> Applicants may base their requests for [H&C] consideration on any number of factors *including, but not limited to*:
>
> (*i*)   establishment in Canada;
>
> (*ii*)   ties to Canada;
>
> (*iii*)   the best interests of any children affected by their application;
>
> (*iv*)   factors in their country of origin (this includes but is not limited to: Medical inadequacies, discrimination that does not amount to persecution, harassment or other hardships that are not described in [the refugee determination test];
>
> (*v*)   health considerations;
>
> (*vi*)   family violence considerations;
>
> (*vii*)   consequences of the separation of relatives;
>
> (*viii*)   inability to leave Canada has led to establishment; and/or
>
> (*ix*)   any other relevant factor they wish to have considered not related to [the refugee determination test].

In terms of health considerations, this is often advanced as risk to life because of lack of access to health care in the country of origin. For this type of H&C argument, the following medical evidence would generally be provided:

- letter from doctor, hospital, or health care provider explaining the diagnosis and medical care required, including for mental health conditions;
- connection to psychiatrist, psychologist, or therapist to conduct an assessment and provide diagnosis and care required when a mental health condition is at issue;
- hospital records;
- prescriptions for medications; and
- letter from a medical professional in the country of nationality or other expert on unavailability of care or proof of exorbitant cost of treatment there.

A number of clear resources[103] are available to assist with H&C applications.

Another key role for health care providers serving people with precarious immigration status is to help address the health concerns that contributed to their falling out of status, which will make it more likely that their H&C application will be accepted. Keep in mind that an H&C application is submitted when someone is inadmissible, has overstayed, or both, so a good H&C would start with a strong narrative of why the individual fell out of status. The reasons are sometimes health related, so including the steps an individual is taking to improve their health can be persuasive in seeking discretionary consideration. Examples include addiction treatment, mental health counselling, diagnosis, medical referrals, and violence prevention programs.

*Medical Documentation to Support a Citizenship Applicant
Who Cannot Pass the Citizenship Test or French- or
English-Language Requirements*

Permanent residents applying for citizenship must

- demonstrate proficiency in English or French (to Language Instruction for Newcomers to Canada Level 4);
- pass a mandatory written citizenship test (which is much harder than its predecessor)[104] in English or French with no interpretation, to establish their knowledge of the rights and responsibilities of Canadian citizenship; and
- pay a $630 fee.[105]

Structural barriers such as these have led to disproportionately higher citizenship refusals for women, refugees, and family class–sponsored immigrants. The requirements do not consider the under-education of women and girls worldwide; interrupted formal schooling resulting from forced displacement; long wait times for government-funded language classes; caregiving or employment responsibilities that make it difficult to attend classes; and trauma interfering with the ability to focus and retain information. Finally, and compellingly, the new written citizenship test is in effect a literacy test.[106]

One can request a waiver of the fee on compassionate grounds, particularly if the applicant is on social assistance.[107] As well, health providers can provide documentation to IRCC to request a waiver from the language and knowledge (i.e., test) requirements on compassionate grounds.[108]

Medical Documentation Setting Out the Health Risks for an Individual in Detention or Facing Inadmissibility or Removal Proceedings

Earlier in this chapter, we briefly surveyed some of the many problems with Canada's immigration detention regime. Too many individuals with precarious or no status are detained, including at times in provincial jails; this may be due to symptoms of mental illness. Appropriate medical care and documentation are not only hard to obtain in immigration detention, but, as a 2021 Human Rights Watch report details,[109] medical documentation needs to be accompanied by access to counsel and procedural checks on CBSA's authority, given CBSA's insufficient oversight to date. Our advice to physicians supporting an individual in immigration detention, as well as through the immigration procedures, is always to work in collaboration with the patient's immigration legal advocate and, if relevant, criminal counsel and to provide letters of support.

Case Scenario Resolution

- *Carlos*: Given Carlos's symptoms, you're concerned about colon cancer. You agree to see him without charge. You also diagnose mechanical back pain and provide him with exercises he can practice at home to relieve his short-term symptoms. You contact the legal aid clinic in Carlos's area and, on a subsequent visit, guided by his new immigration lawyer, you write a letter of support for his H&C application, outlining his suspected diagnosis. You connect him with several community organizations that support migrants, which offer him food supports and emergency funds because he cannot work. You connect him to a community health centre so his investigations can be covered. Unfortunately, he is diagnosed with colon cancer and requires surgery and chemotherapy. His counsel will then submit updated medical documentation for his H&C application.
- *Maria*: You help to connect Maria to a midwife for her prenatal, delivery, and postpartum care, which is covered in Ontario regardless of immigration status. You also offer to connect her with a local organization that supports survivors of sexual assault and intimate partner violence and is sensitive to the needs of migrants, which includes free legal counsel. One pathway to permanent residence that could be available to Maria is the Temporary Resident Permit for Victims of Family Violence;[110] another could be an application for restoration of Maria's study permit. A six-month

TRP would give Maria access to discretionary IFHP and the ability to apply for a work permit. After a certain period of time, TRP holders can become eligible to apply for PR. In short, there could be options for Maria to regularize her status; connecting her to a skilled advocate is key.

- *Elias*: After being turned away from the other walk-in clinic, Elias feels humiliated and excluded and withdraws further. However, one of his shelter workers learns of the situation and calls your clinic. You are registered with IFHP, and your clerical staff are well acquainted with the IFHP documentation and billing process. You schedule an appointment for him the following week. Elias's symptoms are consistent with posttraumatic stress disorder, and you offer to refer him to an IFHP-covered psychotherapist for counselling. During your physical exam, you also note several scars, which he explains were caused by knife wounds when he was attacked in his country of origin. At his request, you contact his refugee lawyer and obtain further details to write a strong medical report for his refugee hearing, detailing both his physical scars and his mental health symptoms, including memory impairments that may affect his ability to testify. You book close follow-up with Elias and continue to support him with comprehensive primary care, including mental health care. You help to connect him with several community organizations serving LGBTQ2S+ newcomers, where he soon finds new friends and a roommate. Nine months later, his claim is accepted, and you note a marked improvement in his mood as he gains a deeper sense of safety and security.

Health Care Providers and Positive Systemic Advocacy for Migrants

Power to the people, no one is illegal!!
We didn't cross the border, the border crossed us![111]

These chants can be heard ringing out during migrant justice demonstrations in cities and towns from coast to coast, challenging the ways in which state-mandated borders create illegality.

Migrant justice organizing, led by migrants themselves, is part of a long history of struggle, with deep connections between anti-colonial, anti-capitalist, Indigenous sovereignty, and anti-poverty organizing. Health providers engage in migrant justice organizing and systemic advocacy with and alongside migrants in many ways, including through demonstrations, direct action, research, writing, community allyship, and other solidarity work.

Starting in 2001, the first chapter of NOII was formed in Montreal,[112(p. 98)] followed by the creation of NOII groups across Canada. NOII is both "an ideological framework to counter border imperialism" and "an extended network of grassroots migrant justice groups without any overarching centralization."[113(p. 98)] Justicia for Migrant Workers, Migrant Workers Alliance for Change, the End Immigration Detention Network, and many more organizations have fought and continue to fight for migrant rights.

Through decades of advocacy efforts and grassroots organizing,[114(p. 76)] some cities across Canada have adopted "don't ask, don't tell" policies, including Toronto, Hamilton, Vancouver, Ajax, Montreal, Edmonton, and London. These policies are intended to ensure the provision of services irrespective of immigration status and are supposed to limit municipal cooperation and interaction with immigration authorities.[115] However, these policies generally offer access only to municipal services, and there are often discrepancies between policy and practice; in many cases, access without fear is not implemented.

Because of the differences on the ground and variable policy environments across provinces and municipalities, health-specific migrant justice organizing has evolved to meet local needs.

In Toronto in 2009, arising from a request by NOII-Toronto, the group Health for All formed, calling for access to health services without fear of debt, denial of service, detention, or deportation; universal health coverage for all people in Canada, and regularization of status for all people in Canada, solely on the basis of their being human. This was followed, in 2016, by the launch of the Ontario-based OHIP (Ontario Health Insurance Plan) for All campaign, calling for access to provincially covered health care for all people across the province. In addition, direct clinical care for people without status in Ontario has been provided by many individuals and organizations over the years: Community Health Centres are able to provide care to a limited number of uninsured people; midwives have fought for and won the ability to provide care to people who are uninsured; and, since 1999, volunteer care has been provided through what is now known as the Canadian Centre for Refugee and Immigrant Health Care in Scarborough. Additionally, for the past 16 years, the Health Network for Uninsured Clients (https://www.hnuc.org) has been advocating for improved access to care for people without OHIP across the Greater Toronto Area.

In British Columbia, Sanctuary Health has been actively advocating for the creation of referral networks for people without status and advocating for access to care. They describe themselves as "a grassroots community group. We deploy direct action, movement-building, community-engagement, and direct support strategies to advocate for access to services for all regardless of immigration status or documentation. We are committed to building cross-sectoral alliances of mutual support to advance the migrant-justice movement on unceded Coast Salish territories."[116]

On the national level, in response to draconian cuts to refugee health care in 2012, a successful cross-country campaign, Canadian Doctors for Refugee Care, fought for the full reinstatement of the IFHP.[117]

Health providers have also been active in calling for an end to immigration detention, amplifying the calls put forward by detained migrants, community organizations, and human rights organizations. Advocacy has included open letters[118] and demonstrations, supported by information gathered through research[119] and news articles.

The COVID-19 pandemic has also led to positive improvements in access to care, following years of community-based advocacy, although significant provincial variability has resulted in unequal access to care. During the pandemic, migrants were disproportionately affected, from early difficulties accessing testing, to inhumane labour conditions resulting in rapid spread of the virus and deaths of agricultural and factory workers, to difficulties accessing vaccines, and to lack of paid sick days, highlighting the dire need for access to care.

In Ontario, at the start of the COVID-19 pandemic in March 2020, the government issued a directive (OHIP Bulletin 4749) allowing individuals access to covered medically necessary care regardless of their insurance status, with all hospital-based care covered and three billing codes for use by community providers.[120] Despite this expanded coverage, many hospitals and providers remained unaware of its existence, and providers seeing uninsured patients still had to advocate to have their patients seen. In March 2023, the provincial government abruptly cancelled the program. At the time of writing, various groups are advocating to reverse these cuts and to establish permanent health care coverage for uninsured people living and working in Ontario.

Conclusion

Health providers have an important role to play in ensuring that all migrants have access to health care. This can occur through direct care provision, through creating clinical spaces that are welcoming and safe, through individual-level advocacy by writing letters and reports, and through system advocacy in allyship with directly affected migrant communities.

NOTES

1 Gagnon M, Kansal N, Goel R, et al. Immigration status as the foundational determinant of health for people without status in Canada: a scoping review. J Immigr Minor Health. 2021 October; 24(4): 1029–44. https://doi.org/10.1007/s10903-021-01273-w.

2 Walia H. Border and rule: global migration, capitalism, and the rise of racist nationalism. Halifax: Fernwood Publishing; 2021.

3 Walia H. Border and rule: global migration, capitalism, and the rise of racist nationalism. Halifax: Fernwood Publishing; 2021.

4 Keung N. Nanny spared deportation with reprieve from immigration minister [Internet]. Toronto Star; 2017 July 12. Available from: https://www.thestar.com/news/immigration/2014/08/22/nanny_spared _deportation_with_reprieve_from_immigration_minister.html.

5 *Immigration and Refugee Protection Act*, SC 2001, c 27.

6 *Citizenship Act*, RSC, 1985, c C-29.

7 Canadian Labour Congress. Sanctuary cities [Internet]. Ottawa: Canadian Labour Congress, n.d. [cited 2023 Apr 8]. Available from: https://canadianlabour.ca/uncategorized/sanctuary-cities/.

8 Macklin A. And just like that, you're an illegal immigrant [Internet]. National Post; 2015 Mar 19. Available from: https://nationalpost.com /opinion/audrey-macklin-poof-now-youre-an-illegal-immigrant.

9 Nyers P. The regularization of non-status immigrants in Canada: limits and prospects. Can Rev Social Policy. 2005; (55):109–14.

10 Lupick T. Metro Vancouver hospitals refer hundreds of immigration cases to border control [Internet]. The Georgia Straight; 2015 Dec 9. Available from: https://www.straight.com/news/593441/metro-vancouver -hospitals-refer-hundreds-immigration-cases-border-police.

11 Amnesty International. Canada: stop incarcerating immigration detainees in provincial jails [Internet]. London: Amnesty International; 2021 October 15. Available from: https://www.amnesty.org/en/latest/news/2021/10 /canada-stop-incarcerating-immigration-detainees-provincial-jails/.

12 Human Rights Watch. Canada: abuse, discrimination in immigration detention [Internet]. New York: Human Rights Watch; 2021 June 17. Available from: https://www.hrw.org/news/2021/06/17/canada-abuse -discrimination-immigration-detention.

13 Note we use the terms *lawyer* and *advocate* interchangeably throughout this chapter for a reason. Having a skilled lawyer who can challenge unfair or incorrect immigration decisions in court (and who can therefore set up the first-instance application to meet legal tests) is always preferable. For example, we know that having a lawyer makes a refugee claimant 275 per cent more likely to be accepted (see Rehaag S. The role of counsel

in Canada's refugee determinations system: an empirical assessment. Osgoode Hall Law J [Internet]. 2011;49[1]. Available from: https://digitalcommons.osgoode.yorku.ca/ohlj/vol49/iss1/3). However, in many communities across Canada, there is a dearth of immigration and refugee lawyers, and the practical reality is that others, such as settlement workers, often play the role of advocate.

14 United Nations. Convention relating to the status of refugees (adopted 1951 July 28, entered into force 1954 Apr 22). Treaty Series, vol. 189, p. 137 [cited 2023 Jan 31]. Available from: https://www.refworld.org/docid/3be01b964.html.

15 Colaiacovo I. Not just the facts: adjudicator bias and decisions of the Immigration and Refugee Board of Canada (2006–2011). J Migr Hum Secur. 2013;1(4):122–47. https://doi.org/10.1177/233150241300100401.

16 Flecker K. The truth about Canada's Temporary Foreign Worker Program [Internet]. Winnipeg: Manitoba Federation of Labour; 2013 Jan 17. Available from: https://mfl.ca/the-truth-about-canadas-temporary-foreign-worker-program/.

17 Walia H. Border & rule: global migration, capitalism, and the rise of racist nationalism. Halifax: Fernwood Publishing; 2021.

18 Walia H. Border & rule: global migration, capitalism, and the rise of racist nationalism. Halifax: Fernwood Publishing; 2021.

19 See Employment and Social Development Canada. Hire a temporary worker through the seasonal agricultural worker program: overview [Internet]. Ottawa: Employment and Social Development Canada; 2022 [modified 2024 Oct 2]. Available from: https://www.canada.ca/en/employment-social-development/services/foreign-workers/agricultural/seasonal-agricultural.html.

20 UFCW Canada. More workers arrested in another immigration raid in SW Ontario [Internet]. Toronto: UFCW Canada; 2009 June 25. Available from: https://www.ufcw.ca/index.php?option=com_content&view=article&id=651&Itemid=6&lang=en.

21 Migrant Workers Alliance for Change. Decent & dignified housing for migrant farmworkers [Internet]. Toronto: The Alliance; 2020 [cited 2020 Apr 24]. Available from: https://migrantworkersalliance.org/wp-content/uploads/2020/12/MRN-Submission_-Decent-Dignified-Housing-for-Migrant-Farmworkers.pdf.

22 See Otero G, Preibisch K. Citizenship and precarious labour in Canadian agriculture. Vancouver: Canadian Centre for Policy Alternatives; 2015.

23 See Tasker JP. In scathing report, auditor general says feds failed to protect foreign farm workers from the pandemic [Internet]. CBC News, 2021 Dec 9. Available from: https://www.cbc.ca/news/politics/ag-foreign-farm-workers-pandemic-1.6279572; Office of the Auditor General of Canada.

Health and safety of agricultural temporary foreign workers in Canada during the COVID-19 pandemic. Ottawa: Office of the Auditor General of Canada; 2021.

24 Hennebry JL, Williams G. Making vulnerability visible: medical repatriation and Canada's migrant agricultural workers. CMAJ. 2015 Apr;187(6):391-2. https://doi.org/10.1503/cmaj.141189.

25 Orkin AM, Lay M, McLaughlin J, et al. Medical repatriation of migrant farm workers in Ontario: a descriptive analysis. CMAJ Open. 2014;2(3):E192–8. https://doi.org/10.9778/cmajo.20140014.

26 See Galerand E, Gallié M, Ollivier-Gobeil J. Domestic labour and exploitation: the case of the Live-In Caregiver Program in Canada (LCP) [Internet]. Montreal: McGill University, Labour Law and Development Research Laboratory; 2015 January. Available from: https://www.mcgill .ca/lldrl/files/lldrl/15.01.09_rapport_en_vu1.1.13.pdf.

27 Immigration, Refugees and Citizenship Canada. Comprehensive Ranking System (CRS) tool: skilled immigrants (Express Entry) [Internet]. Ottawa: Government of Canada; 2022 [modified 2024 Feb 27]. Available from: https://www.cic.gc.ca/english/immigrate/skilled/crs-tool.asp.

28 Triandafyllidou A, Nalbandian L. Can the COVID-19 crisis be an opportunity for Canada's migrant farmworkers? [Internet]. openDemocracy; 2020 Aug 5. Available from: https://www.opendemocracy.net/en /pandemic-border/can-the-Covid-19-crisis-be-an-opportunity-for-canadas -migrant-farmworkers/.

29 *Immigration and Refugee Protection Act*, SC 2001, ss 108–109. Note that the automatic loss of permanent residence flowing from a former refugee's re-availment of the protection of their home country is currently being challenged in Federal Court on *Charter* grounds. See *Gnanapragasam v Canada (IRCC)*, Federal Court File No. IMM-8433-22.

30 See Immigration, Refugees and Citizenship Canada. Medical inadmissibility [Internet]. Ottawa: Government of Canada; 2022 Jan 4 [modified 2024 Jan 8]. Available from: https://www.canada.ca /en/immigration-refugees-citizenship/services/immigrate-canada /inadmissibility/reasons/medical-inadmissibility.html.

31 For approximate sponsorship wait times, see Government of Canada. Family sponsorship [Internet]. Government of Canada; 2022 [last modified 2024 Nov 18]. Available from: https://eservices.cic.gc.ca/epay/order .do?category=15.

32 Canadian Council for Refugees. Family reunification: practical guide [Internet]. Montreal: Canadian Council for Refugees; 2015 [cited 2023 Apr 8]. Available from: https://ccrweb.ca/files/frguide.pdf.

33 This rule was challenged unsuccessfully in a Supreme Court of Canada decision called *Canada (Attorney General) v Mavi*, 2011 SCC 30.

34 *Hilewitz v Canada (Minister of Citizenship and Immigration)*, 2005 SCC 57.

35 The Social Rights Advocacy Centre posts any developments relating to *Toussaint v. Canada* on its website: https://www.socialrights.ca/Toussaint.html.

36 Toussaint v. Attorney General of Canada, 2024 ONSC 69.

37 Dauvergne C. How the Charter has failed non-citizens in Canada. McGill Law J. 2013;58:3.

38 Sultana A. Citizenship and health: what role can citizenship play in the social determinants of health? [Internet]. Toronto: Wellesley Institute; 2017. Available from: https://www.wellesleyinstitute.com/publications/citizenship-and-health/.

39 Immigration, Refugees and Citizenship Canada. Language classes funded by the Government of Canada. Immigration, Refugees and Citizenship Canada; 2018 May 30 [modified 2024 May 15]. Available from: https://www.canada.ca/en/immigration-refugees-citizenship/services/new-immigrants/new-life-canada/improve-english-french/classes.html.

40 *Citizenship Act*, s 5(1)(d); *Citizenship Regulations*, SOR/93-246, s 14.

41 Bill C-24, *An Act to amend the Citizenship Act and to make consequential amendments to other Acts*, 2nd Sess, 41st Parl, 2014 (assented to 19 June 2014); later amended by Bill C-6, *An Act to amend the Citizenship Act and to make consequential amendments to another Act*, 1st Sess, 42nd Parl, 2017 (assented to 19 June 2017).

42 Nakache D, Stone J, Winter E. Aiming at civic integration? How Canada's naturalization rules are sidelining refugees and family class immigrants [Internet]. Rev Eur Migr Int. 2020 [cited 2024 Jan 8];36(24):77–97. Available from: https://journals.openedition.org/remi/17205?lang=en.

43 Gagnon M, Kansal N, Goel R, et al., "Immigration Status as the Foundational Determinant of Health for People Without Status in Canada: A Scoping Review," *Journal of Immigrant and Minority Health*, 2022;24:1029–44. https://doi.org/10.1007/s10903-021-01273-w.

44 Chen BYY. 2021. Protecting refugees' health: how is the reinstated interim federal health program working? Ottawa: Pathways to Prosperity.

45 Immigration, Refugees and Citizenship Canada. Interim federal health program: what is covered [Internet]. Ottawa: Immigration, Refugees and Citizenship Canada; 2022 Apr 28 [modified 2024 Aug 13]. Available from: https://www.canada.ca/en/immigration-refugees-citizenship/services/refugees/help-within-canada/health-care/interim-federal-health-program/coverage-summary.html.

46 The provinces vary, but many have recommendations or even requirements for principles that must be complied with in charging for uninsured services, sometimes including suggested rates; see, for example, Alberta (College of Physicians & Surgeons of Alberta. Charging

for uninsured professional services [Internet]. Edmonton: College of Physicians & Surgeons of Alberta; 2014 Sep 9. Available from: https://cpsa.ca/physicians/standards-of-practice/charging-for-uninsured-professional-services/); Ontario (Ontario Medical Association. Physician's guide to uninsured services: a guide for Ontario physicians [Internet]. Toronto: The Association; 2019 Jan. Available from: https://swpca.ca/Uploads/ContentDocuments/2019-Physicians-Guide-to-Uninsured-Services-10Jan19%20(004).pdf); and Nova Scotia (Doctors Nova Scotia. Non-insured services [Internet]. Dartmouth [NS]: Doctors Nova Scotia; n.d. Available from: https://doctorsns.com/contract-and-support/non-insured-services).

47 Garasia S. Clinical outcomes and healthcare use in provincially medically uninsured populations in Canada: a descriptive systematic review [Internet]. Hamilton (ON): Centre for Health Economics and Policy Analysis, 2019 February 4. Available from: https://chepa.mcmaster.ca/wp-content/uploads/2022/12/19-01-clinical-outcomes-and-healthcare-use-in-provincially-medically-uninsured-populations-in-canada-a-descriptive-systematic-review.pdf.

48 Hynie M, Ardern CI, Robertson A. Emergency room visits by uninsured child and adult residents in Ontario, Canada: what diagnoses, severity and visit disposition reveal about the impact of being uninsured. J Immigr Minor Health. 2016;18(5):948–56. https://doi.org/10.1007/s10903-016-0351-0.

49 In Alberta you can get midwifery care without Alberta Health Care coverage (Lucina Midwives. Can I get midwifery care if I don't have Alberta Health Care coverage? [Internet]. Edmonton: Lucina Midwives; n.d. Available from: https://lucinamidwives.ca/midwives/faqs/), but there is a billing cap on each individual midwife, limiting how much care each can give per year (Mack E. Midwifery care in Alberta highly sought after, although rural communities face shortages [Internet]. Calgary Journal; 2022 June 30. Available from: https://calgaryjournal.ca/2022/06/30/midwifery-care-in-alberta-highly-sought-after-although-rural-communities-face-shortages/). Everywhere else seems to need provincial health plan coverage or has no midwife registry.

50 Ontario Women's Justice Network. What does mandatory charging mean? [Internet]. Toronto: Ontario Women's Justice Network; 2023. Available from: http://owjn.org/2016/01/what-does-mandatory-charging-mean/.

51 Tabibi J, Ahmad S, Baker L, et al. Intimate partner violence against immigrant and refugee women [Internet]. London (ON): Centre for Research & Education on Violence Against Women & Children; 2018. Available from: https://www.vawlearningnetwork.ca/our-work/issuebased_newsletters/issue-26/Plain-Text-Issue-26.pdf.

52 Mattoo D. Race, gendered violence, and the rights of women with precarious immigration status [Internet]. Toronto: Barbra Schlifer Commemorative Clinic; 2017. Available from: https://schliferclinic.com/wp-content/uploads/2018/03/Race-Gendered-Violence-and-the-Rights-of-Women-with-Precarious-Immgration-Status.pdf.

53 Bhuyan R, Osborne B, Zahraei S, et al. Unprotected, unrecognized Canadian immigration policy and violence against women, 2008–2013. Toronto: University of Toronto; 2014.

54 Bhuyan R, Osborne B, Zahraei S, et al. Unprotected, unrecognized Canadian immigration policy and violence against women, 2008–2013. Toronto: University of Toronto; 2014.

55 City of Toronto. City of Toronto launches new "Toronto For All" campaign to support undocumented residents [Internet]. Toronto: City of Toronto, 2021 Aug 24. Available from: https://www.toronto.ca/news/city-of-toronto-launches-new-toronto-for-all-campaign-to-support-undocumented-residents/.

56 Carolino B. Refugee lawyers say Toronto police have no legal duty to inquire into immigration status. Canadian Lawyer; 2020 Aug 28. Available from: https://www.canadianlawyermag.com/practice-areas/immigration/refugee-lawyers-say-toronto-police-have-no-legal-duty-to-inquire-into-immigration-status/332824.

57 Moffette D. Often asking, always telling: the Toronto Police Service and the sanctuary city policy. Toronto: No One Is Illegal; 2015; Hudson G, Atak I, Manocchi M, et al. (No) access T.O.: a pilot study on sanctuary city policy in Toronto, Canada. Toronto: Ryerson Centre for Immigration and Settlement; 2017 [cited 2023 Apr 8]. RCIS Working Paper No. 2017/1. Available from: https://ssrn.com/abstract=2897016.

58 Deshman A. To serve some and protect fewer: the Toronto Police Services' policy on non-status victims and witnesses of crimes. J Law Soc Policy. 2009;22(1):209–35. https://doi.org/10.60082/0829-3929.1007.

59 Government of Canada. Language classes funded by the Government of Canada [Internet]. Ottawa: Government of Canada; 2024 May 15. Available from: https://www.canada.ca/en/immigration-refugees-citizenship/services/new-immigrants/new-life-canada/improve-english-french/classes.html.

60 Government of Ontario. Adult learning: English as a second language [Internet]. Ottawa: Government of Ontario; 2019 Aug 29 [updated 2024 Apr 3]. Available from: https://www.ontario.ca/page/adult-learning-english-second-language.

61 Kalvapalle R. Canadian children being held as "guests" in immigration detention centres: report [Internet]. Global News; 2017 Feb 23. Available from: https://globalnews.ca/news/3269654/canadian-children-immigration-detention-centres-report/.

62 CBC News. Toronto school board pushes "don't ask, don't tell" policy on immigration status. CBC News; 2007 May 3. Available from: https://www .cbc.ca/news/canada/toronto/toronto-school-board-pushes-don-t-ask -don-t-tell-policy-on-immigration-status-1.633747.

63 *Education Act of Ontario*, RSO 1990, c E2.

64 *Education Act*, s 21(1)(a): "every person who attains the age of six years on or before the first school day in September in any year shall attend an elementary or secondary school on every school day from the first school day in September in that year until the person attains the age of 18 years."

65 Law Union of Ontario. TDSB finally delivers on its promise of a don't ask don't tell policy [Internet]. Toronto: Law Union of Ontario; 2007 May 18. Available from: https://www.lawunion.ca/2007/tdsb-finally-delivers-on -its-promise-of-a-dont-ask-dont-tell-policy/.

66 See Wiens M. York first Canadian university to give "Dreamers" a chance at a degree. CBC News, 2018 Jan 16. Available from: https://www.cbc.ca /news/canada/toronto/canadian-dreamers-york-university-1.4488252.

67 Bruser D. She's one of Canada's dreamers. They said she had "limitless" potential. But now her future is on hold [Internet]. Toronto Star; 2020 July 25. Available from: https://www.thestar.com/news /investigations/2020/07/25/shes-one-of-canadas-dreamers-they-said-she -had-limitless-potential-but-now-her-future-is-on-hold.html#:~:text=At%20 U%20of%20T%2C%20tuition,due%20to%20lack%20of%20money.

68 Government of Canada. Financial assistance for protected persons [Internet]. Ottawa: Government of Canada; 2019 July 17. Available from: https://www.canada.ca/en/services/benefits/education/student-aid /protected-persons.html.

69 See Immigration, Refugees and Citizenship Canada. CIMM – undocumented populations – March 3, 2022 [Internet]. Ottawa: Immigration, Refugees and Citizenship Canada; 2022 Mar 3 [updated 2022 June 15. Available from: https://www.canada.ca/en/immigration -refugees-citizenship/corporate/transparency/committees/cimm -mar-03-2022/undocumented-populations.html; Tomlinson K. False promises: foreign workers are falling prey to a sprawling web of labour trafficking in Canada [Internet]. Globe and Mail; 2019 Apr 6. Available from: https://www.theglobeandmail.com/canada/article-false-promises -how-foreign-workers-fall-prey-to-bait-and-switch/.

70 See Canada Border Services Agency. Removal from Canada. Ottawa: Canada Border Services Agency; 2022 Feb 24 [modified 2024 Sep 27]. Available from: https://www.cbsa-asfc.gc.ca/security-securite/rem-ren -eng.html. At the time of writing, CBSA is not deporting individuals to Iraq, Afghanistan, Democratic Republic of Congo, certain regions in Somalia (Middle Shabelle, Afgoye, and Mogadishu), the Gaza Strip,

Ukraine, Syria, Mali, the Central African Republic, South Sudan, Libya, Yemen, Burundi, Venezuela, and Haiti.

71 Access Alliance Multicultural Community Health Centre. Racialised groups and health status: a literature review exploring poverty, housing, race-based discrimination and access to health care as determinants of health for racialized groups. Toronto: The Centre; 2005.

72 See City of Toronto. Acceptable documentation of Canadian status [Internet]. Toronto: City of Toronto; n.d. [cited 2023 Apr 9]. Available from: https://www.toronto.ca/community-people/employment-social -support/housing-support/rent-geared-to-income-subsidy/acceptable-id/.

73 Schizophrenia Society of Ontario. Double jeopardy: deportation of the criminalized mentally ill. Toronto: Schizophrenia Society of Ontario; 2010; Bernhard JK, Goldring L, Young J, et al. Living with precarious legal status in Canada: implications for the well-being of children and families. Refuge. 2007;24(2):101–14 https://doi.org/10.25071/1920-7336.21388.

74 "The fundamental rights to liberty and security of person and freedom of movement are expressed in all the major international and regional human rights instruments, and are essential components of legal systems built on the rule of law … These rights apply in principle to all human beings, regardless of their immigration, refugee, asylum-seeker or other status. In accordance with these principles, the detention of asylum-seekers 'should be a measure of last resort' and the detention of other migrants must be exceptional and scrupulously justified" (UN Refugee Agency. Guidelines on the applicable criteria and standards relating to the detention of asylum-seekers and alternatives to detention. Geneva: The Agency; 2012).

75 The prohibition of arbitrary detention presupposes that immigration detention must only ever be used as a last resort. The Working Group on Arbitrary Detention has reiterated regarding deprivation of liberty of migrants that "any form of administrative detention or custody in the context of migration must be applied as an exceptional measure of last resort, for the shortest period and only if justified by a legitimate purpose, such as documenting entry and recording claims or initial verification of identity if in doubt" (UN Working Group on Arbitrary Detention. Revised deliberation no. 5 on deprivation of liberty of migrants. Geneva: UN Human Rights Council; 2018).

76 See Human Rights Watch. Legal analysis of agreements allowing immigration detention in Canadian provincial jails [Internet]. New York: Human Rights Watch; 2022. Available from: https://www.hrw.org /news/2022/04/04/legal-analysis-agreements-allowing-immigration -detention-canadian-provincial-jails.

77 Human Rights Watch. Canada: abuse, discrimination in immigration detention [Internet]. New York: Human Rights Watch; 2021. Available

from: https://www.hrw.org/news/2021/06/17/canada-abuse
-discrimination-immigration-detention.

78 *Immigration and Refugee Protection Act*, SC 2001, s 57.

79 Immigration and Refugee Board of Canada. Report of the 2017/2018 external
audit (detention review) [Internet]. Ottawa: Immigration and Refugee Board of
Canada; 2018. Available from: https://irb-cisr.gc.ca/en/transparency
/reviews-audit-evaluations/Pages/ID-external-audit-1718.aspx. Note that the
Immigration Division has taken active steps to reform in response to this report.

80 Human Rights Watch. Joint Submission to the Committee on the Rights of
the Child's review of Canada [Internet]. Human Rights Watch; 2020 Mar 4.
Available from: https://www.hrw.org/news/2020/03/04/joint
-submission-committee-rights-childs-review-canada.

81 Bureau B. CBSA backtracks on commitment to track all children separated
from a parent [Internet]. CBC News; 2022 June 17. Available from: https://
www.cbc.ca/news/canada/ottawa/ottawa-cbsa-backtracks-pledge-to
-track-number-1.6489901.

82 Gros H, Muscati S. Death of immigration detainee an urgent wake-up
call for Canada [Internet]. New York: Human Rights Watch; 2022 Feb 4.
Available from: https://www.hrw.org/news/2022/02/04/death
-immigration-detainee-urgent-wake-call-canada#:~:text=What%20we%20
do%20know%20is,detention%2C%20most%20in%20provincial%20jail s.

83 Bill C-20, which establishes an independent complaints and oversight
body for CBSA, received royal assent on 31 October 2024 (Bill C-20, *An
act establishing the Public Complaints and Review Commission and amending
certain acts and statutory instruments*, 1st Sess, 44th Parl, 2021. Available
from: https://www.parl.ca/LegisInfo/en/bill/44-1/c-20).

84 Human Rights Watch. Canada: British Columbia to end immigration
detention in jails [Internet]. New York: Human Rights Watch; 2022.
Available from: https://www.hrw.org/news/2022/07/21/canada-british
-columbia-end-immigration-detention-jails.

85 As an example of how a criminal charge can be life-altering, consider this
real-life example. A migrant worker, previously under the SAWP and
then issued a temporary resident permit (TRP) after being found to be a
victim of human trafficking for labour exploitation (giving him a pathway
to PR under the Permit Holder Class), was then in a fight and in self-
defence injured his attacker. He was charged but ultimately not convicted.
However, although the criminal case was cleared, he was detained for
a few weeks in jail, and during this time his TRP expired. A subsequent
TRP was approved, but it came with a note about the criminal charge and
potential inadmissibility. He is no longer eligible under the Permit Holder
Class for PR. Although this can be legally challenged, it will create undue
delay and difficulty for this individual's status in Canada.

86 Substance Abuse and Mental Health Services Administration. SAMHSA's concept of trauma and guidance for a trauma-informed approach. Rockville (MD): Substance Abuse and Mental Health Services Administration; 2014.

87 Laher N, Sultana A, Aery A, et al. Access to language interpretation services and its impact on clinical and patient outcomes: a scoping review [Internet]. Toronto: Wellesley Institute; 2018. Available from: https://www.wellesleyinstitute.com/wp-content/uploads/2018/04/Language-Interpretation-Services-Scoping-Review.pdf.

88 Sultana A, Aery A, Kumar N, et al. Language interpretation services in health care settings in the GTA [Internet]. Toronto: Wellesley Institute; 2018. Available from: https://www.wellesleyinstitute.com/wp-content/uploads/2018/04/Language-Interpretation-Services-in-the-GTA.pdf.

89 Royal Children's Hospital Melbourne. Working with interpreters [Internet]. Parkville (VIC): Royal Children's Hospital Melbourne; n.d. Available from: https://www.rch.org.au/immigranthealth/clinical/Working_with_interpreters/; Migrant & Refugee Health Partnership. Guide for clinicians working with interpreters in healthcare settings [Internet]. Kingston (ACT): Migrant & Refugee Health Partnership; 2019. Available from: https://culturaldiversityhealth.org.au/wp-content/uploads/2019/10/Guide-for-clinicians-working-with-interpreters-in-healthcare-settings-Jan2019.pdf.

90 211. About 211 [Internet]. Ottawa: 211; n.d. [cited 2023 Apr 9]. Available from: https://211.ca/about-211/.

91 Rehaag S. The role of counsel in Canada's refugee determinations system: an empirical assessment. Osgoode Hall Law J. 2011;49(1): 71–116. Available from: https://doi.org/10.60082/2817-5069.1073.

92 Smith CD, Rehaag S, Farrow TCQ. Access to justice for refugees: how legal aid and quality of counsel impact fairness and efficiency in Canada's asylum system [Internet]. Toronto: Canada Excellence Research Chair in Migration and Integration, Centre for Refugee Studies, Canadian Forum on Civil Justice; 2021. https://www.torontomu.ca/cerc-migration/Research/projectbriefs/A2J_Refugee_Claimaints_Dec_2021.pdf.

93 Sunderji N, Powles K, Tau M, et al. Understanding the complexity of treatment of mental illness and addictions in Ontario [Internet]. Toronto: Department of Psychiatry and Department of Family and Community Medicine, University of Toronto; 2017 [cited 2023 Apr 8]. Available from: https://incomesecurity.org/wp-content/uploads/2020/04/Understanding-the-complexity-of-treatment-of-mental-illness-and-addictions-in-Ontario-w-2-headers-updated-May-2018-_2.pdf.

94 Refugee hearing preparation: a guide for refugee claimants [Internet]. Vancouver (BC): Kinbrace Community Society [cited 2023 Apr 9]. Available from: https://kinbrace.ca/wp-content/uploads/2014/06/RHP-Vancouver-%E2%80%93-English-150.pdf .

95 Immigration and Refugee Board of Canada. Chairperson guideline 8: procedures with respect to vulnerable persons appearing before the IRB [Internet]. Ottawa: The Board; 2012. Available from: https://irb.gc.ca /en/legal-policy/policies/Pages/GuideDir08.aspx#a4.

96 Immigration and Refugee Board of Canada. Chairperson Guideline 8: procedures with respect to vulnerable persons appearing before the IRB [Internet]. Ottawa: The Board; 2012. Available from: https://irb.gc.ca /en/legal-policy/policies/Pages/GuideDir08.aspx#a4.

97 Immigration and Refugee Board of Canada. Backlog and wait times (refugee claims and appeals [Internet]. Ottawa: The Board; 2021 Sep 9. Available from: https://www.irb-cisr.gc.ca/en/transparency/pac -binder-nov-2020/Pages/pac8.aspx#:~:text=Projected%20wait%20 times%20are%20approximately,12%20months%20for%20refugee%20appeals.

98 Canadian Council for Refugees. Processing times for family reunification have reached absurd new lengths [Internet]. Montreal: Canadian Council for Refugees; 2021 June 17. Available from: https://ccrweb.ca/en /processing-times-family-reunification-39-months.

99 Hvidtfeldt C, Petersen JH, Norredam M. Waiting for family reunification and the risk of mental disorders among refugee fathers: A 24-year longitudinal cohort study from Denmark. Soc Psychiatr Psychiatr Epidemiol 2022;57:1061–72. https://doi.org/10.1007/s00127-021-02170-1.

100 Löbel L-M, Jacobsen J. Waiting for kin: a longitudinal study of family reunification and refugee mental health in Germany. J Ethn Migr Stud. 2021;47(13):2916–37 https://doi.org/10.1080/1369183X.2021.1884538.

101 Section 11.3, relating to children at risk, of Immigration, Refugees and Citizenship Canada (IRCC). Overseas processing of family members of in-Canada applicants for permanent residence [Internet]. Ottawa: IRCC; 2021. Available from: https://www.canada.ca/en/immigration-refugees -citizenship/corporate/publications-manuals/operational-bulletins -manuals/permanent-residence/non-economic-classes/overseas-family -members.htm; Immigration, Refugees and Citizenship Canada (IRCC). Temporary resident permits [Internet]. Ottawa: IRCC; 2024. Available from: https://www.canada.ca/en/immigration-refugees-citizenship /corporate/publications-manuals/operational-bulletins-manuals /temporary-residents/permits.html; Canadian Council for Refugees. Family reunification: practical guide [Internet]. Montreal: Canadian Council for Refugees; 2015 [cited 2023 Apr 8]. Available from: https:// ccrweb.ca/files/frguide.pdf.

102 Unfortunately, IRCC's full IP-5 Manual has been taken offline by IRCC. It has been replaced with this reference: Immigration, Refugees and Citizenship Canada. Humanitarian and compassionate consideration [Internet]. Ottawa: Immigration, Refugees and Citizenship Canada; 2014.

Available from: https://www.canada.ca/en/immigration-refugees
-citizenship/corporate/publications-manuals/operational-bulletins
-manuals/permanent-residence/humanitarian-compassionate
-consideration.html.

103 See Community Legal Education Ontario (CLEO). Making a
humanitarian and compassionate (H&C) application [Internet].
Toronto: CLEO; 2019. Available from: https://www.cleo.on.ca/en
/publications/handc; Barbra Schlifer Commemorative Clinic. Gathering
evidence for humanitarian and compassionate (H&C) applications: a
toolkit for advocates supporting women survivors [Internet]. Toronto:
Barbra Schlifer Commemorative Clinic; 2018. Available from:
https://schliferclinic.com/wp-content/uploads/2018/05/HC
-Toolkit-2018-Update.pdf; and Barbra Schlifer Commemorative Clinic.
H&C assessment or support letter checklist – health professionals
and therapists [Internet]. Toronto: Barbra Schlifer Commemorative
Clinic; 2017. Available from: https://refugeeclaims.files.wordpress.
com/2017/08/hc-assessment-or-support-letter-checklist.pdf.

104 The pass rate is now 75 per cent, compared with the previous 60 per cent.

105 *Regulations Amending the Citizenship Regulations*, PC 2014-1453, (1997)
C Gaz II, 3479 (*Citizenship Act*).

106 Tarone E, Bigelow M. Alphabetic print literacy and processing of
oral corrective feedback in L2 interaction. In: Mackey A, editor.
Conversational interaction in second language acquisition. Oxford:
Oxford University Press; 2007; Tarone E, Bigelow M. Alphabetic literacy
and adult SLA. In: Herschensohn J, Young-Scholten M, editors. The
Cambridge handbook of second language acquisition. Cambridge:
Cambridge University Press; 2013.

107 *Tammie Lynn Mayes and Justice for Children and Youth v Minister of
Citizenship and Immigration* (22 January 2019), Ottawa T-797-18 (Can FC).

108 *Citizenship Act*, RSC 1985, c C-29, s 5(3).

109 Gros H. "I didn't feel like a human in there": immigration detention
in Canada and its impact on mental health [Internet]. Toronto: Human
Rights Watch and Amnesty International; 2021. Available from: https://
www.hrw.org/report/2021/06/17/i-didnt-feel-human-there
/immigration-detention-canada-and-its-impact-mental.

110 Immigration, Refugees and Citizenship Canada (IRCC). Temporary
resident permit (TRP) for victims of family violence [Internet]. Ottawa:
IRCC; 2021. Available from: https://www.canada.ca/en/immigration
-refugees-citizenship/corporate/publications-manuals/operational
-bulletins-manuals/temporary-residents/permits/family-violence.html.

111 Fortier C. No one is illegal, Canada is illegal! Negotiating the
relationships between settler colonialism and border imperialism through

political slogans [Internet]. Decolonization: Indigeneity, Education & Society (blog); 2015 Sep 21. Available from: https://decolonization. wordpress.com/2015/09/21/no-one-is-illegal-canada-is-illegal -negotiating-the-relationships-between-settler-colonialism-and-border -imperialism-through-political-slogans/.

112 Walia H. Undoing border imperialism. Chico (CA): AK Press; 2013.

113 Walia H. Undoing border imperialism. Chico (CA): AK Press; 2013.

114 Gardner KS. From sanctuary to abolition: migrant justice organizing in Toronto, Vancouver, Montreal, and Ottawa. PhD [dissertation] [Internet]. Toronto: York University; 2021. Available from: https://yorkspace.library .yorku.ca/xmlui/bitstream/handle/10315/39105/Gardner_Karl_2021 _PhD.pdf?sequence=2&isAllowed=y.

115 Paquet M, Benoit N, Atak I, et al. Sanctuary cities and Covid-19: the case of Canada. In: Triandafyllidou A, editor. Migration and pandemics. Cham, Switzerland: Springer; 2022. p. 85–102. IMISCOE Research Series. https://doi.org/10.1007/978-3-030-81210-2_5.

116 Community victory: refugee claimants' Canadian babies get health care from birth [Internet]. Sanctuary Health (blog); 2024 May 8. Available from: http://sanctuaryhealth.blogspot.com/.

117 *Canadian Doctors for Refugee Care v. Canada (Attorney General)*, 2014 FC 651

118 Beder M, Cohen M, Hui K, et al. End immigration detention: an open letter. Lancet. 2018;392(10145):P381–2. https://doi.org/10.1016/S0140 -6736(18)31567-8.

119 Kronick R, Rousseau C, Cleveland J. Asylum-seeking children's experiences of detention in Canada: a qualitative study. Am J Orthopsychiatry. 2015;85(3):287–94.

120 Ontario Ministry of Health. COVID-19 expanding access to OHIP coverage and funding physician and hospital services for uninsured patients [Internet]. Toronto: Ontario Ministry of Health and Ministry of Long-Term Care; 2020. OHIP Bulletin 4749. Available from: https:// www.ontario.ca/document/ohip-infobulletins-2020/bulletin-4749-covid -19-expanding-access-ohip-coverage-and-funding.

8 Family Law and Health

ANITA VOLIKIS, JAMIE AHN, AND KATHLEEN DOUKAS

Consider the following scenario: Sari and Jason, a married couple living in Toronto, Ontario, have been your patients for the past 10 years. They have recently decided to separate, with a plan for divorce.

Sari has come to the office today to ask you for medication to help her sleep. Since the plan to separate became final, she has been having increasing difficulty with insomnia.

She tells you that she has hired a lawyer to help with the separation but feels anxious about how much it costs. She has not worked in several years because Jason made a salary that they could both live on comfortably.

Most worrying for Sari is the fact that they have two small children, ages 3 and 7. She has been their primary caregiver since giving up working outside of the home. She is not sure how the separation will affect her ability to parent the children.

She is tearful and looks to you for guidance.

When patients are experiencing separation or divorce, the repercussions in their lives can be far reaching and serious. Beyond the emotional turmoil that often accompanies the end of a relationship, separating spouses such as Sari and Jason must confront difficult questions, such as "Who will take care of the children?" "Where will I live?" and "Will I have to pay support?" Combine this with the fact that answering these questions often involves navigating costly, complex, and slow-moving family law systems, and patients may quickly feel overwhelmed and turn to their health care providers for guidance and support, just as Sari has done in the preceding scenario.

This chapter is intended to inform health care providers about four overarching topics that can help guide their discussions with separating patients: first, a brief introduction to family law; second, the relationship between family law issues and health; third, the most common legal issues affecting patients; and fourth, resources that health care providers can direct patients to for further assistance. Sari and Jason's scenario is used throughout the chapter to illustrate how health care providers can provide support to their patients as they navigate various legal issues.

A Family Law Primer

Family law refers to the legal system that governs relationships between spouses and between parents and their children.[1] It deals with issues such as marriage, cohabitation, divorce, separation, decision-making responsibility, parenting time, support, property division, and domestic contracts. These issues are described briefly here, and many are explored in greater depth in the "Common Issues Affecting Patients Navigating a Separation" section of this chapter.

Formation and Dissolution of the Spousal Relationship:
Marriage, Cohabitation, and Separation

Marriage is the lawful union between two persons to the exclusion of all others.[2] To be married in Canada, both partners

- must meet minimum age requirements (18 or 19 years, depending on the province or territory, with exceptions for younger individuals if they have the consent of their parents or legal guardians; children younger than age 16, however, are not allowed to get married anywhere in Canada);[3]
- cannot be too closely related by blood or adoption;[4]
- cannot already be married;
- must consent to being married; and
- must understand what it means to get married.[5]

A marriage that occurs outside of Canada will generally be recognized if it is legal according to the laws of the place where it occurred and if it complies with Canada's federal laws on marriage.[6]

Cohabitation, however, refers to living together in a marriage-like relationship without being married.[7(p. 4)] Cohabiting couples, like married spouses, are afforded certain rights and responsibilities upon the breakdown of the relationship if they meet specific requirements. For example, couples in Ontario will qualify as spouses for the purposes of spousal support under the *Family Law Act* if they have cohabited (a) continuously for a period of three years or more or (b) in a relationship of some permanence if they have a child together.[8]

Separation occurs when partners live apart from each other because the relationship has broken down. A *divorce* is a court order that ends a marriage.[9(p. 6)] If a separated individual wants to remarry, they must obtain a divorce.

Separated couples may choose to address corollary issues such as parenting, child or spousal support, and property division in one of three general ways:

1. via application in court, where a judge will be the decision-maker and issue legally binding orders regarding the issues before them;
2. by using an alternative dispute resolution (ADR) process, such as mediation (in which parties engage a neutral third party to assist them in resolving a dispute)[10(p. 10)] or arbitration (in which a neutral third party renders a binding decision, referred to as an *award*, after conducting a hearing);[11] or
3. via a negotiation between the parties, ideally through their respective lawyers, typically resulting in a resolution of the issues formalized in a separation agreement.

It is important to seek and obtain legal advice promptly after separation because of the limitation periods related to certain claims. For example, in Ontario, a party must commence a court action asserting a claim for equalization of net family property within six years of the date of separation, within two years of a divorce, or within six months of the other spouse's death (whichever of these is sooner).[12]

Parenting after Separation: Decision-Making Responsibility and Parenting Time

Decision-making responsibility (formerly called *custody*) refers to the responsibility assigned to one or more parent that allows them to make significant decisions about a child's life and well-being, such as those relating to health, education, and religion. Decision-making responsibility can be sole (one parent makes important decisions alone), joint (parents consult each other and make decisions together), or divided (one parent is responsible for some decisions, and the other parent is responsible for others).[13]

Parenting time (formerly called *access*) is the time that a child spends in a parent's care, regardless of whether the child is physically with that parent during that time. If, for example, the child is at school for a portion of the day, that time will still be considered as part of parenting time. Parenting time arrangements can be shared (a child lives at least 40 per cent of the time with each parent) or split (parents have more than one child, and each parent has one or more children living with them most of the time).[14] A parent may also have the majority of parenting time, which refers to situations in which a child spends more than 60 per cent of the time with that parent.[15]

The overarching principle when determining decision-making responsibility and parenting time regimes is the best interests of the child.[16] It would not be in the best interests of the child, for example, for a court to grant joint decision-making responsibility to parents who have an antagonistic relationship because this may result in the child being exposed to greater parental conflict, as well as cause delays in important decisions being made. Parenting concepts, as well as the intersection of parenting issues and the duties of health care professionals, are explored further in the "Family Law and Health" and "Common Issues Affecting Patients Navigating a Separation" sections of this chapter.

Income Security after Separation: Support

The financial consequences of separation can be significant and even overwhelming for a patient, regardless of whether they are the partner paying support or the partner receiving support. *Spousal support* (also commonly referred to as *alimony* or *maintenance*) refers to money paid by one spouse to financially support the other after they separate or divorce.[17] *Child support*, however, is money that a parent pays to support their children financially after a separation or divorce.[18] Entitlement to both forms of support, as well as the considerations of quantum and duration, are also explored further in the "Common Issues Affecting Patients Navigating a Separation" section of this chapter.

Other Issues in Family Law

A patient may have to address several other issues when they separate that are not explored in depth in this chapter. In Ontario, for example, married couples who are separating must address the division of property. Property is not physically divided between separated spouses; rather, each spouse must first value their net family property (the value of all the property that a spouse owns on the date of separation after deducting the spouse's debts and other liabilities, as well as the value of property that the spouse owned on the date of marriage; see, e.g., section 4 of the Ontario *Family Law Act* for a more fulsome definition of net family property). Thereafter, a calculation is performed (known as *equalization*) whereby the spouse whose net family property has the lesser value of the two net family properties is generally entitled to a payment equalling one-half the difference between them.[19] For further information about property division, refer to https://www.justice .gc.ca/eng/fl-df/divorce/prop.html.

Whether a patient has entered a domestic contract with their partner is also an important consideration in determining their rights and responsibilities upon separation. *Domestic contracts* (such as cohabitation agreements; marriage agreements, commonly referred to as pre-nups or post-nups; and separation agreements) are written agreements between partners that outline their rights and responsibilities during the relationship, when the relationship ends, or both.[20] Again, this issue is not discussed in a fulsome manner in this chapter, and readers should refer to other sources for further information.

Family Law and Health

Family law, particularly in the areas of relationships between parents and children, marital issues, and separation or breakdown of the marital home, is highly relevant to family medicine. Family physicians typically care for the entire family unit (and often an extended family unit) throughout the life span. Thus, when this unit is disrupted, patients often seek care at their family physician's office early on in the process. Many family physicians will be asked to support one or more family members through separation, divorce, financial issues arising from dissolution of a relationship, property issues, and even child decision-making and parenting time issues. Managing the health of children in the case of relationship breakdown is also a frequent issue encountered by family physicians.

Clinicians can support patients through the scenarios outlined here in numerous ways. They can recognize acute medical issues while linking them to the underlying psychosocial factors at play (e.g., mental health diagnoses that arise, such as depression, posttraumatic stress disorder, and anxiety). They can recognize that counselling regarding areas of law and rights is out of their scope but can confidently refer to and provide resources for patients to use. In addition, because legal processes surrounding separation, divorce, and associated issues are often lengthy, the family physician can serve as an advocate and support the patient throughout this process. Finally, in certain situations (e.g., violence in the home when minors are involved), physicians will be required by mandatory reporting obligations to act on and report what they come to know.

Most commonly, patients will present to the family medicine office with an acute health concern. Family law issues may contribute to or exacerbate existing illness, which is well borne out in the literature. For example, the experience of separation or divorce confers risk for poor health outcomes, including a 23 per cent higher mortality rate. Although most individuals cope well after a relationship ends and resilience is the most common response, a full 10–15 per cent of individuals will suffer significantly; overall elevated adverse health risks are driven by this poorly functioning group.[21] Studies have also found that recent divorce is associated with smoking; poor quality of life; and high degrees of psychological distress, anxiety, and depression, but these associations are attenuated with time.[22]

In addition to mental health outcomes, physical health is also affected by divorce. Divorce is known to be a significant risk factor for acute myocardial infarction. One study that looked at adults ages 45–80 years found a consistent increased risk of myocardial infarction among patients who had ever been divorced, and this risk was greatest in women who had experienced multiple divorces.[23]

During any marital breakdown, the treating physician should be alert to the possibility of family violence. Depending on the particular situation, there may be a duty to report (i.e., if children are in the home). Family violence may include physical abuse, sexual abuse, threats of violence or death, harassment, neglect, and psychological or financial abuse. Unfortunately, the risk of family violence is higher soon after a separation.[24] Clinicians can screen for each of these types of risk, but they must do so in a sensitive way and seek to ensure patient safety. Ensuring patients are alone when asking screening questions and having appropriate follow-up supports available is paramount. Creating a safety plan when needed is a key component of keeping patients safe, and being aware of province-specific guidelines regarding mandatory reporting of different types of family violence is a professional responsibility. In situations of physical violence (including sexual assault or abuse), the family physician will need to serve as a supportive presence while also assessing and treating injuries, and if patients are agreeable, they should consider referring them to specialized centres, such as sexual assault and domestic violence teams (Ontario has 37 such hospital-based Sexual Assault/Domestic Violence Treatment Centres).

Further information about these centres can be found at https://www
.sadvtreatmentcentres.ca/healthcare-options.html. These topics are
also explored in a more fulsome manner in the "Common Issues Affecting Patients Navigating a Separation" section of this chapter.

Patients may also bring their children to their family physician for
evaluation during stressful life transitions. Turning our focus to the paediatric population, divorce can be a traumatic experience for some children, and it is an adverse childhood experience (ACE) for many. ACEs
are potentially traumatic events that occur in childhood. They have
been linked to chronic health problems, mental illness, and substance
use in adolescence and adulthood.[25] However, the ability to mitigate the
effects of divorce is significant. Research has shown that particular interventions can improve outcomes for children and families of divorce.[26]
Divorce education classes for parents, which are common in the United
States, are designed to inform parents about how to minimize negative
effects of divorce on their children. Studies have found that attendees
report decreased conflict with their ex-partners and less court involvement to resolve disagreements.[27] Community-based programs for children that encourage supportive listening and exploration of feelings and
that offer a place for children to access social supports have also been
found to reduce negative feelings about divorce, reduce school-related
behavioural issues, and increase competence.[28] Finally, mediation has
been found to result in more contact between children and fathers after
divorce, as well as less conflict between divorced parents.[29] Mediation,
however, is often inappropriate in cases involving family violence in
light of the safety issues and power imbalances that may be in play.[30]

Family physicians can serve as powerful advocates for their paediatric patients. They can advocate for mediation (when appropriate)
and specific programming for children to mitigate the negative effects
of divorce, as well as foster resiliency and open communication about
challenges they are facing. This is critical particularly because children
can often feel confused, anxious, and at fault when parents divorce;
they require careful and consistent reassurance and support during this
challenging transitional period.

Thus, the family physician has a critical role to play when patients
are experiencing separation or divorce. It is paramount to recognize
that although this is a transitional life experience for all involved, there
are steps clinicians can take to mitigate negative outcomes for both
adult and paediatric patients. Key points include screening for mental and physical health conditions, offering supportive counselling and
resources to address these conditions, directing patients to appropriate legal resources, and being aware of the importance of screening for
safety in case of family violence.

Common Issues Affecting Patients Navigating a Separation

Income Security

When a patient goes through a separation, there are financial repercussions that arise upon the splitting of their household. Patients who were the primary income earners for the household may suddenly be obligated to pay child and spousal support. Alternatively, support from ex-partners may become a critical financial resource for patients who were stay-at-home parents who stepped away from the workforce to raise their children. These patients may not know how to deal with errant payors or the remedies available to them. Separating patients should receive assistance in addressing and stabilizing their new financial circumstances as soon as possible.

Child Support

Child support is the money that a parent pays to financially support their dependent child or children after a separation or divorce. Child support may be mandated by a court order or agreed to through a domestic contract or agreement. A child's right to child support arises from federal and provincial or territorial legislation.[31]

Each parent has an obligation to provide support for dependent children. Dependent children are usually those who are younger than age 18. In Ontario, a child younger than age 18 is not dependent if they marry or if they are at least 16 years old and have withdrawn from parental control.[32] Dependent children may also be older than age 18 if they (a) are going to school full time (the obligation to pay child support typically continues until the child gets one university- or college-level degree, although this is not necessarily always the case) or (b) have a disability, illness, or some other cause that makes them unable to leave the care of their parents.[33]

WHO PAYS CHILD SUPPORT?

Child support is typically paid by the parent who spends less time with the child to the parent who takes care of the child most of the time.[34] The parent who pays child support is commonly referred to as the *payor parent* and the parent who receives the child support as the *payee* or *recipient parent*. Child support, however, is not the right of the recipient parent: it remains the right of the child, who can seek support from a payor parent through the recipient parent as long as need is demonstrated.[35]

In some Canadian jurisdictions, including Ontario, a parent includes a person who has demonstrated a settled intention to treat a child as a child of his or her family, except in foster care situations.[36] Therefore, the payor parent does not necessarily have to be a birth parent: an adoptive parent, a step-parent, or a person who has a parent–child relationship with the child may be obligated to pay child support after separation. Parents must support their children even if they do not see the children or have other children from a previous or new relationship.[37(pp. 1–2)]

WHAT DETERMINES THE AMOUNT OF CHILD SUPPORT?
The amount of child support payable has two main components: first, a basic monthly amount called the *table amount* and second, an amount for special or extraordinary expenses.[38]

Table Amount
The basic monthly amount of child support is often referred to as the *table amount* because it is usually determined in accordance with leg-islated support tables. These tables take into consideration the payor parent's gross annual income and the number of children entitled to support from the payor parent.[39] The table amount is meant to cover basic monthly expenses, such as clothing, food, and school supplies.[40]

Each province and territory has its own legislated support tables. If the payor parent lives in another Canadian province or territory from the one in which the recipient parent lives, the support table for the province or territory where the payor parent lives applies.[41]

Special or Extraordinary Expenses
In addition to the basic table amount of child support, parents may also have to help pay for certain special or extraordinary expenses relating to their children. In Ontario, these expenses are commonly referred to as *section 7 expenses* because they are governed by section 7 of the *Federal Child Support Guidelines* and Ontario's *Child Support Guidelines*.[42] These expenses are as follows:

(a)   child care expenses incurred as a result of the employment, illness, disability or education or training for employment of the spouse/partner who has the majority of parenting time;

(b)   that portion of the medical and dental insurance premiums attribut-able to the child;

(c)   health-related expenses that exceed insurance reimbursement by at least $100 annually, including orthodontic treatment, professional counselling provided by a psychologist, social worker, psychiatrist or any other person, physiotherapy, occupational therapy, speech therapy and prescription drugs, hearing aids, glasses and contact lenses;

   (d)   extraordinary expenses for primary or secondary school education or for any other educational programs that meet the child's particular needs;

   (e)   expenses for post-secondary education; and

   (f)   extraordinary expenses for extracurricular activities.[43]

Special or extraordinary expenses must be reasonable – that is, affordable – to the parents, as well as necessary for the child's best interests.[44] Thus, a particular expense may be considered special or extraordinary for one family but not for another family. When a particular expense is found to be special or extraordinary, it is typically shared by the parents based on their respective incomes.[45]

DETERMINING THE PAYOR PARENT'S INCOME

The *Federal Child Support Guidelines* set out how a payor parent's income is calculated. First, the payor parent's annual income is determined using the sources of income included under the heading "Total income" on the T1 General form issued by the Canada Revenue Agency. This amount is then adjusted in accordance with Schedule III of the *Federal Child Support Guidelines.*[46]

In some cases, additional considerations, such as whether the payor parent has incurred a non-recurring capital gain or business investment loss, may apply to the determination of income. Other scenarios in which a court could make certain adjustments and attribute income to the payor parent to arrive at a fair determination of income include the following:

- where the payor parent is a shareholder of a company and what they are being paid is not reflective of what is available to them;
- if a payor parent is found to be intentionally under-employed or unemployed;
- where a payor parent is found to have diverted income; and
- if a payor parent is a non-resident and is taxed differently than they would be taxed if they resided in Canada.[47]

ENFORCING CHILD SUPPORT

In most Canadian jurisdictions, legislation sets out automatic or mandatory filing of support orders with a government body that is responsible for enforcing the order. In Ontario, for example, the Family Responsibility Office (FRO) is responsible for collecting child support directly from the payor parent, keeping a record of the amounts paid, and then paying that amount to the recipient parent.[48]

If a payor parent misses a payment, the government can enforce the child support owing in several ways, such as

- deducting payments automatically from their income;
- registering a charge against their personal property or real estate; or
- garnishing their bank account.[49]

Other methods that the FRO can use to incentivize payor parents to pay include suspending their driver's licence, cancelling their passport, and reporting them to credit bureaus.[50]

SOCIAL ASSISTANCE AND CHILD SUPPORT

If a recipient parent is receiving social assistance from the Ontario Disability Support Program (ODSP) or Ontario Works (OW), they must report child support payments to the appropriate program. It should be noted that as of 2017, child support payments do not affect a person's eligibility for ODSP or OW.[51] However, payor parents receiving social assistance from ODSP or OW may still be obligated to pay child support.

Spousal Support

Spousal support is money paid by one partner to the other after they separate or divorce. Spousal support is almost always paid by the partner with the higher income to the partner with the lower income.[52] Time limits for initiating spousal support claims vary by jurisdiction.[53] These are outlined in Table 8.1.

The determination of the issue of spousal support generally occurs in two steps. First, the proposed recipient partner's entitlement to spousal support must be determined. Second, the quantum and duration of support must be determined.

Whether a partner is entitled to support or not after separation depends on several factors, including

- the financial means and needs of both partners;
- the length of the relationship;
- the roles of each partner during the relationship;
- the effect of those roles and the breakdown of the relationship on their current financial positions;
- the care of the children;
- the goal of encouraging a partner who receives support to be self-sufficient; and
- any other orders, agreements, or arrangements already made about spousal support.[54]

Table 8.1. Time Limits for Initiating Spousal Support Claims by Province or Territory

Province or territory	Limitation period[a]
Alberta, Manitoba, New Brunswick, Nova Scotia, Ontario, Quebec, Saskatchewan, and Yukon	No time limit
British Columbia	Married spouses must initiate spousal support claims within two years of divorce. Unmarried partners must bring a claim within two years of separation.
Newfoundland and Labrador, Northwest Territories, Nunavut, and Prince Edward Island	Proceeding may not be commenced for married or unmarried spouses more than two years after the day the spouses separate.

[a] Lenkinski EL, Carr A. HFA-202 limitation periods. In: Halsbury's laws of Canada – infants and children (2022 reissue). Toronto: Lexis Nexis Canada; 2022.

There are three general conceptual bases for entitlement to spousal support in Canada:

1. compensatory (recognizes that when a relationship ends, partners are entitled to be compensated for contributions to the family and for economic losses sustained as a result);
2. contractual (domestic agreements between partners may either create or negate a spousal support obligation, under appropriate circumstances); and
3. non-compensatory (recognizes that marriage is a joint endeavour premised on mutual support and that spouses may have an obligation to meet or contribute to the needs of their former partners if they have the capacity to pay, even in the absence of contractual or compensatory grounds for a spousal support obligation).[55]

Once entitlement to spousal support is established, the next issues to be determined are the quantum and duration of support. In determining these, a judge may again consider factors such as the length of the relationship, the parenting arrangements for any children, the roles of the partners during the relationship, and the age of each partner. The Spousal Support Advisory Guidelines (SSAGs) are a guide for determining the appropriate amount and duration of spousal support.[56] Further information about the SSAGs can be accessed at https://www.justice.gc.ca/eng/fl-df/spousal-epoux/ssag-ldfpae.html.

SOCIAL ASSISTANCE AND SPOUSAL SUPPORT

In Ontario, separated partners on social assistance must try to get any spousal support that they might be entitled to. If the recipient partner does not already have a support agreement or order, they are usually expected to get one. If the recipient partner does not make a reasonable effort to get spousal support, they may get less or no social assistance. The recipient partner, however, does not need to make such efforts if there is a history of IPV, if the payor partner cannot be found, or if the payor partner is not working and cannot pay support.[57(pp. 5–6)]

CHANGING SUPPORT ARRANGEMENTS

Child and spousal support arrangements can be determined and changed by agreement, through ADR, or by a judge in the court process. When a party wants to change a support arrangement (e.g., the quantum or duration) and they are unable to come to an agreement with their ex-partner, that party may decide to initiate a court action. In Ontario, a judge will only change a spousal support order if there has been a significant or material change in circumstances sufficient to warrant a variation. For example, a judge may change a spousal support arrangement if

- either partner's income has gone up or down;
- the child or children's living arrangements have changed; or
- the judge thinks that the recipient parent should now be self-supporting.[58(p. 11)]

Consider the following: Sari informs you that Jason has told her that she needs to find a job as soon as possible because he is certain that he will not owe her any support once the divorce is final. She is very concerned about this because she is currently unable to work as a result of the effects of long COVID, and she has no income streams. Sari is worried that she will not be able to financially support herself and her children without child and spousal support.

What Steps Would You Suggest Sari Consider Taking at This Time?

Sari should see her lawyer about her entitlement to spousal support and obtain their opinion. Factors such as whom the children live with after Sari and Jason separate will affect child support, whereas spousal support will depend on Sari's needs and the career sacrifices that she has made to care for the family. Her health care provider should also provide support to Sari as she recovers from long COVID, including informing her about income support programs for those unable to work for medical reasons, such as the Ontario Disability Support Program.

Housing Security

It can be critical for health care providers to support patients who may be facing housing instability in the case of separation. The loss of access to the family home may mean the loss not only of physical shelter for patients, but also their community connections and supports.

MATRIMONIAL HOME

The *matrimonial home* (also referred to as the *marital home, family home,* and *family residence* in various Canadian jurisdictions) can generally be described as the residence around which a couple's normal family life revolves.[59] For many Canadians, this is the primary and often sole residence in which the family lives.

Given the centrality of the matrimonial home in the lives of families, these properties are treated differently from others both during the relationship and upon separation. An important caveat, however, is that the default rights regarding the matrimonial home and the legal mechanisms by which these rights are enforced and protected vary depending on jurisdiction and marital status. For example, in Ontario, the matrimonial property statutes apply only to married spouses. In jurisdictions in which unmarried cohabiting partners are not covered by these statutes, they must seek to establish their rights regarding the matrimonial home through other means, such as domestic contracts and trust claims, which can be difficult.[60] It can be important for health care providers to clarify whether the patient was married to their partner or not in order to inform clients about the proper avenues for further support.

POSSESSORY RIGHTS

A belief that patients may have regarding the matrimonial home is that whoever legally owns the home (i.e., is on the title to the home) has the right to remove inhabitants at will. This is not always true. Under matrimonial property statutes, married spouses (and, in some jurisdictions, unmarried cohabiting partners) generally have an equal right to stay in the matrimonial home throughout the relationship and after separation.[61] This right is known as the possessory right.

The possessory right applies whether the matrimonial home is leased or owned outright (except in Newfoundland and Labrador and Nova Scotia, where matrimonial homes must be owned by either one or both spouses).[62] If the property is owned, the possessory right is independent of legal ownership.[63] In other words, the spouse who owns the property cannot, for example, evict the other spouse or change the locks to the property.

In the case of married spouses in Ontario, their possessory rights generally continue until one of the following events occurs:

- a court order regarding possession of the matrimonial home is made;
- the parties come to a separation agreement that says a spouse cannot live there;
- the matrimonial home is sold or, in the case of rented properties, the lease ends; or
- the parties get divorced.[64]

In Ontario, unmarried partners do not have an automatic right to stay in the family home if it is not in their name.[65] If they want to stay, they may try to come to an agreement with the titled party to stay in the home or make a claim for ownership of the home by asserting equitable principles and remedies.[66] For example, a non-titled cohabiting partner may assert that they contributed to the acquisition, retainment, or upkeep of the property.[67]

Consider the following: Sari notes that currently, she and Jason are living in a rental home, and Jason is the only person named on the lease agreement. She is terrified that Jason will make good on his threats to kick her out of the home and keep the children from her if she does not agree to his requests for the separation and eventual divorce.

How Could You Support Sari at This Time?

Given the laws surrounding possessory rights in Ontario, Jason cannot legally remove Sari from the rental home. Until a court orders Sari to leave, Sari agrees to leave, the lease ends, or Jason and Sari go through with a divorce, Sari is entitled to stay in the matrimonial home.

This, however, does not mean that it would necessarily be beneficial for Sari to stay. For example, you may be concerned about escalating conflict or violence in the home. You may want to ask Sari whether she is able to stay with a local friend or family member as the litigation unfolds. If she is able to do so, she should be directed to her lawyer regarding the parenting implications that would arise from taking the children out of the matrimonial home. You may also want to provide Sari with safety planning resources, which are discussed further in the "Family Violence" section of this chapter.

It may also be prudent to link Sari to housing supports in her area or to agencies that work with women and children to secure temporary and permanent housing when leaving relationships.

Parenting

The issues of decision-making responsibility and parenting time can be among the most difficult for patients to deal with upon separation. The determination of which parents have decision-making responsibility (the right to make important decisions for their child or children) and of parenting time (the time that their child or children spends in their care) can become a lengthy, hard-fought process if parties are unable to agree on these matters.[68]

If children are drawn into the parental conflict, such as by being bystanders, passive weapons, communication channels, or active participants who collect evidence or communicate threats or insults, the effects can be devastating. Researchers have found that behavioural problems among children are associated with the duration and animosity of their parents' legal battles and that parental conflict can have long-lasting and serious consequences for children, including effects on children's self-esteem, ability to adjust and cope, and social competence.[69] In the case of parenting disputes in particular, children may be subject to loyalty binds by parents vying for their favour. Separating parents and their children should be encouraged to get appropriate support as soon as possible.

In Canada, the governing principle in the determination of parenting issues is the best interests of the child. In general terms, the best interests of the child is a legal test used to decide what would best protect a child's physical, psychological, and emotional safety, security, and well-being.[70] In determining the decision-making parent or parents and the parenting time schedule, courts may consider several factors in tailoring a decision that is in the best interests of the child, including

(a)   the child's needs, given the child's age and stage of development, such as the child's need for stability;

(b)   the nature and strength of the child's relationship with each spouse, each of the child's siblings and grandparents and any other person who plays an important role in the child's life;

(c)   each spouse's willingness to support the development and maintenance of the child's relationship with the other spouse;

(d)   the history of care of the child;

(e)   the child's views and preferences, giving due weight to the child's age and maturity, unless they cannot be ascertained;

(f)   the child's cultural, linguistic, religious and spiritual upbringing and heritage, including Indigenous upbringing and heritage;

(g)   any plans for the child's care;

(h)   the ability and willingness of each person in respect of whom the order would apply to care for and meet the needs of the child;

(i)   the ability and willingness of each person in respect of whom the order would apply to communicate and cooperate, in particular with one another, on matters affecting the child;

(j)   any family violence and its impact on, among other things,

   (i)   the ability and willingness of any person who engaged in the family violence to care for and meet the needs of the child, and

   (ii)   the appropriateness of making an order that would require persons in respect of whom the order would apply to cooperate on issues affecting the child; and

(k)   any civil or criminal proceeding, order, condition, or measure that is relevant to the safety, security and well-being of the child.[71]

Courts may also enlist the assistance of government offices such as the Office of the Children's Lawyer (in Ontario), social workers, and counselling professionals in determining the best interests of the child.

In some situations, including those in which there are concerns about the needs of the children and the parents' ability to meet those needs and to overcome presenting challenges, a parenting capacity assessment may assist in the determination of decision-making responsibility and parenting time regimes that are in the best interests of the child.[72] A parenting capacity assessment is conducted by a clinician who has the requisite technical or professional skill to determine the child's needs and the ability and willingness of the parents to satisfy those needs.[73] The clinician may make recommendations regarding decision-making and parenting time, but the judge hearing a parenting matter remains responsible for making the final order.[74]

PARENTING AND DISCLOSURE OF A CHILD'S MEDICAL INFORMATION

For health care professionals, it is critical to consider whether a patient has decision-making responsibility for their child when the child needs medical treatment. The disclosure of a child's medical records or information to a parent can also be a complex issue requiring court intervention. Factors such as whether the parent has decision-making responsibility or parenting time rights, the ability of the child to consent to the disclosure of information, and the statutory mechanisms in play can all complicate disclosure matters. For example, section 20(5) of Ontario's *Children's Law Reform Act* states, "The entitlement to parenting time with respect to a child includes the right to visit with and be visited by the child, and includes the same right as a parent to *make inquiries and to be given information about the child's well-being, including in relation to the child's health and education* [emphasis added]."[75] The judiciary has explained that the purpose of section 20(5) is to recognize that parents, regardless of whether they have decision-making responsibility or not, should be fully informed on issues affecting the welfare of a child in order to ensure that they at all times act in the child's best interests.[76]

Section 20(5) of the *Children's Law Reform Act*, as it relates to the entitlement of a parent to obtain information directly from health care providers, appears to conflict with privacy legislation, such as Ontario's *Personal Health Information Protection Act (PHIPA)*,[77] which governs the collection, use, and disclosure of personal health information by health care providers. Under *PHIPA*, there is no general right to access another individual's personal health information, including that of children.[78]

The courts in Ontario have resolved this apparent conflict between family law legislation and privacy legislation by stating that the right to information under family law legislation is not absolute; for example, it is subject to alteration by court order or by separation agreement. The right must be interpreted through the lens of the best-interests-of-the-child principle, as are all decisions affecting children.[79]

Whether a child has the capacity to consent to the disclosure of their medical information under *PHIPA* may also affect a health care provider's ability to disclose the same. If a child lacks capacity under section 21 of *PHIPA*, then a substitute decision-maker may act on their behalf provided that they meet the conditions under section 26(2).[80]

PHIPA prescribes a hierarchy of substitute decision-makers in section 26(1), with parents having decision-making responsibility taking precedence over parents who have parenting time but do not have decision-making responsibility. When two parents have joint decision-making responsibility, they are equally ranked and must agree on the decision to disclose information. If a health care provider is dealing with two equally ranked substitute decision-makers, then neither parent can act independently of the other. They would have to agree, return to court to alter the arrangement respecting decision-making, or obtain another appropriate order.[81]

Whether a child has the capacity to consent to the disclosure of medical information is a determination made by the health care provider.[82] If the child in question has the capacity to consent, only they may give or withhold consent to the disclosure of health information, pursuant to section 23(1) of *PHIPA*. If, however, the person is a child younger than age 16, a parent may give or withhold consent on the child's behalf, unless the information sought relates to treatment within the meaning of the *Health Care Consent Act* about which the child themself has made a decision on their own.[83,84]

If there is any question regarding what a health care provider may disclose based on provincial or territorial health privacy legislation, they can call the regional medical protection agency (in Canada, the CMPA) to ask them what they are legally required to disclose.

SUPERVISED PARENTING TIME

Supervised parenting time refers to parenting time when a parent is under the supervision of a third party. It is generally ordered if it is believed that a child stands to gain some benefit from a parent maintaining an ongoing role in their life, but there are concerns about the parent's risk of harm to the child. For example, if there is a risk of child abduction or emotional or physical harm to the child, parenting time may be supervised. Supervision is generally intended to be a transitional measure while the parent proves that they are able to have safe contact with their child.[85]

Supervision arrangements can vary in degree of formality. Informal arrangements may involve a family member, neighbour, or volunteer acting as the third-party supervisor. More formal supervision may occur in supervised access centres or through the use of professionals such as childcare workers or social workers. It is important that there be clear expectations and contracts between the supervisor, court, counsel, and parents for supervision, especially in cases in which there is a history of sexual abuse. There can be a great degree of variability in the training of third-party supervisors and mandates for programs in supervised access centres. If required, the supervisor should have appropriate training to recognize subtle forms of abuse.[86]

OFFICE OF THE CHILDREN'S LAWYER

The Office of the Children's Lawyer (OCL) is an independent law office in Ontario's Ministry of the Attorney General that delivers justice programs on behalf of children in Ontario. Similar offices can be found across Canadian jurisdictions. The OCL represents the interests of children younger than age 18 in matters involving parenting time, contact, and decision-making responsibility; child protection; and more.[87]

Parties to a family law matter involving the determination of parenting issues may ask the judge to make an order requesting the involvement of the OCL. A judge may also independently decide to request the involvement of the OCL. Within 14 days of the court making the order, the parties must complete the OCL intake forms. If the OCL accepts the case, they may assign a lawyer (to act as the legal representative of the child or children), clinician, or both to the matter. The representatives of the child may then

- meet with the child's parents or anyone asking for parenting time or decision-making responsibility in respect to the child;
- meet with the child as many times as they believe is necessary;
- determine the child's wishes, when possible;
- contact relevant sources of information, such as teachers, doctors, day care providers, therapists, and so forth;
- meet with the parents or other parties to provide feedback and, where appropriate, suggest ways to resolve the issues between the parties;
- take a legal position that includes the child's wishes and other important information regarding the family; and
- tell the court what position they are taking on behalf of the child.[88]

If a physician is contacted by the OCL, they must provide collateral information as requested. Generally, the physician will receive a signed consent form from the parties involved.

Child Protection

Child protection issues may arise when addressing parenting after separation. Child protection laws across Canada establish a system of state intervention into the privacy of the family in circumstances in which caretakers are unable or unwilling to provide a minimum standard of care for their children.[89]

Generally, a child will be found to be in need of protection if (a) the child is neglected, left alone, or uncared for; (b) has been abused or is likely to be abused; or (c) sees abuse or violence between adults in the home. Abuse includes physical, sexual, and emotional abuse.[90]

The primary purpose of Canadian child protection laws is to promote the best interests, protection, and well-being of children.[91] Additional purposes are to recognize and promote the following:

1. While parents may need help in caring for their children, that help should give support to the autonomy and integrity of the family unit and, wherever possible, be provided on the basis of mutual consent.

2. The least disruptive course of action that is available and appropriate in a particular case to help a child, including the provision of prevention services, early intervention services and community support services, should be considered.
3. Services to children and young people should be provided in a manner that respects a child's or young person's need for continuity of care and for stable relationships within a family and cultural environment, takes into account physical, emotional, spiritual, mental and developmental needs and differences among children and young persons, takes into account a child's or young person's race, ancestry, place of origin, colour, ethnic origin, citizenship, family diversity, disability, creed, sex, sexual orientation, gender identity and gender expression, takes into account a child's or young person's cultural and linguistic needs, provides early assessment, planning and decision-making to achieve permanent plans for children and young persons in accordance with their best interests, and includes the participation of a child or young person, the child's or young person's parents and relatives and the members of the child's or young person's extended family and community, where appropriate.
4. Services to children and young persons and their families should be provided in a manner that respects cultural, religious and regional differences, wherever possible.
5. Services to children and young persons and their families should be provided in a manner that builds on the strengths of the families, wherever possible.
6. First Nations, Inuit and Métis peoples should be entitled to provide, wherever possible, their own child and family services, and that all services to First Nations, Inuit and Métis children, young people and families should be provided in a manner that recognizes their cultures, heritages and traditions, connection to their communities and the concept of the extended family.
7. Appropriate sharing of information, including personal information, in order to plan for and provide services is essential for creating successful outcomes for children and families.[92]

In Ontario, the government pays for child welfare agencies called Children's Aid Societies (CAS) to help children younger than age 18 in need of protection. Once a report is made to the CAS, a child protection worker will conduct an initial screening. The CAS may then decide to initiate an investigation, which involves the CAS caseworker visiting the child's home and speaking with the parents and the child. The investigation may also involve interviews with individuals outside the home, such as other family members, neighbours, teachers, and health care providers.[93]

If a child is determined to be in need of protection and is removed from the home, parents should be urged to immediately seek and obtain legal advice and representation. The CAS may remove a child from a parent even if they are not the alleged abuser if the CAS believes that they are not sufficiently protecting the child from harm.[94]

If an agreement cannot be reached between the parent and the CAS about where the child will be placed, a child protection trial must occur. There are five possible results from a child protection trial:

1. *Dismissal*: the court decides that no child protection order is needed.
2. *Supervision order*: the child stays at the home of a parent, family, or community member, but the CAS is involved in their supervision.
3. *Interim society care*: the child is placed into time-limited custody of CAS with foster parents.
4. *Extended society care*: the child is permanently in the custody of the CAS and may be adopted.
5. *Custody order*: a parent, relative, or community member is given custody of the child.[95]

The CAS also has the power to remove children at birth if there are significant concerns for their safety. The CAS may be concerned about a child's safety if

- the patient has previous children who have been taken by the CAS;
- the patient is homeless or living in an unsafe environment;
- the patient has a serious drug or alcohol problem; or
- the patient is experiencing other types of instability, including emotional and mental health concerns.[96]

Family Violence and Intimate Partner Violence

The recognition and understanding of family violence and its harmful effects continues to evolve in both health care and family law. In the legal sphere, both the legislature and the judiciary have recently taken steps to acknowledge and address the epidemic of family violence. For example, the *Divorce Act* was amended in 2021 to define *family violence* in the context of the best interests of the child. This new definition recognizes that family violence can be perpetrated in many forms that can cause significant harm to both victims and witnesses in family law cases.[97]

WHAT IS FAMILY VIOLENCE AND INTIMATE PARTNER VIOLENCE?
Family violence (also known as *domestic violence*) is broadly defined in the *Divorce Act* as conduct, whether or not the conduct constitutes a criminal offence, by a family member towards another family member that is violent or threatening, that constitutes a pattern of coercive and controlling behaviour, or that causes that other family member to fear for their own safety or for that of another person. In the case of a child, family violence also includes direct or indirect exposure to such conduct.[98] IPV (also known as *spousal violence*) is a type of family violence and specifically refers to multiple forms of harm caused by a current or former intimate partner or spouse. Examples of family violence and IPV include

- physical abuse;
- sexual abuse;
- forced confinement;
- threats of harm to others or oneself;
- harassment;
- name calling;
- preventing contact with friends and family;
- financial abuse;
- stalking; and
- cyber-violence.[99]

IPV affects people of all genders; ages; and socio-economic, racial, educational, ethnic, and religious backgrounds; women, however, account for the vast majority of people who experience IPV, and it is most often perpetrated by men. According to police-reported data from 2019, for example, of the 107,810 people aged 15 years and older who experienced IPV in Canada in 2019, 79 per cent were women. Indigenous women in Canada were more likely to have experienced IPV in their lifetime (61 per cent) compared with non-Indigenous women (44 per cent).[100] Family violence also has a particular impact on racialized immigrant women, who may be dependent on their spouse for immigration status, have limited proficiency in English, or come from a culture in which greater emphasis is placed on the family.[101]

The destructive effects of family violence on the physical, emotional, and mental well-being of an individual are well documented. Children who are exposed to family violence are at risk of long-term psychological distress, and they may experience longitudinal effects on physical health, substance abuse, interpersonal violence, and self-harm.[102] Beyond its direct impact on the health of victims and witnesses, IPV can also play an insidious role in family law proceedings. For example, perpetrators of family violence have been shown to use legal proceedings as a way to control or punish their former partners.[103] Women who sustain brain injury from IPV may also be at risk of having their diagnosis used against them in disputes about parenting.[104]

DUTY TO WARN AND DUTY TO REPORT

Physicians have a duty to maintain strict confidentiality about health matters with their patients. In a select few cases, this confidentiality can be broken and information disclosed to a specific third party; in these cases, it is generally permitted and sometimes mandated through legislation, legal policies, or by-laws.

A duty to report requires physicians to disclose confidential health information to a third party; each province and territory has different legislation regarding what constitutes a duty to report. A specific example of this is a physician's duty to report a suspicion of child abuse or abuse in the home where a child resides. Generally, physicians will never be held at fault for breaching confidentiality if such reports are made in good faith.

A duty to warn is not mandated by Canadian courts; however, the Supreme Court of Canada notes that physicians are permitted to warn authorities (i.e., police) when they have been made aware of significant threats towards another person or group that could cause imminent danger. Physicians should seek clarification and advice from the CMPA in such cases.[105]

DISCLOSURE OF ABUSE AND SCREENING

Patients may not be forthcoming in disclosing the abuse they may experience at home for several reasons. Victims may be fearful of others' judgment, perpetrator retaliation, and adverse police or judicial responses. In the case of victims of long-standing patterns of family violence, they may view coercive and controlling behaviours as a normal part of the relationship or not consider the violence as being sufficiently serious to warrant disclosure.[106]

Legal practitioners and health care providers alike may be assisted by domestic violence screening tools in cases involving family violence, IPV, or both. One such tool is the Government of Canada's HELP Toolkit, which is intended to help family lawyers with identifying and responding to family violence. More information about the HELP Toolkit can be found at https://www.justice.gc.ca/eng//fl-df/help-aide /toc-tdm.html.

When patients approach health care providers with information about abuse, it is important that they carefully document the incidents, because independent evidence of family violence can be critical if the patient becomes involved in litigation. In the case of sexual abuse, a referral to a Sexual Assault/Domestic Violence Treatment Centre should be offered as a confidential resource for patients that can assist with documenting abuse in a sensitive and legally robust manner. Patients should be reassured that police will not be called without their express consent unless there are children in the home and their safety is felt to be at risk.

SAFETY PLANS

A particularly dangerous time for victims of IPV is when they separate from their partner. Multiple studies have demonstrated that the risk of lethal violence is particularly high after parental separation, especially in the first few months.[107] A CBC News investigation regarding intimate partner homicides across Canada between January 2015 and June 2020 revealed that a recent separation was involved in 22 per cent of the domestic homicide cases studied.[108]

When a patient is facing safety issues in the process of separating, it is important that they have a safety plan for leaving the relationship. A safety plan lays out step by step how an individual will leave their partner and includes information such as where they will go and what they will take with them. The goal of a safety plan is to minimize the risk of harm.[109(p. 7)] If a patient is contemplating leaving an abusive intimate partner, they should be referred to a counselling agency, crisis helpline, or a local shelter to discuss what is happening and to learn how to create a safety plan tailored to their situation. They should also be encouraged to obtain legal advice about their situation as soon as possible, especially if the patient has children that they want to take with them. More information about how patients can escape family violence can be found at https://www.justice.gc.ca/eng/cj-jp /fv-vf/help-aide.html and https://www.cleo.on.ca/en/publications /handbook.

RESTRAINING ORDERS

A restraining order is a court order that limits where someone can go, what someone can do, and whom they can contact. The conditions of a restraining order can be general (e.g., a person must stay away from their partner and their children) or specific (e.g., a person cannot go within 500 metres of their partner's home or workplace or their children's school). The conditions of a restraining order are generally tailored to the specific situation, and breaching the conditions of a restraining order is a crime.[110]

In Ontario, an individual may apply for a restraining order against their partner if (a) the parties were married or lived together for any period of time or (b) the parties have a child together.[111] Restraining orders can be particularly important in cases involving family violence. The party seeking the restraining order will generally have to prove that there are reasonable grounds to fear for their own safety or the safety of their children.[112]

If the court is of the view that a restraining order is not required, there are other orders that can be made to constrain a party's behaviour. For example, Ontario's *Children's Law Reform Act* enables the court to make orders limiting the duration, frequency, manner, or location of contact or communication between the parties or between a party and a child.[113]

EXCLUSIVE POSSESSION ORDERS

When a patient is separated and engaged in high-conflict litigation or there are concerns regarding family violence, it can be critical for health care providers to inform them about exclusive possession orders. As the name suggests, these are court orders granting one of the spouses the right to stay in or return to the matrimonial home to the exclusion of the other spouse.[114] These orders are not routinely granted and can be difficult to obtain. In Ontario, exclusive possession orders may come with certain conditions, such as that the party given exclusive possession must pay for household expenses.[115] In considering whether to grant an exclusive possession order, the court must consider the following factors:

- the best interests of the children affected;
- any existing orders regarding family property and existing support orders or other enforceable support obligations;
- the financial position of both spouses;
- any written agreement between the parties;

- the availability of other suitable and affordable accommodation; and
- any violence committed by a spouse against the other spouse or the children.[116]

Benefits of an exclusive possession order for a spouse include that they will not have to deal with moving. The simple fact of physical separation may also be a protective measure for victims of family violence.

RELOCATION

As the Supreme Court of Canada recently affirmed, family violence is an important factor for judges to consider in relocation cases.[117] *Relocation* refers to a change in the place of residence of a child or parent who has parenting time, decision-making responsibility, or both that is likely to have a significant impact on the child's relationships with those who have parenting time, decision-making responsibility, or contact.[118] The grave implications of family violence for the positive development of children makes it an influential factor in relocation cases.[119] Other factors that a court must take into consideration to determine whether a proposed relocation is in the best interests of the child include

(a) the reasons for the relocation;

(b) the impact of the relocation on the child;

(c) the amount of time spent with the child by each person who has parenting time or a pending application for a parenting order and the level of involvement in the child's life of each of those persons;

(d) whether the person who intends to relocate the child complied with any applicable notice requirement …, provincial family law legislation, an order, arbitral award, or agreement;

(e) the existence of an order, arbitral award, or agreement that specifies the geographic area in which the child is to reside;

(f) the reasonableness of the proposal of the person who intends to relocate the child to vary the exercise of parenting time, decision-making responsibility or contact, taking into consideration, among other things, the location of the new place of residence and the travel expenses; and

(g) whether each person who has parenting time or decision-making responsibility or a pending application for a parenting order has complied with their obligations under family law legislation, an order, arbitral award, or agreement, and the likelihood of future compliance.[120]

A patient who has decision-making responsibility or parenting time with respect to a child and who intends to relocate must notify any other person who has parental rights of their intention at least 60 days before the expected date of the proposed relocation, unless the court dispenses with or modifies this requirement because of factors such as family violence. The notice must set out

- the expected date of the relocation;
- the address of the new place of residence and contact information of the person or child; and
- a proposal as to how parenting time and/or decision-making responsibility could be exercised.[121]

If a parent objects to the proposed location, they must complete within 30 days of receiving notice of the proposed move a form setting out their objection that includes

- a statement that they object the proposed relocation;
- the reasons for the objection; and
- their views on the proposal for the exercise of parenting time, decision-making responsibility, or both.[122]

Consider the following: at a follow-up encounter with Sari, she discloses that although she initially told you that the reason for her separation was "growing apart," she had in fact thought about leaving her marriage almost as soon as it began. Jason could be charming at work and to family members, but at home he struggled with drinking too much and at times with anger management. You ask Sari more about life at home, and she discloses that in the past, Jason has hurt her by pushing her down and striking her. She is sure these were isolated incidents and tells you that he would never hurt their children. Jason, in fact, initiated the separation because he has been seeing another woman at work, and he has told Sari that he wants to move in with this person.

What Else Might You Screen for in This Situation, Now That This New Information Has Been Disclosed?

It would be important to screen for specific types of intimate partner violence, including further physical abuse, sexual abuse, and financial and emotional abuse. A screen for sexually transmitted infections would also be appropriate. It is prudent to examine Sari, with her consent, and to document any physical signs of abuse you note. If sexual abuse is disclosed, you should discuss a referral to a specialized sexual assault and domestic violence centre with Sari.

Do You Have Any Duties as a Physician Now That You Know That Jason Has Been Physically Violent towards Sari?

When a child younger than age 16 has been exposed to violence in the home, regardless of whether or not the child themself has been reported to be harmed, the physician must report this to child protection authorities. Further questioning is needed to determine whether this call is required with the information given earlier. Note that legislation in all provinces and territories requires physicians to report to child protection authorities when there are reasonable grounds to believe or suspect a child has been abused, is being abused, or is at risk of being abused. This includes being a witness to domestic violence in the home. It is important to review this information with Sari, because it may be important to make this call together to discuss the situation from a safety perspective. Initially, clinicians can speak to a child protective worker anonymously to see whether they feel a report is warranted.

What Advice or Supports Should You Provide Sari at This Encounter?

Creating a safety plan is paramount. Encouraging Sari to have a safe haven to get to quickly with her children and important belongings (health cards, passports, medications) is important. Knowing about particular resources for her mental health to support her through this challenging time is also important, because Sari and her children may benefit from professional counselling support (see the "Resources for Health care Providers and Patients" section).

Resources for Health Care Providers and Patients

As discussed in this chapter, patients navigating separation may face numerous complex issues. Tables 8.2, 8.3, and 8.4 present practical and informational resources that health care providers can share with their patients.

Table 8.2. Child and Spousal Support Resources

Organization and resource	Description	Source
Government of Canada's *Federal Child Support Guidelines: Step-by-Step*	Step-by-step guide regarding child support; includes general information and sample scenarios and calculations	https://www.justice.gc.ca/eng/rp-pr/fl-lf/child-enfant/guide/index.html
2017 Simplified Federal Child Support Tables	PDFs of simplified child support tables	https://www.justice.gc.ca/eng/fl-df/child-enfant/fcsg-lfpae/2017/index.html
2017 Child Support Table Look-up	Tool to look up table support payable on the basis of annual gross income, number of children, and payor parent's province of residence	https://www.justice.gc.ca/eng/fl-df/child-enfant/2017/look-rech.aspx
Government of Canada's Spousal Support Advisory Guidelines page	Introduces the Spousal Support Advisory Guidelines and contains tools such as Steps to Using the Spousal Support Advisory Guidelines and the Revised User's Guide	https://www.justice.gc.ca/eng/fl-df/spousal-epoux/ssag-ldfpae.html
My Support Calculator	Online child and spousal support calculator	https://www.mysupportcalculator.ca/

Table 8.3. Parenting Resources

Organization and resource	Description	Source
Government of Canada's Parenting Plan Tool	Interactive tool that helps develop a personalized parenting plan	https://www.justice.gc.ca/eng/fl-df/parent/plan.html
Ontario Women's Justice Network's Applying for Decision-Making Responsibility and Parenting Time resource	Provides definitions and a step-by-step guide for applying for decision-making responsibility and parenting time	https://www.owjn.org/2012/05/01/applying-for-child-custody/
Association of Family and Conciliation Courts Ontario's Parenting Plan Guide and Template	Guide for creating parenting plans	https://afccontario.ca/parenting-plan-guide-and-template/

Table 8.4. Family Violence and Intimate Partner Violence Resources

Organization and resource	Description	Source or contact number
Community Legal Education Ontario's *Do You Know a Woman Who Is Being Abused? A Legal Rights Handbook*	A guide to the legal system for women in Ontario whose partners abuse them	https://www.cleo.on.ca/en /publications/handbook
Steps to Justice's My Safety Plan	Fill-in-the-blank safety plan PDF	https://www.cleo.on.ca /wp-content/uploads/plan-1 .pdf
Government of Canada's Family Violence Resources	Lists family violence resources and services in specific areas	https://www.canada.ca/en /public-health/services /health-promotion/stop -family-violence/services .html
Assaulted Women's Helpline	Ontario crisis line that is free of charge, available 24/7; can assist with counselling, safety planning, and providing information about urgent moves	1-866-863-7868
Anishinabe Women's Crisis Home & Family Healing Agency – Talk4Healing	Help, support, and resources for Indigenous women, by Indigenous women, across Ontario	https://www.beendigen .com/programs /talk4healing/
Family Court Support Workers	Ontario service that provides support to victims of family violence involved in family court processes	https://www.ontario.ca/page /family-court-support -workers
Barbara Schlifer Commemorative Clinic	Counselling and other support services, such as advocacy and legal support	https://www.schliferclinic.com 1-416-323-9149
Luke's Place	Family law support centre for abused women; provides direct services to women and children in Durham region	https://www.LukesPlace.ca
Luke's Place Tech Safety Guide	Assists victims of abuse with creating a plan to use technology in a strategic and safe way	https://www.LukesPlace.ca /tech-safety
Shelter Safe	Online resource regarding shelters across Canada	https://www.sheltersafe.ca
Shelter Movers of Toronto	Assists with urgent moves from home or from a shelter; includes police assistance	https://www.sheltermovers .com 1-416-320-4232

NOTES

1 Davies C, Bissett-Johnson A, Grey J. Family law in Canada [Internet]. The Canadian Encyclopedia; 2013 July 30, 2013 [last modified 2015 Feb. 23]. Available from: https://www.thecanadianencyclopedia.ca/en/article /family-law.

2 *Civil Marriage Act*, SC 2005, c 33, s 2. Available from: https://laws-lois .justice.gc.ca/eng/acts/c-31.5/page-1.html.

3 *Civil Marriage Act*, SC 2005, c 33, s 2. Available from: https://laws-lois .justice.gc.ca/eng/acts/c-31.5/page-1.html.

4 *Marriage (Prohibited Degrees) Act*, SC 1990, c 46. https://laws-lois.justice .gc.ca/eng/acts/M-2.1/page-1.html.

5 Ontario Women's Justice Network. Getting married in Ontario [Internet]. Toronto: Ontario Women's Justice Network; 2022 [cited 2023 July 12]. https://owjn.org/2022/09/03/getting-married-in-ontario/.

6 Settlement.org. Will the Canadian government recognize my foreign marriage? [Internet]. Toronto: Settlement.org; 2021 [modified 2021 June 2]. Available from: https://settlement.org/ontario/daily-life/life-events /marriage/will-the-canadian-government-recognize-my-foreign-marriage/.

7 Community Legal Education Ontario (CLEO). An introduction to family law in Ontario. Toronto: CLEO; 2019.

8 *Family Law Act*, RSO 1990, c F3, ss 29–30. https://www.ontario.ca/laws /statute/90f03.

9 Community Legal Education Ontario (CLEO). An introduction to family law in Ontario. Ontario: CLEO; 2019.

10 Glaholt D, Rotterdam M. The law of ADR in Canada: an introductory guide. Markham (ON): LexisNexis Canada; 2011.

11 Family Law Education for Women. Family law arbitration [Internet]. Family Law Education for Women; n.d. [cited 2023 July 12]. Available from: https://onefamilylaw.ca/family-law-resources/family-law-arbitration/.

12 *Family Law Act*, RSO 1990, c F3, s. 7(3). Available from: https://www .ontario.ca/laws/statute/90f03.

13 Government of Ontario. Parenting time, decision-making responsibility and contact [Internet]. Toronto: Government of Ontario; 2021 [modified 2023 Nov 2]. Available from: https://www.ontario.ca/page/parenting -time-decision-making-responsibility-and-contact.

14 Government of Ontario. Parenting time, decision-making responsibility and contact [Internet]. Toronto: Government of Ontario; 2021 [modified 2023 Nov 2]. Available from: https://www.ontario.ca/page/parenting -time-decision-making-responsibility-and-contact.

15 Government of Canada. Making plans: A guide to parenting arrangements after separation or divorce [Internet]. Ottawa: Government of Canada;

2024 [modified 2024 May 17]. Available from: https://www.justice.gc.ca
/eng/fl-df/parent/mp-fdp/p5.html.

16 *Divorce Act*, RSC 1986, c 3 (2nd Supp), s 16(1). Available from: https://
laws-lois.justice.gc.ca/eng/acts/d-3.4/.

17 Community Legal Education Ontario. What is spousal support? [Internet].
Toronto: Community Legal Education Ontario; 2022 [cited 2024 Jan 30].
Available from: https://www.cleo.on.ca/en/publications/spousalsupport
/what-spousal-support.

18 Ontario Women's Justice Network. Child support [Internet]. Toronto:
Ontario Women's Justice Network; n.d. [cited 2023 July 12]. Available
from: https://owjn.org/2022/09/01/child-support/.

19 *Family Law Act*, RSO 1990, c F3, s 5. Available from: https://www.ontario
.ca/laws/statute/90f03.

20 Ontario Women's Justice Network. Separation agreements and other
domestic contracts [Internet]. Toronto: Ontario Women's Justice Network;
2017 [cited 2023 July 12]. Available from: https://owjn.org/2017/07/20
/separation-agreements-and-other-domestic-contracts/.

21 Sbarra DA. Divorce and health: current trends and future directions.
Psychosom Med. 2015; 77(19):227–36. https://doi.org/10.1097/PSY
.0000000000000168.

22 Ding D, Gale J, Bauman A, et al. Effects of divorce and widowhood on
subsequent health behaviours and outcomes in a sample of middle-aged
and older Australian adults. Sci Rep. 2021;11(1):15237. https://doi
.org/10.1038/s41598-021-93210-y.

23 Dupre ME, George LK, Liu G, et al. Association between divorce and
risks for acute myocardial infarction. Circ Cardiovasc Qual Outcomes.
2015;8(3):244–51. https://doi.org/10.1161/CIRCOUTCOMES.114.001291.

24 Government of Canada. Fact sheet – divorce and family violence
[Internet]." Ottawa: Government of Canada; 2022 [modified 2024 May 17].
Available from: https://www.justice.gc.ca/eng/fl-df/fsdfv-fidvf.html.

25 Centers for Disease Control and Prevention. Fast facts: preventing adverse
childhood experiences [Internet]. Atlanta: Centers for Disease Control and
Prevention; 2024. Available from: https://www.cdc.gov/aces/prevention
/index.html.

26 Amato PR. The consequences of divorce for adults and children: an
update. Druš Istraž. 2014;23(1):5–24. https://doi.org/10.5559/di.23.1.01.

27 Criddle MN, Allgood SM, Piercy KW. The relationship between mandatory
divorce education and level of post-divorce parental conflict. J Divorce
Remarriage. 2003;39(3–4):99–111. https://doi.org/10.1300/J087v39n03_05.

28 Pedro-Carroll J. Fostering resilience in the aftermath of divorce: the role of
evidence-based programs for children. Fam Court Rev. 2005;43(1):52–64.
https://doi.org/10.1111/j.1744-1617.2005.00007.

29 Emery RE, Sbarra D, Grover T. Divorce mediation: research and reflections. Fam Court Rev. 2005;43(1):22–37. https://doi.org/10.1111/ j.1744-1617 .2005.00005.x.

30 Government of Canada. Best practices for representing clients in family violence cases: part II: managing the file [Internet]. Ottawa: Government of Canada; 2022. Available from: https://justice.gc.ca/eng/rp-pr/fl-lf /famil/bpfv-mpvf/viol2b.html.

31 Hudani F. HIC-77 statute based right. In: Halsbury's laws of Canada – infants and children (2022 reissue). Toronto: Lexis Nexis Canada; 2022.

32 *Family Law Act*, RSO 1990, c F3, s 31(2). https://www.ontario.ca/laws /statute/90f03.

33 *Family Law Act*, RSO 1990, c F3, s 31(1). https://www.ontario.ca/laws /statute/90f03.

34 Community Legal Education Ontario (CLEO). What is child support? [Internet]. Toronto: CLEO; 2024 [cited 2024 Jan 30]. Available from: https://www.cleo.on.ca/en/publications/childsupport/what-child -support.

35 Hudani F. HIC-77 statute based right. In: Halsbury's laws of Canada – infants and children (2022 reissue). Toronto: Lexis Nexis Canada; 2022.

36 Hudani F. HIC-82 Divorce Act: in the place of a parent. In: Halsbury's laws of Canada – infants and children (2022 reissue). Toronto: Lexis Nexis Canada; 2022.

37 Community Legal Education Ontario (CLEO). What is child support? [Internet]. Toronto: CLEO; 2024 [cited 2024 Jan 30]. Available from: https://www.cleo.on.ca/en/publications/childsupport/what-child -support.

38 Community Legal Education Ontario (CLEO). How is child support calculated? [Internet]. Toronto: CLEO; 2021 [cited 2024 Jan 30]. Available from: https://www.cleo.on.ca/en/publications/childsupport/how-are -basic-child-support-amounts-calculated.

39 Community Legal Education Ontario (CLEO). What is child support? [Internet]. Toronto: CLEO; 2024 [cited 2024 Jan 30]. Available from: https://www.cleo.on.ca/en/publications/childsupport/what-child -support.

40 Community Legal Education Ontario. (CLEO) How is child support calculated? [Internet]. Toronto: CLEO; 2021 [cited 2024 Jan 30]. Available from: https://www.cleo.on.ca/en/publications/childsupport/how-are -basic-child-support-amounts-calculated.

41 Government of Canada. The federal child support guidelines: step by step. Ottawa: Government of Canada; 2022. Available from: https://www .justice.gc.ca/eng/rp-pr/fl-lf/child-enfant/guide/step4-etap4.html.

42 *Child Support Guidelines*, O. Reg. 391/97, s 7. Available from: https://www
.ontario.ca/laws/regulation/970391.

43 *Federal Child Support Guidelines*, SOR/97-175, s 7. Available from: https://
laws-lois.justice.gc.ca/eng/regulations/SOR-97-175/index.html.

44 Community Legal Education Ontario (CLEO). How is child support
calculated? [Internet]. Toronto: CLEO; 2021 [cited 2024 Jan 30]. Available
from: https://www.cleo.on.ca/en/publications/childsupport/how-are
-basic-child-support-amounts-calculated.

45 Community Legal Education Ontario (CLEO). How is child support
calculated? [Internet]. Toronto: CLEO; 2021 [cited 2024 Jan 30]. Available
from: https://www.cleo.on.ca/en/publications/childsupport/how-are
-basic-child-support-amounts-calculated.

46 *Federal Child Support Guidelines*, SOR/97-175, s. 16. Available from: https://
laws-lois.justice.gc.ca/eng/regulations/SOR-97-175/index.html.

47 *Federal Child Support Guidelines*, SOR/97-175, ss. 17–20. Available from:
https://laws-lois.justice.gc.ca/eng/regulations/SOR-97-175/index.html.

48 Community Legal Education Ontario (CLEO). How is spousal support
enforced? [Internet]. Toronto: CLEO; 2022. Available from: https://www
.cleo.on.ca/en/publications/spousalsupport/how-spousal-support
-enforced.

49 Community Legal Education Ontario (CLEO). How is spousal support
enforced? [Internet]. Toronto: CLEO; 2022. Available from: https://www
.cleo.on.ca/en/publications/spousalsupport/how-spousal-support
-enforced.

50 Community Legal Education Ontario (CLEO). How is spousal support
enforced? [Internet]. Toronto: CLEO; 2022. Available from: https://www
.cleo.on.ca/en/publications/spousalsupport/how-spousal-support
-enforced.

51 Government of Ontario. 5.15 – Spousal and child support [Internet].
Toronto: Government of Ontario; 2022. Available from: https://www
.ontario.ca/document/ontario-disability-support-program-policy
-directives-income-support/515-spousal-and-child.

52 Community Legal Education Ontario (CLEO). What is spousal support?
[Internet]. Toronto: CLEO; 2022 [cited 2024 Jan 30]. Available from:
https://www.cleo.on.ca/wp-content/uploads/spousalsupport.pdf.

53 Lenkinski EL, Carr A. HFA-202 limitation periods. In: Halsbury's laws of
Canada – infants and children (2022 reissue). Toronto: Lexis Nexis Canada;
2022.

54 Government of Canada. About spousal support [Internet]. Ottawa:
Government of Canada; 2022 [modified 2024 May 17]. Available from:
https://www.justice.gc.ca/eng/fl-df/spousal-epoux/ss-pae
.html?wbdisable=true.

55 Lenkinski EL, Carr A. HFA-203 conceptual grounds for entitlement. In: Halsbury's laws of Canada – infants and children (2022 reissue). Toronto: Lexis Nexis Canada; 2022.

56 Government of Canada. Spousal support advisory guidelines [Internet]. Ottawa: Government of Canada; 2022 [modified 2024 May 17]. Available from: https://www.justice.gc.ca/eng/fl-df/spousal-epoux/ssag-ldfpae.html.

57 Community Legal Education Ontario (CLEO). What is spousal support? [Internet]. Toronto: CLEO; 2022 [cited 2024 Jan 30]. Available from: https://www.cleo.on.ca/wp-content/uploads/spousalsupport.pdf.

58 Community Legal Education Ontario (CLEO). What is spousal support? [Internet]. Toronto: CLEO; 2022 [cited 2024 Jan 30]. Available from: https://www.cleo.on.ca/wp-content/uploads/spousalsupport.pdf.

59 See, for example, e.g. *Taylor v Taylor*, 34 RFL (2d) 377, 149 DLR (3d) 461 (ONSC) at para. 54.

60 Lenkinski EL, Carr A. HFA-177 law in various jurisdictions. In: Halsbury's laws of Canada – infants and children (2022 reissue). Toronto: Lexis Nexis Canada; 2022.

61 See, for example, *Family Law Act*, RSO 1990, c F3, s 19 (1). Available from: https://www.ontario.ca/laws/statute/90f03.

62 Lenkinski EL, Carr A. HFA-168 criteria. In: Halsbury's laws of Canada – infants and children (2022 reissue). Toronto: Lexis Nexis Canada; 2022; Lenkinski EL, Carr A. HFA-176 right of equal possession. In: Halsbury's laws of Canada – infants and children (2022 reissue). Toronto: Lexis Nexis Canada; 2022.

63 Lenkinski EL, Carr A. HFA-176 right of equal possession. In: Halsbury's laws of Canada – infants and children (2022 reissue). Toronto: Lexis Nexis Canada; 2022.

64 Community Legal Education Ontario (CLEO). Right to stay in the family home [Internet]. Toronto: CLEO; 2024 [cited 2024 Jan 30]. Available from: https://www.cleo.on.ca/en/publications/property-division-married -couples/right-to-stay-in-the-family-home-2.

65 Community Legal Education Ontario (CLEO). Right to stay in the family home [Internet]. Toronto: CLEO; 2024 [cited 2024 Jan 30]. Available from: https://www.cleo.on.ca/en/publications/property-division-married -couples/right-to-stay-in-the-family-home-2.

66 Lenkinski EL, Carr A. HFA-177 law in various jurisdictions. In: Halsbury's laws of Canada – infants and children (2022 reissue). Toronto: Lexis Nexis Canada; 2022.

67 See, for example, *Kerr v Baranow*, 2011 SCC 10, at paras. 1–2. Available from: https://canlii.ca/t/2fs3h.

68 Government of Ontario. Parenting time, decision-making responsibility and contact [Internet]. Toronto: Government of Ontario; 2021 [modified

2023 Nov 2]. Available from: https://www.ontario.ca/page/parenting
-time-decision-making-responsibility-and-contact.

69 Research and Statistics Division. The effects of divorce on children
[Internet]. Ottawa: Department of Justice Canada [cited 2024 Jan 30].
Available from: https://www.justice.gc.ca/eng/rp-pr/fl-lf/divorce
/wd98_2-dt98_2/wd98_2.pdf.

70 *Divorce Act*, RSC 1986, c 3 (2nd Supp), s 16(2). Available from: https://
laws-lois.justice.gc.ca/eng/acts/d-3.4/; Government of British Columbia.
What does the law mean by "best interests of the child"? [Internet].
Government of British Columbia; 2024 [updated 2024 Aug 1; cited 2023
July 12]. Available from: https://www2.gov.bc.ca/gov/content
/life-events/divorce/family-justice/family-law/parenting-apart
/best-interests#:~:text=The%20%E2%80%9Cbest%20interests%20of%20
the,%2C%20security%20and%20well%2Dbeing.

71 *Divorce Act*, RSC 1986, c 3 (2nd Supp), s 16(3). Available from: https://
laws-lois.justice.gc.ca/eng/acts/d-3.4/.

72 Navigating Onward. Parenting Capacity Assessment (PCA) [Internet].
London (ON): NavOn; n.d. [cited 2024 Jan 30]. Available from: https://
navigatingonward.com/services/parenting-capacity-assessment-pca/.

73 See, for example, *Children's Law Reform Act*, RSO 1990, c C12, s 30. Available
from: https://www.ontario.ca/laws/statute/90c12.

74 Navigating Onward. Parenting Capacity Assessment (PCA) [Internet].
London (ON): NavOn; n.d. [cited 2024 Jan 30]. Available from: https://
navigatingonward.com/services/parenting-capacity-assessment-pca/.

75 *Children's Law Reform Act*, RSO 1990, c C12, s 20(5). Available from:
https://www.ontario.ca/laws/statute/90c12. https://www.ontario.ca
/laws/statute/90c12.

76 L.S. v. B.S, 2022 ONSC 5796 at para. 73. Available from: https://canlii
.ca/t/jscj7.

77 *Personal Health Information Protection Act*, 2004, SO 2004, c 3, Sched. A.

78 *L.S. v. B.S*, 2022 ONSC 5796 at para. 61. Available from: https://canlii.ca/t/jscj7.

79 *L.S. v. B.S*, 2022 ONSC 5796 at paras. 75–77. Available from: https://canlii
.ca/t/jscj7.

80 *L.S. v. B.S*, 2022 ONSC 5796 at paras. 68–70. Available from: https://canlii
.ca/t/jscj7.

81 *L.S. v. B.S*, 2022 ONSC 5796 at paras. 68–69. Available from: https://canlii
.ca/t/jscj7.

82 *L.S. v. B.S*, 2022 ONSC 5796 at para. 65. Available from: https://canlii
.ca/t/jscj7.

83 *L.S. v. B.S*, 2022 ONSC 5796 at para. 66. Available from: https://canlii
.ca/t/jscj7.

84 *Health Care Consent Act*, 1996, SO 1996, c 2, Sched. A.

85 Jaffe PG, Crooks CV, Bala N. Making appropriate parenting arrangements in family violence cases: applying the literature to identify promising practices [Internet]. Ottawa: Government of Canada; 2005 [modified 2022 Dec 28]. Available from: https://www.justice.gc.ca/eng/rp-pr/fl-lf/parent/2005_3/p5.html.

86 Jaffe PG, Crooks CV, Bala N. Making appropriate parenting arrangements in family violence cases: applying the literature to identify promising practices [Internet]. Ottawa: Government of Canada; 2005 [modified 2022 Dec 28]. Available from: https://www.justice.gc.ca/eng/rp-pr/fl-lf/parent/2005_3/p5.html.

87 Government of Ontario. Office of the Children's Lawyer [Internet]. Toronto: Government of Ontario; 2021 [updated 2023 Dec 4]. Available from: https://www.ontario.ca/page/office-childrens-lawyer.

88 Government of Ontario. The Office of the Children's Lawyer in family law [Internet]. Toronto: Government of Ontario; 2021 [updated 2024 Mar 1]. Available from: https://www.ontario.ca/page/office-childrens-lawyer-family-law.

89 Hudani F. HIC-173 child protection legislation. In: Halsbury's laws of Canada – infants and children (2022 reissue). Toronto: Lexis Nexis Canada; 2022.

90 Family Law Education for Women. Child protection and family law [Internet]. Family Law Education for Women; n.d. [cited 2024 Jan 30]. Available from: https://onefamilylaw.ca/family-law-topics/child-protection-and-family-law/.

91 See, for example, *Child, Youth, and Family Services Act, 2017*, S.O. 2017, c. 14, Sched. 1, s. 1.

92 Hudani F. HIC-174 purposes of child protection legislation. In: Halsbury's laws of Canada – infants and children (2022 reissue). Toronto: Lexis Nexis Canada; 2022; *Child, Youth, and Family Services Act, 2017*, s. 1(2).

93 Family Law Education for Women. Child protection and family law [Internet]. Family Law Education for Women; n.d. [cited 2024 Jan 30]. Available from: https://onefamilylaw.ca/family-law-topics/child-protection-and-family-law/.

94 Family Law Education for Women. Child protection and family law [Internet]. Family Law Education for Women; n.d. [cited 2024 Jan 30]. Available from: https://onefamilylaw.ca/family-law-topics/child-protection-and-family-law/.

95 Family Law Education for Women. Child protection and family law [Internet]. Family Law Education for Women; n.d. [cited 2024 Jan 30]. Available from: https://onefamilylaw.ca/family-law-topics/child-protection-and-family-law/.

96 Family Law Education for Women. Child protection and family law [Internet]. Family Law Education for Women; n.d. [cited 2024 Jan 30]. Available from: https://onefamilylaw.ca/family-law-topics/child-protection-and-family-law/.

97 Government of Canada. The *Divorce Act* changes explained [Internet]. Ottawa: Government of Canada; 2022 [modified 2024 May 17]. Available from: https://www.justice.gc.ca/eng/fl-df/cfl-mdf/dace-clde/div15.html.

98 *Divorce Act*, RSC 1986, c 3 (2nd Supp), s 2(1). Available from: https://laws-lois.justice.gc.ca/eng/acts/d-3.4/.

99 Government of Canada. Fact sheet: Intimate partner violence [Internet]. Ottawa: Government of Canada; 2022 [modified 2024 July 31]. Available from: https://women-gender-equality.canada.ca/en/gender-based-violence/intimate-partner-violence.html.

100 Government of Canada. Fact sheet: Intimate partner violence [Internet]. Ottawa: Government of Canada; 2022 [modified 2024 July 31]. Available from: https://women-gender-equality.canada.ca/en/gender-based-violence/intimate-partner-violence.html.

101 George P, Medhekar A, Chaze F, et al. In search of interdisciplinary, holistic and culturally informed services: the case of racialized immigrant women experiencing domestic violence in Ontario. Fam Court Rev. 2022;60(3):530–45. https://doi.org/10.1111/fcre.12653.

102 Lloyd M. Domestic violence and education: examining the impact of domestic violence on young children, children, and young people and the potential role of schools. Front Psychol. 2018;9:2094. https://doi.org/10.3389/fpsyg.2018.02094.

103 Jaffe P, Campbell M, Straatman A-L, et al. Risk factors for children in situations of family violence in the context of separation and divorce [Internet]. Ottawa: Government of Canada; 2021. Available from: https://www.justice.gc.ca/eng/rp-pr/cj-jp/fv-vf/rfcsfv-freevf/p4.html.

104 Wyton M. Brain injury from abuse puts women at risk in court [Internet]. The Tyee; 2023 Feb 10 . Available from: https://thetyee.ca/News/2023/02/10/Brain-Injury-Abuse-Women-Risk-Court/.

105 Canadian Medical Protective Association. When to disclose confidential information [Internet]. Ottawa: Canadian Medical Protective Association; 2015 [revised October 2023]. Available from: https://www.cmpa-acpm.ca/en/advice-publications/browse-articles/2015/when-to-disclose-confidential-information.

106 National Domestic and Family Violence Bench Book. Impact on consent and disclosure [Internet]. Sydney (NSW): National Domestic and Family Violence Bench Book, Australasian Institute of Judicial Administration; 2023 [updated July 2024]. Available from: https://dfvbenchbook.aija.org.au/article/1080250.

107 Jaffe P, Campbell M, Straatman A-L, et al. Risk factors for children in situations of family violence in the context of separation and divorce [Internet]. Ottawa: Government of Canada; 2021. Available from: https://www.justice.gc.ca/eng/rp-pr/cj-jp/fv-vf/rfcsfv-freevf/p4.html.

108 Carman T, Ivany K, Uguen-Csenge E. Warning signs present in 1 in 3 homicides of intimate partners, CBC investigation finds [Internet]. *CBC News*, 2021 Dec 10. Available from: https://www.cbc.ca/news/canada /warning-signs-intimate-partner-homicide-1.6269761.

109 Community Legal Education Ontario (CLEO). Do you know a woman who is being abused? [Internet]. Toronto: CLEO; 2022 . Available from: https://www.cleo.on.ca/wp-content/uploads/handbook.pdf.

110 Government of Ontario. Getting a restraining order [Internet]. Toronto: Government of Ontario; 2021 [updated 2024 Feb 29]. Available from: https://www.ontario.ca/page/getting-restraining-order.

111 Government of Ontario. Getting a restraining order [Internet]. Toronto: Government of Ontario; 2021 [updated 2024 Feb 29]. Available from: https://www.ontario.ca/page/getting-restraining-order.

112 *Family Law Act*, RSO 1990, c F3, s 46. https://www.ontario.ca/laws /statute/90f03.

113 *Children's Law Reform Act*, RSO 1990, c C12, s 28(1)(c).

114 Steps to Justice. 4. Go to court to get an order for exclusive possession [Internet]. Toronto: Steps to Justice; 2021. Available from: https://stepstojustice.ca/steps /family-law/3-go-court-get-order-exclusive-possession/.

115 *Family Law Act*, RSO 1990, c F3, s 24(1). https://www.ontario.ca/laws /statute/90f03.

116 *Family Law Act*, RSO 1990, c F3, s 24(3). https://www.ontario.ca/laws /statute/90f03.

117 *Barendregt v Grebliunas*, 2022 SCC 22 at para. 147. Available from: https:// canlii.ca/t/jpbbg.

118 *Divorce Act*, RSC 1986, c 3 (2nd Supp), s 16(1). Available from: https:// laws-lois.justice.gc.ca/eng/acts/d-3.4/.

119 *Barendregt v Grebliunas*, 2022 SCC 22 at paras. 142–143. Available from: https://canlii.ca/t/jpbbg.

120 *Divorce Act*, RSC 1986, c 3 (2nd Supp), s 16.92(1). Available from: https:// laws-lois.justice.gc.ca/eng/acts/d-3.4/.

121 *Divorce Act*, RSC 1986, c 3 (2nd Supp), s 16.9(1)-(3). Available from: https://laws-lois.justice.gc.ca/eng/acts/d-3.4/.

122 *Divorce Act*, RSC 1986, c 3 (2nd Supp), ss. 16.91(1)(b) and 16.91(2). Available from: https://laws-lois.justice.gc.ca/eng/acts/d-3.4/.

Indigenous Legal Expert Reflection on Chapter 8

CAITLYN E. KASPER

As an Anishinaabekwe from the Chippewas of Georgina Island First Nation who holds an Honours Specialist in Political Science from the University of Toronto and a Juris Doctor from Osgoode Hall, I have spent more than a decade as an Indigenous person practicing in Western institutions and systems that have historically had and continued to have profound negative effects on Indigenous families.

I began the practice of law in northern Ontario for a private law firm that specialized in criminal law, and shortly thereafter it expanded to include family law, child protection, and mental health law for Indigenous people and communities that included remote fly-in First Nations reserves. I spent five years litigating in these areas before joining Aboriginal Legal Services (ALS) in Toronto as legal counsel in 2014.

Today, as a senior lawyer and manager at ALS, I have had the opportunity to use my legal expertise in appellate court law reform and test case litigation in criminal, child welfare, and civil rights and the privilege of representing Indigenous interests at every level of court in the country, including the Supreme Court of Canada.

In my role as advocate, I am reminded on a daily basis of the unique nature of Indigenous culture, history, and challenges across Canada. I am also reminded of the importance of humility in recognizing that the complex and multifaceted struggles faced by Indigenous people demand continuous unbiased and nonjudgmental interactions that foster genuine relationships of trust.

In each of the four overarching topics discussed in this chapter, there are nuances in how Indigenous people are treated under the law that, once identified and understood, can be used by a health care provider to more fully support the patient during this difficult time in their life.

A Family Law Primer

In this section, there is a focus on common terminology in the area of family law. This is an excellent place to begin, because using the correct terminology for Indigenous people, communities, and so forth can be elusive. Historically, the use of Indian status as a means of determining Indigenous identity has relied on the narrow definition of who is – and ergo who is not – an "Indian" under the *Indian Act*, first enacted in 1857.[1] Given that this piece of legislation was meant to extinguish Indigenous rights and identity through colonization, the under-inclusive nature of this term in its failure to acknowledge Métis, Inuit, and non-status Indian families is unsurprising.

Today, the emphasis for Indigenous and non-Indigenous service providers is on self-identification and inclusiveness. This is reflected, for example, in the 2018 child welfare legislation amendments in Ontario (through the *Child Youth and Family Services Act*)[2] that define a First Nations, Inuit, or Métis child or youth as one that self-identifies or has a parent that self-identifies as such.

It should also be noted that within the Indigenous community, there is a complicated relationship with organized religion that should be handled gently. Although some Indigenous individuals and communities remain largely within the Christian faith, others have decidedly not and do not refer to their beliefs or ceremonial practices as a religion. Rather, they are more commonly considered a person's spirituality or way of life.

Family Law and Health

Although the subject of child protection is mentioned only briefly in the chapter, it is imperative for health care providers to recognize the direct connection between inter-generational trauma as an aspect of psychosocial factors that can greatly contribute to mental health diagnosis and individual and family capacity to navigate crisis in both the short and the long terms.

The legal system in Canada has been used as a cruel instrument towards Indigenous people, and more specifically with respect to deconstruction of the family unit, the legislation of Section 88 of the *Indian Act* during the 1950s acted as a catalyst for overwhelming harm for generations of Indigenous children, youth, families, and communities. This section permitted Canada to enter into agreements with the provinces and territories to provide child welfare services on reserve (despite the status of reserve land as a federal responsibility and within federal jurisdiction). The result was a systematic and forceful removal of generations of Indigenous children, the details of which are more fully explained in numerous commission reports and studies nationwide, particularly the report of the Truth and Reconciliation Commission,[3] which has identified the large-scale child welfare removals of Indigenous children as cultural genocide.

This disruption in families was designed to prevent the transmission of traditional cultural values and identity from one generation to the next. Designated as the Sixties Scoop and, more recently, the Millennial Scoop, the consequences of this government action have been described by Canadian courts as leaving children fundamentally disoriented, with a reduced ability to lead healthy and fulfilling lives, and resulting in psychiatric disorders, substance abuse, and higher rates of unemployment, violence, and suicide.[4]

As such, the ability of a health care provider to provide resources and referrals that are Indigenous-specific, offered by Indigenous service providers, or both is invaluable. Although not every Indigenous patient will request Indigenous services, it is my experience that individuals are more likely to access and continue working with community organizations and programs that connect healing with culture and community.

Common Issues Affecting Patients Navigating Separation

Income security can often be a central concern for Indigenous patients, who are over-represented in lower-income households and, as such, are more likely to experience poverty and unstable housing. In situations in which financial support is a contentious issue between parties, it is helpful for the health care provider to have a general understanding of the type of legal aid available in their jurisdiction and include this as an important resource for referral.

It should be noted that for Indigenous families with children undergoing separation, if the payor parent lives or works on reserve and is not taxed on their income, this will fall under the scenario in which a court may make an adjustment and impute income to the payor parent, thereby increasing the amount of support received by the recipient parent. Likewise, matrimonial homes located on reserve are also treated differently under the law with a specific piece of legislation dedicated to this area. A patient in this situation should definitely be advised to speak with a lawyer who has working knowledge of the differences in family law that can arise for Indigenous families.

Although there is certainly legal precedent in family law concerning the best interests of the Indigenous child with respect to parental separation, parenting time, and parental decision-making that emphasizes the importance of fostering and maintaining connection with Indigenous community and culture, this has been especially developed in the area of child protection law.

It cannot be emphasized enough that there are fundamentally different approaches to child protection for Indigenous communities and families in comparison with every other non-Indigenous group in Canada. Child protection for Indigenous families is a complex web of provincial legislation, regulations, policy guidelines, federal legislation, and constitutional rights.[5] I briefly noted some of the history of child removal in Indigenous communities by government and the consequences of unchecked provincial involvement in Indigenous child apprehension. In fact, the final report of the Truth and Reconciliation Commission in 2015 included in its Calls to Action the creation of national Indigenous child welfare legislation. This call was answered with the *Act respecting First Nations, Inuit and Métis children, youth and families*.[6] On 1 January 2020, this new federal legislation came into effect for all provinces and territories in Canada and created a comprehensive reform of Indigenous child and family services.

The rules, norms, and standards outlined in this federal act must be considered and applied in every instance in which the child, youth, or family is Indigenous. It overrides provincial and territorial law and recognizes the inherent jurisdiction of First Nations over their own children and families. Furthermore, the federal act confirms the best interests of the Indigenous child as those within their cultural identity and connection to traditional territory.

There are also different time limits and different types of placement options for Indigenous children, with the focus on keeping the child within their family and community. Legal standing has been legislated for First Nations bands and communities to participate in child protection matters in which the child is a member of the First Nations. Use of customary or kinship care agreements are often an alternative to apprehension and support reconnection as the best type of planning.

These are just some of the ways in which Indigenous families and children are treated differently under the law as a direct result of the invasive colonial violence that has been inflicted on Indigenous people for generations. Although the underlying purpose of much of this legislation is to try and repair the harms that have occurred, it has been my professional experience that acting as a source of support for Indigenous people to understand the factors involved in family-related legal issues and providing encouragement for them to exercise as much control as possible over their legal process is absolutely vital as they navigate this foreign system.

Resources for Health Care Providers and Patients

As mentioned earlier, these resources should be routinely updated and expanded to include the Indigenous-specific services in each jurisdiction.

NOTES

1 *Indian Act*, RSC 1985, c I-5.
2 *Child Youth and Family Services Act*, SO 2017, c 14, Sched 1.
3 Canada, Truth and Reconciliation Commission. Canada's residential schools: the legacy. vol. 5. Montreal and Kingston (ON): McGill-Queen's University Press; 2015.
4 *Brown v Canada (Attorney General)*, 2013 ONSC 5637 at paras. 3–9.
5 Specifically, s. 7 of the *Charter of Rights and Freedoms* (*Canadian Charter of Rights and Freedoms*, Part I of the *Constitution Act, 1982*, being Schedule B to the *Canada Act 1982* (UK), 1982, c 11) and s. 35 of the *Constitution Act, 1982* (*Constitution Act, 1982*, being Schedule B to the *Canada Act 1982* (UK), 1982, c 11).
6 *Act respecting First Nations, Inuit and Métis children, youth and families*, SC 2019, c 24.

9 Health, Social, and Structural Determinants of Health in the Context of Traumatic Brain Injury and the Criminal-Legal System in Canada

FLORA I. MATHESON, PROMISE HOLMES SKINNER, AND CHRISTINE CARTHEW

This chapter provides an overview of the Canadian criminal-legal system and suggests key points of intervention for primary care providers to support their patients who become entangled in this system. The chapter focuses on a specific health issue that is highly prevalent among people who become involved with the criminal-legal system: traumatic brain injury (TBI), which has a prevalence that can reach 90 per cent. Although there are many ways the topic of health and the criminal-legal system can be understood and addressed, in our experience, brain injury provides a crucial opportunity for health providers to make a difference for their patients who are entangled with the criminal-legal system.

Patients with symptoms of TBI (e.g., poor memory and concentration, psychiatric concerns, easily frustrated or angered, sensitive to light and noise) have unique needs, do not fare well in the criminal-legal system, and require support from primary care providers at critical points in the criminal-legal process. The chapter also reviews the key health and social–structural determinants of health experienced by people who are involved with the criminal-legal system. Quality of life among these people is affected by physical and mental illnesses and substance use. Structural determinants of health among those who are involved with the criminal-legal system include poverty, homelessness, and systemic racism, the latter exemplified by the extreme over-incarceration of people from Black and Indigenous communities.

The chapter provides details on the criminal-legal process, beginning with an overview of the Canadian criminal-legal system and followed by an introduction to bail, sentencing, and parole. As you read this chapter, you will be introduced to the case of Amara, who gets entangled in the system. The chapter provides practical guidance on how primary care providers can support their patients with TBI during critical junctures in the criminal-legal process.

Amara's Story, Part 1

Dr. X is a primary care doctor who works in the downtown core of a large city. Many of their patients are involved with the criminal-legal system. Dr. X sees Amara, a 28-year-old woman who engages in sex work, about an unrelated issue, when Amara shares that she recently suffered a head injury, taking an elbow to the temple during a date, and she has now had a headache and nausea for more than 24 hours. Dr. X notices signs of confusion and is very concerned. Dr. X assesses Amara and determines she has a concussion, which is considered a TBI (see Appendix 2 for a head injury screener). Amara and her doctor agree to meet again in one week to follow up on her concussion symptoms. Unfortunately, two nights before her appointment, Amara is arrested and is not able to see her doctor.

Two nights before her doctor's appointment, Amara responds to a knock at her apartment door and is met by two police officers. Surprised and afraid, Amara pulls the door close to her body, leaving the door only slightly ajar, speaking to the officers from inside her apartment. Officers say they are responding to a call from a concerned neighbour who heard banging and yelling between a man and a woman coming from Amara's apartment. Amara does not respond, and police observe that she looks afraid and in distress. The officers ask Amara to let them into her apartment. She says no (as is her right), but the officers persist. Amara, now even more afraid, says no again. The officers continue to insist. Amara now feels cornered, trapped, and unsafe. She is starting to panic, feels overwhelmed by the situation, and finds herself unable to control her emotions. This is not usual for Amara, but since the concussion she has been quick to react to stressful situations, going into fight-or-flight mode and feeling as though she's watching herself be overtaken by her concussion symptoms.

Without her usual impulse control, Amara yells at the officers, which causes her to become more afraid, feeling uncharacteristically out of control of her emotions. An officer grabs her tightly by the arms and forces her into the hallway. In a swift reactionary motion, Amara yanks her arms from the officer's grip and accidentally strikes the officer in the face. Both officers immediately grab hold of her and slam her against the wall. She screams, terrified, and one officer slams her head against the wall again, contributing to a second head injury and aggravating her current TBI. He forces his arm around her neck, telling her to shut up and stop resisting. The other officer forces her hands behind her back and places cold, heavy metal handcuffs on her wrists and tells her she is under arrest for assaulting a police officer and resisting arrest. This further terrifies and infuriates her. She cries, yells, and begs for an explanation: "How could I resist arrest when I wasn't even under arrest?!" Met with silence, she asks if she can at least step inside to get shoes or a coat. Police ignore her pleas and drag her down the hallway and outside to the police cruiser, without shoes or a coat.

Note to primary care providers: It is important for physicians to be aware that this example is not unusual; it is not an anomaly, nor is it exceptional or dramatized. This is a common set of disturbing circumstances in an all-too-common unnecessary arrest of a person in a vulnerable situation. It is important for physicians to understand that Amara and many people in this country are routinely arrested for things that have no reasonable prospect of a criminal conviction – and therefore, many people, including Amara, experience physical and psychological harm initiated and exacerbated by the justice system, where the end result will eventually be the charges being set aside. Unfortunately, it is often a very long and painful road for the patient. We implore physicians to keep this in mind when assisting patients who find themselves wrapped up in Canadian courts. Particularly for Indigenous patients and members of racialized communities who are over-represented in the justice system, it is now well understood by lawyers and judges that a person's criminal record says just as much about the person being the target of a discriminatory justice system as it does about their propensity to commit crimes.

Traumatic Brain Injury as a Public Health Concern

The US Centers for Disease Control and Prevention define TBI as a bump, blow, or jolt to the head or a penetrating head injury that disrupts the normal function of the brain.[1] TBI is an important worldwide public health concern that is primarily an invisible impairment.[2] The global incidence of TBI is approximately 20 per 100,000 persons.[3] The worldwide annual incidence rate is 295 per 100,000,[4] and the lifetime global prevalence is 8.4 per cent.[5] Over the past 10 years the number of TBI-related emergency department visits and hospitalizations in Canada and the United States have dramatically increased; in the latter, the increase was more than 50 per cent.[6] Reports suggest that between 1.5 per cent and 2.0 per cent of the American, European, and Australian populations are living with a TBI-related disability.[7] TBI negatively affects quality of life and can lead to broad and diverse behavioural and cognitive impairments.[8]

Traumatic Brain Injury in the Criminal-Legal System

The sheer prevalence of TBI among those ensnared in the criminal-legal system is striking, with estimates of up to 10 times greater than among the general population and rates between 20 and 90 per cent.[9] Four longitudinal studies reported that TBI was associated with both non-violent criminal behaviour (i.e., arrests) and violent crime.[10] The sequelae of TBI, such as memory problems, aggression, and impulsivity, may explain why people with TBI have more involvement in the criminal-legal system, which is ill-equipped to address these health challenges and may thus perpetuate them.[11] People with TBI may have trouble in four primary domains: communication (reading, thinking), emotional dysregulation (heightened or blunted response), behavioural (impulse control), and cognitive functioning (attention, memory, reasoning).[12] TBI can negatively affect a range of aspects of cognitive functioning, for example, memory acquisition and retrieval; planning, judgment, cognitive, and emotional aspects of decision-making; and motivation and impulsivity. Cognitive and behavioural executive functioning deficits are common among people who experience mild, moderate, and severe TBI.[13] TBI can be associated with personality changes, posttraumatic stress disorder, anxiety, major depression, and substance use.[14]

Social and Structural Determinants of Health and Criminal-Legal Involvement

It is well established that the health of people incarcerated in detention centres, jails, and prisons is poor and much worse than that of the general population.[15] People who experience incarceration are at greater risk of physical and mental illnesses, substance use disorders, communicable and infectious illnesses, TBI, and developmental disabilities.[16] For example, a Canadian study reported that men newly admitted to federal penitentiaries self-reported substantial health concerns, including head injuries (34.1 per cent), back pain (19.3 per cent), asthma (14.7 per cent), and hepatitis C virus infection (9.4 per cent).[17] People involved with the criminal-legal system often experience mental illnesses, addictions, and chronic illnesses (e.g., HIV/AIDS) that are co-morbid with TBI; thus, their burden of illness is greater, as are barriers to their care. A recent Canadian review article found that the prevalence of childhood abuse was 66 per cent among incarcerated women and 36 per cent among incarcerated men.[18] The prevalence of substance use and mood, anxiety, and psychotic disorders is from 5 to 11 times higher, respectively, among people who are incarcerated relative to the general population.[19]

Racial and ethnic disparities, sex and gender inequities, poor educational attainment, poverty and homelessness, and early life abuse and neglect are abundant among people who are incarcerated.[20] They experience difficulty accessing social and health services for myriad reasons, such as discrimination, long wait lists, no fixed address, and financial insecurity.[21] Pre–COVID-19 research indicates that those released from Ontario correctional facilities have higher rates of emergency department use and hospitalization than the general population.[22] Morbidity and mortality are also high among people who have recently been released,[23] and mortality is particularly high among women and Indigenous persons.[24] A significant proportion of fatalities among people recently released from custody in Ontario are due to drug toxicity, and 22 per cent of those deaths occur within the first week of re-entry.[25] We know from previous research that people who have previously come into contact with the criminal-legal system are often refused care by family doctors and experience discrimination when they access the emergency department.[26] People with a history of incarceration tend to be younger and more likely to face income, housing, and employment precarity relative to the general population.[27]

In Canada, Black, Indigenous, and People of Colour (BIPOC) are over-represented in the criminal-legal system. Black people in Canada are subject to heightened police surveillance; are more likely to be stopped and questioned, charged, severely sentenced, and incarcerated; and are less likely to be granted parole, relative to the general population.[28(p. 83)] To exemplify, although persons from Black communities represent only 3.5 per cent of the Canadian population,[29] they represented 8 per cent of all people in federal custody in 2018–19.[30]

Likewise, the over-representation of Indigenous people, and especially Indigenous women, in the criminal-legal system in Canada is a long-standing issue. In 1991, the final report of the Aboriginal Justice Inquiry of Manitoba revealed that Indigenous people in Manitoba had been arrested and imprisoned in grossly disproportionate numbers.[31] The report stated, "Aboriginal people who are arrested are more likely than non-Aboriginal people to be denied bail, spend more time in pre-trial detention and spend less time with their lawyers, and, if convicted, are more likely to be incarcerated … It is not merely that the justice system has failed Aboriginal people; justice has also been denied to them."[32(p. 1)] This issue persists and extends to Indigenous people across Canada. Indeed, in 2017–18, Indigenous adults in Canada represented 30 per cent of admissions to provincial and territorial custody and 29 per cent of admissions to federal custody, despite representing only 4 per cent of the adult population.[33] Indigenous women in Canada are particularly over-represented in custody. In 2017–18, Indigenous females accounted for 42 per cent of female admissions to provincial and territorial custody, and Indigenous males accounted for 28 per cent of male admissions.[34] It is important to note, too, that more than 90 per cent of federally sentenced Indigenous women in Canada report a lifetime mental health and substance use diagnosis.[35]

The Truth and Reconciliation Commission of Canada (TRC) calls on all Canadians to advance and contribute to reconciliation in Canada. The TRC focused on the over-representation of Indigenous people in Canada's criminal-legal system in their final report, "Honouring the Truth, Reconciling for the Future." It made 18 calls to action to address the continued failure of the justice system with respect to Indigenous people in Canada, including their disproportionate imprisonment.[36]

Amara's Story, Part 2

We return to Amara, who, as we know from her encounter with the police, has sustained another head injury and missed her doctor's appointment.

Amara is taken to the local police station, where she is processed for assaulting a police officer and resisting arrest. She asks if she will be released from the police station. Officers refuse to release her from the station because they claim they intervened in an intimate partner violence situation, and therefore she cannot go back home because that would put her partner in danger. Amara insists that the person at her apartment is (a) not in danger, (b) not her partner, and (c) does not live there. Amara begs officers to release her from the station and asks for their help in removing the person, whom she does not know well, from her home. Amara is concerned about the safety of her home and herself when she returns. Police ignore her pleas and proceed with the booking process, which includes a series of invasive questions.

Because of her concussion, Amara has difficulty processing the questions. She becomes agitated and embarrassed. The officers perceive her to be intentionally uncooperative. Again, the officers escalate the situation rather than defuse it. They insist, unlawfully, that she be strip searched. Amara is humiliated and afraid. She waits for them to offer her a call to a lawyer, but they never do. She knows this is illegal, but she feels raising it will only cause her problems. She tries her best to sleep under the painful fluorescent lights, lying on a metal cot with no blanket, shoes, or coat.

The next morning, Amara is taken from the police station to the courthouse after an overnight stay, more than 12 hours after police took her from her apartment. She is transported to the courthouse in the back of a cargo van with other women picked up from other police stations and jails. They all ride with their hands cuffed behind their backs. When they arrive at the courthouse, Amara and the other women are paraded to an area officers disgracefully call the bullpen before they each speak with a legal aid defence lawyer in a cell that offers no privacy.[37] She is exhausted, hungry, and thirsty, with a headache so severe she cannot concentrate and it physically hurts her to speak (symptoms of her concussion). When it is her turn to see a lawyer, she is taken to a very loud area. She sits on a cold stool and faces a stranger in a suit. The stranger is yelling over all the other strangers in suits seated behind a row of plexiglass across from other accused people. The stranger introduces themself as a legal aid defence lawyer, but Amara cannot hear what they're saying over the yelling in the cells and the commotion from the bullpen. Amara is frustrated and afraid and feels herself becoming angry and irritable. The lawyer repeats their question: "WHAT'S YOUR NAME?!"

Amara manages to answer the first few questions posed to her by the legal aid lawyer, including her name, but becomes confused and triggered when asked what she was arrested for. Amara's anger and irritability are interpreted as rudeness. The legal aid lawyer questions Amara's ability to continue the interview respectfully. Amara becomes fearful that she will not get the help she needs and will be stuck in custody another night. Her fear comes across as aggression before she completely shuts down. The lawyer decides to stop the interview and does not ask Amara whether she requires medical attention. When Amara's name is called in court, the lawyer tells the court they have not been able to prepare a release plan to propose to the prosecutor, and the presiding justice adjourns Amara to the following day. Amara is taken to the women's jail for an overnight stay, a few hours' drive in the back of the cargo van. Amara is strip searched again upon arriving at the jail. By the time she arrives, she has been in custody close to 24 hours. All she has eaten is a cheese sandwich and a juice box. If someone were to ask her, she would rate her headache a 20 out of 10. She silently cries, which worsens her headache. She finally falls asleep before being awoken at 4:30 a.m. when guards rush her to breakfast before getting back in the van for court. At least, she thinks, she'll get to the courthouse before it gets loud and busy. Not so. Amara, and the other women in her van, arrive at the courthouse after 10:00 a.m., and court has already started.

Amara is taken to the cells and waits for someone to show up on the other side of the plexiglass. In the cells, the fluorescent lights aggravate Amara's severe headache. The noises bouncing off the hard surfaces and the banging of the heavy steel doors cause her head to be so painful that she throws up. A different lawyer appears. Amara is determined to keep her cool this time around to get the help she needs to get out of there. She tells the lawyer she needs to keep her eyes closed for the interview. The lawyer asks why, and Amara shares the details of her concussion, missing her doctor appointment, and the police slamming her head against the wall during the arrest and talks about the severe headache and sensitivity to light brought on by the head injuries. Amara answers all the questions during the interview, including the name and address of her doctor, and signs a release form allowing the lawyer to speak with Dr. X.

She shares that she has no family in the city to call and her friends engage in the same kind of work she does and are therefore targets of the criminal-legal system and won't be able to help either.

The lawyer says they will contact her doctor and will come back to speak with her when they've been able to reach Dr. X.

Six hours later, Amara is taken into the courtroom and sees the lawyer from that morning. Amara sees the clock on the wall, which shows that it is 4:30 p.m. Court is ending as she hears the lawyer telling the court that Amara's doctor has not responded, and so there is no release plan to propose. The justice adjourns Amara to the next day.

Amara breaks down in tears at facing another night in custody. She feels helpless – an unfamiliar feeling. The presiding justice sees Amara's distress and orders that she receive medical attention at the jail. Hours later, Amara sees a nurse at the jail who agrees that Amara has a concussion and suspects she sustained a second concussion during her arrest, but there's no way to know for sure. The nurse gives Amara ibuprofen and water and recommends rest. Her symptoms persist because of the constant loud noises from metal bars and doors, people yelling and fighting, and fluorescent lights she cannot hide from.

Note to primary care providers: It is important for physicians to be aware that this is a common scenario for newly arrested patients. Patients routinely spend more days in custody than is necessary because of backlog in the courts, and this contributes to the over-incarceration of vulnerable people.

Introduction to the Canadian Criminal-Legal System

The Canadian criminal-legal system aims to ensure public safety from those who violate criminal law. This includes objectives of preventing crime and enforcing criminal law, protecting the public, delivering justice to the victims of crime and their families, and supporting people to return to their communities after custody to become law-abiding citizens.

Sections 91 and 92 of the *Constitution Act, 1867*[38] set out federal and provincial powers with respect to the criminal-legal system. Federal powers, pursuant to section 91 of the *Constitution Act*, include the legislative power to make criminal laws and the establishment, maintenance, and management of penitentiaries. Provincial powers, pursuant to section 92 of the *Constitution Act*, include the establishment, maintenance, and management of prisons in and for the province; the administration of justice in the province, including maintenance and organization of provincial courts; and the legislative power to make quasi-criminal offences, which relate to regulatory or administrative law (e.g., *Highway Traffic Act*). Said another way, the federal government is solely responsible for enacting the criminal law, and the provincial and territorial governments are responsible for administering the criminal law.

The *Criminal Code*, together with other federal statutes, including, for instance, the *Controlled Drugs and Substances Act* and the *Youth Criminal Justice Act*, form the basis of criminal law and procedure in Canada.[39] That is, these legislative frameworks set out what constitutes a criminal offence (or crime) in Canada.

The Criminal-Legal Process

The criminal-legal process in Canada begins with the investigation of a crime. If the police reasonably believe that a person has committed a crime, they may charge the individual with that crime. When a person is charged with a crime, that person may be held in police custody for a bail hearing or released with an order to appear in court.[40] A person charged with a criminal offence is referred to as *the accused*.

It is important to note that the police have discretion to lay a charge or not. *Discretion* refers to the ability to exercise personal judgment to apply, or not, a power vested by the legal system. This is important in the context of racial bias (conscious and unconscious) in policing in Canada. It is well established that anti-BIPOC racism and racial discrimination are pervasive in policing in Canada. For instance, an inquiry by the Ontario Human Rights Commission into the racial profiling of and racial discrimination against Black people in Toronto confirmed that Black people are more likely than White people to be arrested, charged, and overcharged by the Toronto Police Service.[41] Specifically, in data from 2013 to 2017, Black people represented 32.4 per cent of the charges examined despite representing only 8.8 per cent of Toronto's population, and they had a charge rate 3.9 times that of White people.[42(p. 5)]

Note to primary care providers: It is important to be aware that although everyone in Canada has a constitutional right to retain a lawyer, that does not guarantee they will have a lawyer. People have a right to hire one, but many people cannot afford a lawyer, and most people make too much money to qualify for a legal aid lawyer or public defender. For example, someone working full time for minimum wage at a fast food restaurant may make too much money to qualify for legal aid. The unfortunate reality of Canada's legal system is that many people are left unrepresented, and many people are without someone to advocate for them. This is another reason why your patients need your help advocating for their health needs.

What Is a Bail or Release Hearing?

A bail hearing, formally called a release hearing, takes place in a court in front of a judge or a justice of the peace. The presiding justice decides whether a person who was arrested after being accused of a crime will be released to the community or detained in custody until their trial. Unfortunately, far too often, people who are not released after a hearing rush to plead guilty without a trial. This may be especially true for people with communications challenges resulting from TBI.[43] For example, a judge may engage a defendant in a conversation to ascertain whether the person is capable of entering a plea to a crime, which may be particularly challenging for persons with TBI, "who may have deficits in cognitive functions necessary to comprehend abstract and complex language."[44(p. 2)]

The lengthy wait times for trial in Canada create a situation in which innocent people (e.g., those on a detention order) can be in custody for a year or more before their trial. As a result of this gross injustice, many people who are innocent plead guilty because it means they will be released from custody and the matter will be resolved. For some people, this reality means they plead guilty and are released within days of being arrested.

During the bail hearing, the Crown prosecutor (or, in some instances, the police) will describe the nature of the offence, evidence against the accused, and any factors that might assist the court to decide whether the accused should be held in custody or released before trial.[45] There is a presumption of release in Canada, pursuant to section 11(e) of the *Canadian Charter of Rights and Freedoms*.[46] This section provides that "any person charged with an offence has the right ... not to be denied reasonable bail without just cause." This means that the accused should be released on bail unless the Crown can show cause as to why that should not be the case.[47]

The court will consider three grounds for detention when deciding whether or not to continue to detain the accused: (a) to ensure that the accused will attend court as required, (b) to protect the public, and (c) to maintain public confidence in the justice system.[48]

The least strict type of release is referred to as an "undertaking without conditions." More often, however, an accused person who is granted bail will be required to follow certain conditions given by the court. It is also possible that the court will require someone to act as surety for the accused. A surety promises the court to supervise the accused and ensure that they adhere to their bail conditions. Moreover, the supervising individual pledges a particular amount of money to the court that they must pay if the accused does not follow their bail conditions. If the accused does not have someone to name as surety, they may be able to use a bail program if one is available at the courthouse. Bail programs assign a caseworker to the accused to provide community supervision and monitor their compliance with bail conditions.

The accused, with support from their lawyer or duty counsel, will prepare a bail plan explaining how they will address the Crown's concerns about release. This might include information about where the accused will live after they are released on bail, how they will be supervised in the community, and, notably, what release conditions are reasonable and necessary in the circumstances.[49]

The Canadian Civil Liberties Association (CCLA), in its report "Set Up to Fail: Bail and the Revolving Door of Pre-Trial Detention" reported that, despite the constitutionally entrenched presumption of release, the bail system operates in a manner contrary to both the spirit and the letter of the law, to the detriment of accused persons.[50(p. 1)] The CCLA described the bail system as unnecessarily risk averse and reported that the system disproportionately penalizes poverty, problematic substance use, and mental illness.[51(p. 1)] Canadian bail courts frequently impose numerous and restrictive conditions that set people up to fail. For instance, abstinence requirements are imposed on individuals addicted to alcohol or drugs, and residency requirements are imposed on those who are unhoused.[52(p. 1)] It is a criminal offence to fail to comply with a bail condition, and criminal charges for violating bail conditions are common.[53(pp. 1–2)] The CCLA asserted that this results in a cycle of detention, restrictive release, and re-arrest that is not justifiable for reasons of public safety or to ensure that an accused person will attend court as required.[54(p. 2)]

Amara's Story, Part 3

The next morning is the same, except Amara does not see a lawyer until lunchtime. She feels hopeless, but the lawyer brings good news. Amara's doctor, Dr. X, called, and is in the process of writing a letter to support Amara's release plan. Dr. X had been quite worried about Amara since she had not shown up to her appointment the previous day and was devastated to learn that Amara had to spend a night in jail because of a delay at their office. Dr. X was not made aware by the clinic staff of Amara's situation until the end of the day yesterday. Dr. X wants Amara to know that this has prompted them to impose a new policy in their office that calls or correspondence from lawyers or staff at the courthouse must be treated as urgent and brought to their attention immediately. This policy change ends up helping many more of Dr. X's patients in the future.

An hour later, the lawyer receives Dr. X's letter. The letter details the relationship between Dr. X and Amara, noting that Amara sees Dr. X on a regular basis and that Amara is candid and forthcoming with Dr. X about her life and health issues. Dr. X describes their relationship as one of mutual respect and trust. Dr. X, of course, cannot act as a surety for Amara, or supervise her on release, nor will Dr. X go out of their way to notify authorities if Amara engages in any criminal conduct; however, Dr. X is prepared to provide the court with insight into some programs that Dr. X can refer Amara to that will help to support her while she is on release, and Dr. X can speak to why they believe these referrals will be of assistance to Amara based on Amara's history and underlying health concerns.

Dr. X is careful not to divulge any incriminating or sensitive information about Amara that could get her into more trouble with the law, especially because that is not what Dr. X has been asked to do. Dr. X was asked to write a letter to the court to provide some insight into Amara as a person (beyond the inflammatory charges she faces) and to confirm that what Amara has said is true, which is that she maintains a good relationship with her doctor, whom she sees regularly, and that Dr. X has seen growth in Amara during the time they worked together. They have observed Amara to be receptive to medical and counselling advice, and Amara has shared positive insights that Dr. X finds encouraging with respect to Amara's interest and ability to apply newly learned coping skills. Dr. X was also asked to confirm that Amara was recently diagnosed with a concussion and to opine that the circumstances in custody – if she was to be sentenced to custody (e.g., fluorescent lights, loud noises, lack of privacy, inability to limit stimuli) – would exacerbate Amara's symptoms, therefore worsening her health and prolonging her recovery, which increases the risk of long-term health issues, such as post-concussion symptoms. Dr. X was also asked to explain what steps Amara will be able to take to treat her concussion symptoms from home, to help the court understand how crucial it is for her to be home, and not in custody, during this time.

Note to primary care providers: It is recommended that physicians familiarize themselves with the conditions of custody that can adversely affect their patients, so they can help advocate for them.

It is recommended that physicians adopt Dr. X's approach and prioritize all inquiries from justice workers and lawyers as urgent, to promote the safety and well-being of their patients at risk of or in custody.

Physicians are also recommended to adopt the following approach when writing letters for patients:

- Avoid discussing unrelated, potentially incriminating information about the patient.

- Identify positives, and do not underestimate the weight that the nature of your relationship with your patient can carry. For example, meeting with you regularly may seem insignificant to you, but to the court it can demonstrate your patient's ability to maintain routine and openness to accountability.
- Highlight accomplishments, growth, and strengths you have observed in your patient during your relationship, understanding that your letter may be the only way the court can learn anything about your patient, aside from the negative information in the arrest report.
- Include relevant or recent diagnoses, symptoms, and treatment plans, explaining how custody can adversely affect your patient's progress.
- If your patient has identified hobbies and interests, please share them.

It is also important to note that at the release hearing stage, what is appropriate for a physician's letter is not the same as what is appropriate and helpful at a later stage of the criminal-legal process, such as sentencing or parole. For now, focusing on the release hearing stage, there are some key things physicians should keep in mind.

At the release (or bail) stage, your patient has only been accused of committing an offence or offences. Canadians pride themselves on preserving the right to be presumed innocent before proven guilty. This means that even though your patient is charged with an offence, they are legally innocent. Later parts of the criminal-legal process will determine whether your patient is factually innocent, but until and unless they plead guilty or are found guilty after trial, your patient, as far as you are concerned, is innocent. So, at the release hearing stage, your patient remains innocent, and you should treat them as innocent.

Because people are presumed innocent at the release stage, your letters of support at the release stage should, generally speaking, not recommend anything rehabilitative. Rehabilitative programs at the release stage betray the right to presumption of innocence and are disproportionately wrongly required by courts for Indigenous accused. Requiring terms of release to address behaviours that your patient is presumed to be innocent of is an outdated approach.

However, in some circumstances, rehabilitative programming will be appropriate for your patient if they are prepared to take responsibility for their charges in some way, either through a guilty plea or an understanding with the prosecutor that the charges will be withdrawn if the patient participates in some form of treatment program. Typically, if your patient has a history of substance dependence and they are prepared to attend substance treatment or cultural programming to address inter-generational trauma, release is sometimes an opportunity for patients to attend treatment. Prosecutors may view your patient's success in treatment in favour of withdrawing the charges, noting that your patient has taken their life in a direction that makes it less likely for them to come before the court again. Convicting them of a criminal offence and giving them a criminal record or sending them to jail would cause more harm than good, not only to your patient but to their community and society generally. However, this type of programming would not be appropriate for a patient charged with possessing one gram of cocaine after a traffic stop that probably resulted in an illegal search of the vehicle. It is important to understand that the majority of charges laid are resolved. Many charges are withdrawn. We urge you to keep in mind that charges laid against patients who experience marginalized statuses may reflect systemic racism in a discriminatory legal system.

What Is Sentencing?

A Note on Language

A person convicted of a crime is referred to as an *offender*. Note there is a growing awareness of the dehumanizing language applied to persons involved with the criminal-legal system, with calls to cease such stigmatizing practices and move towards person-centred and respectful language.[a] For example, the American Bar Association recently released a report to the House of Delegates with a resolution adopted "to eliminate the use of stigmatizing or dehumanizing labels in documents and communications and promote and facilitate the use of 'people-centered language' as well as other non-stigmatizing and humanizing terms when referring to people currently or formerly within the criminal legal system."[b(p. 1)]

a. Tran NT, Baggio S, Dawson A, et al. Words matter: a call for humanizing and respectful language to describe people who experience incarceration. BMC Int Health Hum Rights. 2018;18(1):1–6.
b. American Bar Association. Report to the House of Delegates resolution 502 (adopted). Chicago: American Bar Association, Criminal Legal Section.

If an accused person pleads guilty or is found guilty at trial, the court must then decide on a sentence.[55]

Section 718 of the *Criminal Code* provides the purpose of sentencing:

The fundamental purpose of sentencing is to protect society and to contribute, along with crime prevention initiatives, to respect for the law and the maintenance of a just, peaceful and safe society by imposing just sanctions that have one or more of the following objectives:

(a)   to denounce unlawful conduct and the harm done to victims or to the community that is caused by unlawful conduct;
(b)   to deter the offender and other persons from committing offences;
(c)   to separate offenders from society, where necessary;
(d)   to assist in rehabilitating offenders;
(e)   to provide reparations for harm done to victims or to the community; and
(f)   to promote a sense of responsibility in offenders, and acknowledgement of the harm done to victims or to the community.[56]

A fair sentence considers the circumstances and seriousness of the offence and the person's blameworthiness. Indeed, a fit sentence must be proportionate to the gravity of the offence and the person's degree of responsibility, pursuant to section 718.1 of the Canadian *Criminal Code*.[57] This is a fundamental principle of sentencing.

Other sentencing principles are provided in section 718.2 of the *Criminal Code* and include, for example, the principle of restraint: that "an offender should not be deprived of liberty, if less restrictive sanctions may be appropriate in the circumstances." The court must also consider any relevant aggravating and mitigating circumstances relating to the offence and the person. Aggravating factors might increase a person's sentence, and mitigating factors might decrease a sentence. There is some evidence to suggest that TBI and its concomitant symptoms and effects are a mitigating factor in sentencing decisions.[58]

Section 718.2(e) of the *Criminal Code* is of particular importance in the context of Indigenous over-representation in the prison system. This section provides that "all available sanctions, other than imprisonment, that are reasonable in the circumstances and consistent with the harm done to victims or to the community should be considered for all offenders, *with particular attention to the circumstances of aboriginal offenders* [emphasis added]."[59] This provision of the *Criminal Code* was interpreted by the Supreme Court of Canada for the first time in the case of *R v Gladue*.[60] In *Gladue*, the court outlined key considerations for sentencing Indigenous persons, including, for example, the unique systemic or background factors that have contributed to the individual's involvement in the criminal-legal system (at para. 93). These considerations are engaged in every case involving an Indigenous person, regardless of whether they live on or off reserve. The court's decision in *Gladue* and subsequent decision in *R v Ipeelee*[61] acknowledge and affirm the historical and ongoing realities of colonialism, their influence on Indigenous over-incarceration, and the pressing need to look to alternatives to incarceration for Indigenous persons.[62]

Note to primary care providers: At the sentencing stage, rehabilitative programming is appropriate to recommend because your patient has now been found guilty of the alleged offence.

In writing a letter for the court at the sentencing stage, here are some helpful points to focus on:

- If applicable, include your patient's history of substance dependence, as long as your patient has or is prepared to admit or disclose it to the court.
- Highlight efforts your patient has made to address any substance dependency.
- Focus on your patient's strengths and the history of what has worked for your patient.
- Focus on insights your patient has gained.
- Suggest that you work with your patient on a particular issue your patient has committed to.
- Take more detailed notes than usual when meeting with patients you know are navigating the justice system. Noting the exact words used by the patient is extremely valuable when it comes time for letter writing; even one or two words can have a big impact when they are included in your letter to show insight or growth by your patient.
- Speak about your patient's hobbies or strengths.
- Speak to the nature of your relationship. If your patient is candid with you, this is valuable information so that the court is aware that there is a professional in the community that your patient trusts and who will disclose pertinent information. If your patient is humorous or particularly polite or respectful towards you, this will go a long way to showing the court that your patient is a human being and not just the charges listed beside their name on the court docket.
- Note whether your patient has taken initiative in the past, even if it was the distant past.
- Be careful with the language you use. For example, if your patient previously attended residential treatment somewhere and managed

to stay for half the time allotted, emphasize the success of your patient making it to treatment and staying for half the time.
- Highlight what your patient learned or accomplished while in treatment, even if they did not stay the entire number of days offered by the program.
- If your client struggles to accomplish certain tasks but is aware of the reasons why, emphasize that, and what your patient is prepared to do to address it. For example, if a client has attention deficit hyperactivity disorder and recognizes that filling out forms is extremely difficult, not because of any lack of interest or effort, note, "Next time they'll bring their forms to my office and they will complete them in the waiting area before our appointment, because they do well with accountability and body doubles."
- Emphasize the waiting period for referrals so the court can be aware to schedule future court dates with enough time to allow for an answer on applications. Without this, courts will require your patient to return to court every two to four weeks. Every appearance for someone with concurrent issues is a potential opportunity for them to mistakenly miss court, which will land them in jail. Providing your expertise to minimize the potential harm is a big help.

At the sentencing stage, keep the following in mind:

- It is not appropriate to mention things that may incriminate or harm your client. This is not an ethical conundrum. This is your duty to confidentiality.
- If your patient attended treatment but did not stay the entire duration, do not phrase it as a failure. It isn't. The fact that they attended is a success, as are the days they stayed. Avoid phrases such as *attended treatment without success* or *did not complete*. Instead use language such as *attended for x number of days* and *attended x days of the y days offered by the program*.

What Is Parole?

Parole refers to a period of conditional release that allows a person to serve part of their prison sentence in the community, under state supervision. Public safety is a primary consideration in all parole decisions. Parole is intended to promote public safety by supporting people to reintegrate into society as law-abiding citizens.

Parole must be ordered by a parole board. The Parole Board of Canada has exclusive authority to grant (and revoke) parole for people serving sentences of two years or more, pursuant to the *Corrections and Conditional Release Act*.[63] The Parole Board of Canada also makes parole decisions for people serving sentences of less than two years in most provinces and territories, with the exceptions of Ontario, Quebec, and Alberta, which have their own parole boards.

People on parole are required to follow standard conditions, including reporting to a parole officer. Parole boards can also impose additional ("special") conditions (e.g., to abstain from the use of drugs and alcohol).[64]

What Is Probation?

Probation comes in the form of court-ordered conditions that your patient has to comply with after the resolution of their charges. Probation may follow a jail sentence, but it is often used to supervise the patient in the community without the need for further sanctions. Probation is intended to be a rehabilitative tool, not a form of punishment. So probationary terms should be helpful to the patient, such as access to free counselling and support from a probation officer; in reality, however, probation is often extremely onerous and makes patients feel like they are still stuck in the threatening shadow of the criminal-legal system. The reporting conditions of a probation can set patients with TBI up for failure because it can be difficult for them to remember to report to their probation officer regularly. And the consequence for failing to report is almost always a criminal charge of failing to comply with a court order. This is a serious offence because the criminal-legal system takes crimes against its administration (arguably too) seriously.

Amara does not face probation, fortunately, because her case ends before sentencing, and her charges are eventually withdrawn by the prosecutor, with the help of the letter from Dr. X explaining her TBI diagnosis and symptoms, and with the help of her lawyer's advocacy. However, there is another pivot point of the criminal-legal system where physicians can assist their patients, and that is probation.

Note to primary care providers: Clinicians can write a letter to provide the prosecutor, or the court, with the intention of informing the decision-maker about what terms and conditions would be reasonable for your patient to be responsible for adhering to and which terms and conditions may be difficult or impossible for your patient to comply with considering their TBI diagnosis and their particular abilities and limitations. For example, some patients will be unable to comply with a reporting condition because of their memory issues. Similarly, some patients may be unable to physically attend a probation officer's office on a weekly basis because it will mean choosing between reporting to probation or attending a medical appointment, simply because their energy levels are so dangerously low they cannot conceivably attend two appointments in the same week. Explaining this in your letter and encouraging decision-makers to draft the terms and conditions in a way that delegates referral for counselling through the physician rather than the probation officer will also go a long way to avoid inviting people to breach their conditions and setting them up for failure. Giving the decision-maker as much information as you can to assist in setting your patient up for success is incredibly helpful to everyone involved.

In writing a letter for the court at this stage, a helpful point to focus on, in addition to the points listed for the sentencing stage, follows:

- Note that if your client is on probation, they are required by the court to sign a release allowing the probation officer to speak with service providers. However, because signing the release with probation is not voluntary, many service providers, including physicians, obviously do not disclose anything to probation without the client signing a release with the service provider.

Practical Guidelines on How to Help Your Patient at Critical Junctures in the Criminal-Legal System

It is recommended that primary care providers adopt this approach when writing letters for clients:

- Avoid discussing unrelated, potentially incriminating information about the patient.
- Identify positives, and do not underestimate the weight that the nature of your relationship with your patient can carry. For example, meeting with you regularly may seem insignificant to you, but to the court it can demonstrate your patient's ability to maintain routine and openness to accountability.
- Highlight accomplishments, growth, and strengths you have observed in your patient during your relationship, understanding that your letter may be the only way the court can learn anything about your patient, aside from the negative information in the arrest report.
- Include relevant or recent diagnoses, symptoms, and treatment plans, explaining how custody can adversely affect your patient's progress.
- If your patient has identified hobbies and interests, please share them.

Conclusion

The criminal-legal system is complex and difficult to understand and navigate, especially for people who have sustained a TBI. This chapter explored the Canadian criminal-legal system and used a case study approach to illustrate how people become entangled with the system and some practical ways that primary care providers can support their patients with TBI at critical junctures in the system. Primary care providers can play a critical role in ensuring that release and sentencing conditions reflect patients' abilities and limitations related to their TBI.

NOTES

1 Centers for Disease Control and Prevention. Rates of TBI-related emergency department visits by age group – United States, 2001–2010 [Internet]. Atlanta: Centers for Disease Control and Prevention; 2014 [cited 2023 July 21]. Available from: http://www.cdc.gov/traumaticbraininjury/data/rates_ed_byage.html; Taylor CA, Bell MJ, Breiding MJ, et al. Traumatic brain injury-related emergency department visits, hospitalizations, and deaths – United States, 2007 and 2013. MMWR Surveill Summ. 2017;66(9):1–16. https://doi.org/10.15585/mmwr.ss6609a1.

2 Traumatic brain injury: time to end the silence. Lancet Neurol. 2010;9(4): 331. https://doi.org/10.1016/S1474-4422(10)70069-7.

3 Bryan-Hancock C, Harrison J. The global burden of traumatic brain injury: preliminary results from the Global Burden of Disease Project. Inj Prev; 2010;16(Suppl. 1):A17.

4 Badhiwala JH , Wilson JR, Fehlings MG. Global burden of traumatic brain and spinal cord injury. Lancet Neurol. 2019;18(1):24–5.

5 Nguyen R, Fiest KM, McChesney J, et al. The international incidence of traumatic brain injury: a systematic review and meta-analysis. Can J Neurol Sci. 2016;43(6):774–85. https://doi.org/10.1017/cjn.2016.290.

6 Centers for Disease Control and Prevention. Rates of TBI-related emergency department visits by age group – United States, 2001–2010 [Internet]. Atlanta: Centers for Disease Control and Prevention; 2014 [cited 2023 July 21]. Available from: http://www.cdc.gov/traumaticbraininjury/data/rates_ed_byage.html; Ng R, Maxwell CJ, Yates EA, et al. Brain disorders in Ontario: prevalence, incidence and costs from health administrative data [Internet]. Toronto: Institute for Clinical Evaluative Sciences; 2015. Available from: http://www.ices.on.ca/flip-publication/BrainDisordersInOntario2015/index.html#4/z

7 Tagliaferri F, Compagnone C, Korsic M, et al. A systematic review of brain injury epidemiology in Europe. Acta Neurochir. 2006;148(3):255–68; Langlois JA, Rutland-Brown W, Wald MM. The epidemiology and impact of traumatic brain injury: a brief overview. J Head Trauma Rehabil. 2006;21(5):375–8.

8 Stéfan A, Mathé J-F. What are the disruptive symptoms of behavioral disorders after traumatic brain injury? A systematic review leading to recommendations for good practices. Ann Phys Rehabil Med. 2016;59(1):5–17. https://doi.org/http://dx.doi.org/10.1016/j.rehab.2015.11.002; Carroll LJ, Cassidy JD, Cancelliere C, et al. Systematic review of the prognosis after mild traumatic brain injury in adults: cognitive, psychiatric, and mortality outcomes: results of the international collaboration on mild traumatic brain injury prognosis. Arch Phys Med Rehabil. 2014;95(3 Suppl):S152–S173. https://doi.org/10.1016/j.apmr.2013.08.300.

9 Gunter TD, Philibert R, Hollenbeck N. Medical and psychiatric problems among men and women in a community corrections residential setting. Behav Sci Law. 2009;27(5):695–711; Allely CS. Prevalence and assessment of traumatic brain injury in prison inmates: a systematic PRISMA review. Brain Inj. 2016;30:1161–80. https://doi.org/10.1080/02699052.2016.11916 74; O'Rourke C, Linden MA, Lohan M, et al. Traumatic brain injury and co-occurring problems in prison populations: a systematic review. Brain Inj. 2016;30(7):839–54. https://doi.org/10.3109/02699052.2016.1146967; Bradley R, Sapp D, Kincaid A. Traumatic brain injury among Indiana state prisoners. J Forensic Sci. 2014;59(5):1248–53. https://doi.org/10.1111/1556 -4029.12466.

10 Fazel S, Seewald K. Severe mental illness in 33 588 prisoners worldwide: systematic review and meta-regression analysis. Br J Psychiatry. 2012;200(5):364–73; Schofield PW, Malacova E, Preen DB, et al. Does traumatic brain injury lead to criminality? A whole-population retrospective cohort study using linked data. PLoS One. 2015;10(7):e0132558; McKinlay A, Corrigan J, Horwood LJ, et al. Substance abuse and criminal activities following traumatic brain injury in childhood, adolescence, and early adulthood. J Head Trauma Rehabil 2014;29(6):498–506; Timonen M, Miettunen J, Hakko H, et al. The association of preceding traumatic brain injury with mental disorders, alcoholism and criminality: the Northern Finland 1966 Birth Cohort Study. Psychiatry Res. 2002;113(3):217–26.

11 See, for example, Bryant RA, O'Donnell ML, Creamer M, et al. The psychiatric sequelae of traumatic injury. Am J Psychiatry. 2010;167(3):312–20; Riggio S, Wong M. Neurobehavioral sequelae of traumatic brain injury. Mt Sinai J Med. 2009;76(2):163–72; Kaba F, Diamond P, Haque A, et al. Traumatic brain injury among newly admitted adolescents in the New

York city jail system. J Adolesc Health 2014;54(5):615–7; Lane KS, St Pierre ME, Lauterbach MD, et al. Patient profiles of criminal behavior in the context of traumatic brain injury. J Forensic Sci. 2017;62(2):545–48; Durand E, Fix M, Weiss JJ, et al. Prevalence of history of traumatic brain injury in prison population: a review. Ann Phys Rehabil Med. 2014;57:e70–e71. https://doi.org/10.1016/j.rehab.2014.03.253; Durand E, Watier L, Fix M, et al. History of traumatic brain injury among prisoners: differences depending on the severity of the reported trauma. Ann Phys Rehabil Med. 2014;57:e71. https://doi.org/10.1016/j.rehab.2014.03.254.

12 Wiseman-Hakes C. Traumatic brain injury: integrating TBI, mental health and addictions research program. Toronto: Neurodevelopmental Disabilities; 2019.

13 Rabinowitz AR, Levin HS. Cognitive sequelae of traumatic brain injury. Psychiatr Clin North Am. 2014;37(1):1–11.

14 Sacks AL, Fenske CL, Gordon WA, et al. Co-morbidity of substance abuse and traumatic brain injury. J Dual Diagn. 2009;5(3–4):404–17; Walker R, Hiller M, Staton M, et al. Head injury among drug abusers: an indicator of co-occurring problems. J Psychoact Drugs 2003;35(3):343–53; Walker R, Staton M, Leukefeld CG. History of head injury among substance users: preliminary findings. Subst Use Misuse. 2001;36(6–7):757–70.

15 Taylor CA, Bell JM, Breiding MJ, et al. Traumatic brain injury-related emergency department visits, hospitalizations, and deaths – United States, 2007 and 2013. MMWR Surveill Summ. 2017;66(9):1–16. https://doi .org/10.15585/mmwr.ss6609a1.

16 Langlois JA, Rutland-Brown W, Wald MM. The epidemiology and impact of traumatic brain injury: a brief overview. J Head Trauma Rehabil. 2006;21(5):375–78; Traumatic brain injury: time to end the silence. Lancet Neurol. 2010;9(4):331. https://doi.org/10.1016/S1474-4422(10)70069-7; Timonen M, Miettunen J, Hakko H, et al. The association of preceding traumatic brain injury with mental disorders, alcoholism and criminality: the Northern Finland 1966 Birth Cohort Study. Psychiatry Res. 2002;113(3):217–26; Hayes MO. The life pattern of incarcerated women: the complex and interwoven lives of trauma, mental illness, and substance abuse. J Forensic Nurs. 2015;11(4): 214–22. https://doi.org/10.1097 /JFN.0000000000000092; Fazel S, Seewald K. Severe mental illness in 33 588 prisoners worldwide: systematic review and meta-regression analysis. Br J Psychiatry. 2012;200(5):364–73.

17 Ng R, Maxwell CJ, Yates EA, et al. Brain disorders in Ontario: prevalence, incidence and costs from health administrative data [Internet]. Toronto: Institute for Clinical Evaluative Sciences; 2015. Available from: http:// www.ices.on.ca/flip-publication/BrainDisordersInOntario2015/index .html#4/z.

18 Bodkin C, Pivnick L, Bondy SJ, et al. History of childhood abuse in
    populations incarcerated in Canada: a systematic review and meta-
    analysis. Am J Public Health. 2019;109(3): e1–e11.

19 Kouyoumdjian FG, Cheng SY, Fung K, et al. The health care utilization
    of people in prison and after prison release: a population-based cohort
    study in Ontario, Canada. PLoS One. 2018;13(8):e0201592. https://doi
    .org/10.1371/journal.pone.0201592; Butsang T, McLuhan A, Keown LA,
    et al. Sex differences in pre-incarceration mental illness, substance use,
    injury and sexually transmitted infections and health service utilization: a
    longitudinal linkage study of people serving federal sentences in Ontario.
    Health Justice. 2023;11(1):19. https://doi.org/10.1186/s40352-023-00218-9.

20 Gunter TD, Philibert R, Hollenbeck N. Medical and psychiatric problems
    among men and women in a community corrections residential setting.
    Behav Sci Law. 2009;27(5):695–711; Hayes MO. The life pattern of
    incarcerated women: the complex and interwoven lives of trauma,
    mental illness, and substance abuse. J Forensic Nurs. 2015;11(4):214–22.
    https://doi.org/10.1097/JFN.0000000000000092; John Howard Society
    of Ontario. Remand in Ontario: a backgrounder [Internet]. Toronto: The
    Society; 2005. Available from: https://johnhoward.on.ca/wp-content
    /uploads/2014/09/remand-in-ontario-a-backgrounder-september-2005.pdf.

21 Frank JW, Wang EA, Nunez-Smith M, et al. Discrimination based on
    criminal record and healthcare utilization among men recently released
    from prison: a descriptive study. Health Justice. 2014;2(2):1–8; Wilper
    AP, Woolhandler S, Boyd JW, et al. The health and health care of US
    prisoners: results of a nationwide survey. Am Journal Public Health.
    2009;99(4):666–72. https://doi.org/10.2105/AJPH.2008.144279; Moschetti
    K, Zabrodina V, Stadelmann P, et al. Exploring differences in healthcare
    utilization of prisoners in the Canton of Vaud, Switzerland. PLoS One.
    2017;12(10):e0187255. https://doi.org/10.1371/journal.pone.0187255;
    Kouyoumdjian FG, Cheng SY, Fung K, et al. The health care utilization of
    people in prison and after prison release: a population-based cohort study
    in Ontario, Canada. PLoS One. 2018;13(8):e0201592. https://doi
    .org/10.1371/journal.pone.0201592; Hawks L, Wang EA, Howell B, et al.
    Health status and health care utilization of US adults under probation:
    2015–2018. Am J Public Health. 2020;110(9):1411–7. https://doi
    .org/10.2105/AJPH.2020.305777.

22 Kouyoumdjian FG, Cheng SY, Fung K, et al. The health care utilization
    of people in prison and after prison release: a population-based cohort
    study in Ontario, Canada. PLoS One. 2018;13(8):e0201592. https://doi
    .org/10.1371/journal.pone.0201592; Butsang T, McLuhan A, Keown LA,
    et al. Sex differences in pre-incarceration mental illness, substance use,
    injury and sexually transmitted infections and health service utilization: a

longitudinal linkage study of people serving federal sentences in Ontario. Health Justice. 2023;11(1):19. https://doi.org/10.1186/s40352-023-00218-9.

23 Kouyoumdjian FG, Cheng SY, Fung K, et al. The health care utilization of people in prison and after prison release: a population-based cohort study in Ontario, Canada. PLoS One. 2018;13(8):e0201592. https://doi .org/10.1371/journal.pone.0201592; Butsang T, McLuhan A, Keown LA, et al. Sex differences in pre-incarceration mental illness, substance use, injury and sexually transmitted infections and health service utilization: a longitudinal linkage study of people serving federal sentences in Ontario. Health Justice. 2023;11(1):19. https://doi.org/10.1186/s40352-023-00218-9.

24 Binswanger IA, Blatchford PJ, Mueller SR, et al. Mortality after prison release: opioid overdose and other causes of death, risk factors, and time trends from 1999 to 2009. Ann Intern Med. 2013;159(9):592–600. https:// doi.org/10.7326/0003-4819-159-9-201311050-00005; Singh D, Prowse S, Anderson M. Overincarceration of Indigenous people: a health crisis. CMAJ. 2019;191(18):E487–E488.

25 Groot E, Kouyoumdjian FG, Kiefer L, et al. Drug toxicity deaths after release from incarceration in Ontario, 2006–2013: review of coroner's cases. PloS One. 2016;11(7):e0157512. https://doi.org/10.1371/journal .pone.0157512.

26 Frank JW, Wang EA, Nunez-Smith M, et al. Discrimination based on criminal record and healthcare utilization among men recently released from prison: a descriptive study. Health Justice. 2014;2(2):1–8.

27 Li M. From prisons to communities: confronting re-entry challenges and social inequality. What makes re-entry into communities challenging? SES Indicat. 2018;11(1):1–9.

28 O'Grady B, Gaetz S. Homelessness, gender and subsistence: the case of Toronto street youth. J Youth Stud. 2004;7(4):397–416; Maynard R. Policing Black lives: state violence in Canada from slavery to the present. Black Point (NS): Fernwood Publishing; 2017.

29 Statistics Canada. Canada's Black population: growing in number and diversity. Ottawa: Statistics Canada; 2019.

30 Office of the Correctional Investigator. Annual report 2018–2019 [Internet]. Ottawa: Office of the Correctional Investigator; 2019. Available from: https://oci-bec.gc.ca/sites/default/files/2023-06/annrpt20182019-eng .pdf.

31 Clark, Scott. 2019. Overrepresentation of indigenous people in the Canadian criminal justice system: causes and responses. Ottawa: Department of Justice Canada; 2019.

32 Clark S. Overrepresentation of indigenous people in the Canadian criminal justice system: causes and responses. Ottawa: Department of Justice Canada; 2019.

33 Malakieh J. Adult and youth correctional statistics in Canada, 2017/2018. Ottawa: Statistics Canada; 2019.

34 Malakieh J. Adult and youth correctional statistics in Canada, 2017/2018. Ottawa: Statistics Canada; 2019.

35 Native Women's Association. Over-incarceration of Indigenous women: policy brief. Gatineau (QC): Native Women's Association of Canada; 2020.

36 Truth and Reconciliation Commission of Canada. Honouring the truth, reconciling for the future. Vol. 1: Summary. Toronto: James Lorimer; 2015.

37 The legal aid defence lawyer may be duty counsel, per diem, or public defender, depending on the jurisdiction.

38 *Constitution Act 1867*, 30 & 31 Victoria, c. 3 (U.K.).

39 *Criminal Code*, RSC 1985, c C-46; *Controlled Drugs and Substances Act*, SC 1996, c 19; *Youth Criminal Justice Act*, SC 2002, c 1.

40 John Howard Society of Ontario. An overview of the bail process. Toronto: John Howard Society of Ontario; 2022.

41 Ontario Human Rights Commission. A disparate impact: second interim report on the inquiry into racial profiling and racial discrimination of Black persons by the Toronto Police Service [Internet]. Toronto: Ontario Human Rights Commission; 2020. Available from: https://www.ohrc.on.ca/sites/default/files/A per cent20Disparate%20Impact%20Second%20interim%20report%20on%20the%20TPS%20inquiry%20executive%20summary.pdf#overlay-context=en/disparate-impact-second-interim-report-inquiry-racial-profiling-and-racial-discrimination-black.

42 Ontario Human Rights Commission. A disparate impact: second interim report on the inquiry into racial profiling and racial discrimination of Black persons by the Toronto Police Service [Internet]. Toronto: Ontario Human Rights Commission; 2020. Available from: https://www.ohrc.on.ca/sites/default/files/A%20Disparate%20Impact%20Second%20interim%20report%20on%20the%20TPS%20inquiry%20executive%20summary.pdf#overlay-context=en/disparate-impact-second-interim-report-inquiry-racial-profiling-and-racial-discrimination-black.

43 Turkstra L, Wszalek J. Comprehension of legal language by adults with and without traumatic brain injury. J Head Trauma Rehabil. 2019;34(3):E55; Williams H, Wszalek JA, Turkstra LS. Language impairments in youths with traumatic brain injury: implications for participation in criminal proceedings. J Head Trauma Rehabil. 2015;30(2):86–93.

44 Turkstra L, Wszalek J. Comprehension of legal language by adults with and without traumatic brain injury. J Head Trauma Rehabil. 2019;34(3):E55.

45 Government of Canada. Bail [Internet]. Ottawa: Government of Canada; 2021. Available from: https://www.justice.gc.ca/eng/cj-jp/victims-victimes/report-signale/bail-liberation.html.

46 *Canadian Charter of Rights and Freedoms,* Part I of the *Constitution Act, 1982,* being Schedule B to the *Canada Act 1982* (UK), 1982, c 11.

47 John Howard Society Ontario. An overview of the bail process. Toronto: John Howard Society Ontario; 2022.

48 John Howard Society Ontario. An overview of the bail process. Toronto: John Howard Society Ontario; 2022.

49 Steps to Justice. What is bail? [Internet]. Toronto: Steps to Justice; 2018. Available from: https://stepstojustice.ca/questions/criminal-law/what -bail-hearing/.

50 Deshman A, Myers N. Set up to fail: bail and the revolving door of pre-trial detention [Internet]. Toronto: Canadian Civil Liberties Association and Education Trust; 2014. Available from: https://ccla.org/wp-content /uploads/2021/07/Set-up-to-fail-FINAL.pdf.

51 Deshman A, Myers N. Set up to fail: bail and the revolving door of pre-trial detention [Internet]. Toronto: Canadian Civil Liberties Association and Education Trust; 2014. Available from: https://ccla.org/wp-content /uploads/2021/07/Set-up-to-fail-FINAL.pdf.

52 Deshman A, Myers N. Set up to fail: bail and the revolving door of pre-trial detention [Internet]. Toronto: Canadian Civil Liberties Association and Education Trust; 2014. Available from: https://ccla.org/wp-content /uploads/2021/07/Set-up-to-fail-FINAL.pdf.

53 Deshman A, Myers N. Set up to fail: bail and the revolving door of pre-trial detention [Internet]. Toronto: Canadian Civil Liberties Association and Education Trust; 2014. Available from: https://ccla.org/wp-content /uploads/2021/07/Set-up-to-fail-FINAL.pdf.

54 Deshman A, Myers N. Set up to fail: bail and the revolving door of pre-trial detention [Internet]. Toronto: Canadian Civil Liberties Association and Education Trust; 2014. Available from: https://ccla.org/wp-content /uploads/2021/07/Set-up-to-fail-FINAL.pdf.

55 In law, a person convicted of a crime is referred to as an *offender.* Although we acknowledge that this is a term used by the legal system, in writing this chapter we prefer to use person-centred language except where we are quoting statues or laws. Person-centred language is central to reducing the stigma experienced by people who are involved with the criminal-legal system (see Harney BL, Korchinski M, Young P, et al. It is time for us all to embrace person-centred languages for people in prison and people who were formerly in prison. Int J Drug Policy. 2022;99:103455. https://doi.org/10.1016/j.drugpo .2021.103455).

56 *Criminal Code* RSC, 1985, c C-46.

57 *Criminal Code* RSC, 1985, c C-46.

58 *R v Jarmulowicz,* 2017 ONCJ 332; *R v Adamo,* 2013 MBQB 225; *R v Randhawa,* 2020 ONCA 38.

59 *Criminal Code* RSC, 1985, c C-46.

60 *R v Gladue* [1999] 1 SCR 688.

61 *R v Ipeelee* (2012 SCC 13).

62 Department of Justice Canada. Spotlight on Gladue: challenges, experiences and possibilities in Canada's criminal justice system. Ottawa: Department of Justice Canada, Research and Statistics Division; 2017; Rudin J. Indigenous people and the criminal justice system. 2nd ed. Toronto: Emond Publishing; 2022.

63 *Corrections and Conditional Release Act*, SC 1992, c 20.

64 Parole Board of Canada. Parole Board of Canada: contributing to public safety. Ottawa: Minister of Public Works and Government Services Canada; 2011.

10 Common Legal Issues Affecting People Living with HIV/AIDS

ROBIN NOBLEMAN, DEBBIE RACHLIS, RYAN PECK,
DEVAN NAMBIAR, AND GORDON ARBESS

There are few examples of the role played by social determinants of health that are clearer than their impacts on people living with HIV.[1] The conditions in which people living with HIV "are born, grow, live, work and age, including the health system"[2(p. 3)] determine their health outcomes to a great extent. The law and legal system affect the social determinants of health in varied ways, and access to justice can itself be considered a social determinant.[3]

This chapter explores and examines some common legal problems facing many of the nearly 63,000 people living with HIV in Canada and how those problems can affect their health.[4] The intersection between legal and health problems is so central in the context of HIV that the US Centers for Disease Control and Prevention has recommended a referral to legal services for people diagnosed with HIV as part of their guidelines for care.[5] But access to legal knowledge and understanding among people living with HIV is not always straightforward. Populations most likely to be living with, and affected by, HIV, including gay, bisexual, and other men who have sex with men (GBMSM); African, Caribbean, and Black communities; Indigenous communities; and people who inject drugs, also face multiple intersecting barriers to health.[6] The effects of trauma, colonization, and systemic discrimination continue to create barriers to accessing legal services for certain populations of people living with, and affected by, HIV. Experiences of discrimination at the hands of various state-run systems may deter people from accessing supports. Addictions and mental health issues, including HIV-related cognitive issues, compound these barriers.

The HIV/AIDS movement has long been driven by the greater and meaningful involvement of people living with HIV.[7] This chapter takes an approach that centres the needs and perspectives of people living with HIV in providing guidance on major legal issues they face. The first section considers human rights and anti-discrimination laws in the context of HIV. The second section explores the related issues of privacy and disclosure, a major concern for many people living with HIV. The third section follows with a discussion of how the criminal law regarding non-disclosure of HIV-positive status exacerbates stigma and creates harm, and the fourth section discusses public health law as it relates to HIV testing, reporting, and the use of public health authorities' coercive powers. The fifth section provides a brief overview of access to medications under public and private programs. The chapter ends with a survey of immigration and refugee law issues related to HIV.

Most of the sections of this chapter, including public health, human rights, privacy law, and access to medications, fall under provincial or territorial jurisdiction and therefore vary across the country. Quebec follows the civil law system, so the law may operate differently there than in provinces that follow the common law system (i.e., law made by courts). Although this chapter is intended to provide an overview that applies to all jurisdictions in Canada, all of the authors practice and work in Ontario. As a result, some examples will draw on the law in Ontario with which we are most familiar.[8]

Experts in Our Own Lives: Devan Nambiar, MSc

I am a cisgender South Asian gay man who has lived with HIV for 33 years. For 25 years, I have worked in the HIV sector with communities and people living with HIV in Canada and abroad. For many people living with HIV, from the early days of HIV to those recently diagnosed, it has been and remains difficult to live with a highly stigmatized virus. The stigma is compounded by poverty, gender inequity, sexual orientation, Indigeneity, race, poverty, intimate partner violence, immigration status, and other factors that comprise the social determinants of health. In more than 40 years of HIV, the treatment of HIV has evolved. Still, little has changed regarding HIV stigma because the virus continues to be linked with sexual orientation, sexual practices, homophobia, death, and social discomfort. People living with HIV also face other challenges that can affect their health.

North America has the largest cohort of aging people living with HIV in the world, many of whom did not start treatment until some time after their HIV diagnosis. How HIV will affect brain functions as people age is not known. Despite advancement in antiretroviral therapy in the early

2000s, HIV-associated neurocognitive disorders (HAND) have increased as the population of people living with HIV ages.[a] Older individuals do not know whether their memory lapses are due to a natural aging process or to HAND.

Some people living with HIV are addicted to various substances. There are multiple motivations for using different substances, such as coping with isolation, stigma, discrimination, feeling good, the trauma of HIV diagnosis, and dealing with life stressors.[b] The cure for HIV is light years away, and people find ways to cope and live with a stigmatized virus. Each person living with HIV is an expert on their life and how they manage the social determinants of health and intersecting identities while navigating multiple ways of being in a global culture that stigmatizes them for a viral infection.

The message for health care providers is to build a therapeutic relationship and to see each person as the expert on their health and life. To provide client-centred care, it is essential to consider all the intersections of the person's life. Do not focus only on the clinical aspects of CD4 and viral load. Beneath the HIV status is a person full of dreams, desires, and ambitions to live a whole life.

[a] Reilly JK, Singh NN, Thomas PF, et al. HIV-associated neurocognitive disorder [Internet]. Medscape; 2022 Feb 17. Available from: https://emedicine.medscape.com/article/1166894-overview.

[b] Community-Based Research Centre. U=U, PrEP, substance use, and HIV self-testing: key findings from Sex Now 2021 [Internet]. Vancouver (BC): The Centre; 2022. Available from: https://www.cbrc.net/u_u_prep_substance_use_and_hiv_self_testing_key_findings_from_sex_now_2021.

Human Rights and Anti-Discrimination Laws

HIV-related stigma arises from fear and ignorance about HIV, hostility towards and existing prejudices about the groups most affected by it (e.g., GBMSM, people who inject drugs, Indigenous communities, and Black persons), or both. HIV-related discrimination is the unfair treatment of people on the basis of their actual or suspected HIV-positive status. Discrimination against people living with HIV also extends to those populations at greater risk of HIV.[9] HIV stigma and accompanying discrimination remain pervasive in Canada. Recent Canadian studies found that 40 per cent of Canadians would not use the services of a dentist or doctor living with HIV, 24 per cent of Canadians would not use the services of a hairstylist or barber living with HIV, and 88 per cent of Canadians believe that people living with HIV can experience difficulty getting housing, health care, and employment because of HIV-related stigma.[10]

This section explores protections against HIV-related discrimination and how health care providers can support people living with HIV in upholding their human rights. The section concludes with a brief exploration of remedies for human rights disputes.

Discrimination means unequal or different treatment causing harm. Only some types of unequal treatment are considered illegal discrimination. One element of illegal discrimination is that a person is treated differently on the basis of a characteristic or ground protected by the relevant human rights statute, such as disability, race, or sexual orientation. The protection against discrimination applies in certain social areas such as services, housing, and employment. Human rights laws do not apply outside of the areas listed in a given human rights statute, such as in private interpersonal interactions. General unfairness that is not based on one of the listed grounds is not considered illegal discrimination. For more detailed information on human rights law, see chapter 2 of this volume.

Protections against HIV-Related Discrimination

Disability is a protected ground under human rights laws in all Canadian jurisdictions. Disability is interpreted broadly in human rights law and includes present and past medical conditions, as well as being perceived as having a disability even if one does not.[11] Although not everyone living with HIV identifies HIV as a disability, human rights laws in Canada do consider HIV and AIDS to be disabilities.[12] This means that different and unequal treatment on the basis of HIV status or an AIDS diagnosis can be discriminatory. Addictions and mental health conditions are also considered disabilities.

People may also face complex discrimination based on intersecting personal characteristics. For example, a Black woman living with HIV or a Two-Spirit person living with HIV might experience different layers of discrimination that cannot be easily separated. In fact, many people living with HIV identify with multiple protected grounds and have lived experience of marginalization and exclusion because of how these identities intersect. Their identities may be highly relevant to understanding how discrimination has affected them.[13] An example of intersectional discrimination is found in a British Columbia case in which the human rights tribunal found that a hotel discriminated against an Indigenous woman by evicting her.[14] Although they had other Indigenous guests and other female guests, the tribunal found that the hotel relied on particular stereotypes about an Indigenous woman renting a room alone (specifically, they assumed she was a sex worker) and found discrimination based on a combination of her race and sex.

Discrimination can be direct or indirect. An example of direct discrimination would be a restaurant firing a chef because they find out the chef is living with HIV, and the restaurant does not want such a person working in their kitchen. Direct discrimination is often based on stereotypes, myths, and biases about people with disabilities. An example of indirect discrimination (also called *constructive* or *adverse effects discrimination*) is if the restaurant had a rule that everyone has to work three late night shifts each week, but those shifts interfered with the chef's ability to take their HIV medications at regular times. The rule itself is neutral, but it has a discriminatory effect on the chef because of their disability. Both types of discrimination are prohibited under human rights law. This is because Canada's human rights laws have been interpreted to take into account the idea that people are differently situated and might require different treatment to be put on equal footing. This is called *substantive equality*.

In the indirect discrimination example, the chef required accommodation for their disability-related needs. The *duty to accommodate* is a legal term that refers to the obligation of employers, housing providers, schools, health care providers, and any other persons or organizations that fall under the social areas covered by human rights legislation (whom we call *accommodation providers*) to remove barriers and make adjustments that allow a person with a disability equal access to services, goods, and facilities.[15] Accommodation needs are specific to the individual and may change over time. In the context of employment, the Supreme Court of Canada has described the goals of accommodation in the following way: "The purpose of the duty to accommodate is to ensure that persons who are otherwise fit to work are not unfairly excluded where working conditions can be adjusted without undue hardship."[16]

Accommodation providers must accommodate people with disabilities to the point of undue hardship.[17] This means they sometimes must incur some inconvenience or cost to accommodate the person's disabilities. Some human rights statutes set out that the only considerations in determining undue hardship are health, safety, and cost.[18] If an accommodation provider has reached the point of undue hardship and the person is still unable to comply with the legitimate or *bona fide* expectations of the accommodation provider (e.g., an employee's basic job duties or a tenant's duty to pay rent), the duty to accommodate ends.[19]

The duty to accommodate to the point of undue hardship applies to health care providers in their roles as employers and service providers, and health care providers and trainees benefit from the right to accommodation for their own disabilities from their employers or educational institutions.

Supporting People Living with HIV in Requesting Accommodations

As discussed in chapter 2, the person requesting accommodation and the accommodation provider each have certain rights and responsibilities in the accommodation process.

A health care provider's main role in the disability accommodation process is to provide appropriate medical evidence to support their patient-client's accommodation request. The employer, housing provider, or service provider from whom the person is requesting accommodation is not entitled to know the person's diagnosis because it is the person's confidential medical information. Disclosing a person's HIV status or other diagnoses in this context can be a breach of privacy and may have significant harmful consequences for the person living with HIV (and may lead to legal action against the health care provider). The mere fact that a person is living with HIV is almost never relevant to the person's ability to do their job or live in their home, for example, and it is generally not relevant to their engagement with a particular service (although it may be for some medical services).[20]

Just as it is inappropriate to disclose an exact diagnosis, neither should a medical note in support of an accommodation request be too vague or ambiguous (e.g., "this patient is ill and cannot attend work"). Medical evidence in support of an accommodation request should instead outline (a) the limitations or restrictions associated with the person's disability and (b) the accommodations needed to enable them to perform the essential duties or requirements of the job (or the requirements of being a service user or tenant).[21] For example, a person with a vision impairment might be unable to read small print (restriction), and it would be appropriate to provide them with large-print training materials (accommodation). See chapter 2 for guiding questions to consider when preparing to support a request for accommodation.

Employment Accommodation Support Letter Tips for HIV

Do

- Refer to a *chronic condition* rather than to HIV or another diagnosis.
- List restrictions and the suggested accommodations.
- Include an estimated return-to-work date or date to re-evaluate.
- Request information from the patient on the nature of their job tasks and work environment.

Don't

- Mention HIV status or any other diagnosis.
- Let the employer contact you directly without specific consent.
- Give medical reports or test results to the employer (the patient should get legal advice if they are asked for them).
- Dictate to the employer the exact form accommodation should take.

Test Yourself: What's Wrong with This Accommodation Letter?

Dear employer,
   This patient has been HIV+ for 15 years and has major depression. He is taking medication that has side effects including insomnia and diarrhoea. You must put him on the afternoon shift indefinitely as he is not able to work early mornings. Please call me to discuss if desired.
Dr. N. Jones

Problems with the Letter

- It includes unnecessary information, including diagnoses and length of time living with HIV.
- It is not necessary to disclose the nature of side effects, only the restrictions they create. For example, write "Due to side effects from medication, this patient may be restricted in length of shifts, require extra breaks, or be unable to start work before 11:00 am."
- Do not dictate what the employer should do. Instead, recommend appropriate accommodation, for example, "a later start time would appropriately accommodate his current restrictions."

- Instead of requiring indefinite accommodation for a problem that may resolve, include a time frame during which the patient will be re-evaluated.
- Do not offer to speak to the employer without the patient's permission.
- If in doubt, refer the patient to a legal clinic or similar service that may be able to work with you to draft a letter.

Remedies for Discrimination

When a person believes they have experienced discrimination, they should ideally receive legal advice as soon as possible because there are often strict deadlines for starting a human rights complaint at a human rights tribunal, commission, or court.

As noted in chapter 2, human rights tribunals generally have the ability to award a broad range of remedies to compensate the complainant and prevent future discrimination.[22] Examples of remedies that might be appropriate in cases of HIV-related discrimination include general or HIV-specific human rights training for the person or organization found liable for discrimination; requiring the organization to accommodate the complainant; reinstating a person who was fired because they are living with HIV; and monetary compensation for the person who experienced the discrimination.

Human rights issues often arise in the midst of other legal matters, such as evictions or social assistance disputes. Because human rights laws are quasi-constitutional and prevail over other laws, all other laws must be interpreted in line with human rights law. For example, if a person is facing eviction because of behaviours related to a mental health disability, the person or their legal representative can argue at their eviction hearing that the landlord is required to accommodate their disability rather than evicting them. Another example is if a social assistance worker asked a client for documents by a deadline and suspended their benefits for not providing the documents. If the person was unable to meet that deadline for a reason related to their disability (e.g., they could not gather the documents because of side effects of medications), they could argue that the neutral application of the deadline had a discriminatory effect on them because of their disability.

The Western legal model of adversarial dispute adjudication is not appropriate or meaningful to all people who have experienced discrimination. Some individuals, including Indigenous persons, may prefer a restorative model that provides an opportunity to repair harm, resolve conflict, and repair relationships among those who were harmed, those who have caused harm, and the community.[23]

Privacy and Disclosure

People living with HIV continue to face discrimination, social exclusion, and even violence across all aspects of their lives. Given the high level of stigma and discrimination that people living with HIV experience, a person's HIV-positive status is extremely sensitive information. Protecting the privacy of a person's health information and helping them determine when they do and do not have to disclose their HIV status can play an important role in reducing the stigma and discrimination they may face. This section explores the legal regulation of privacy in Canada; when a person living with HIV must disclose their status; health care providers' legal obligations with respect to the confidentiality of a patient's HIV status and other personal health information; and legal remedies for breach of privacy.

Legal Regulation of Privacy

Privacy is the right to control or consent to how one's personal information is handled by others. The duty of confidentiality imposes a legal obligation on some professionals not to reveal personal information without consent, which is one way to protect individuals' privacy.[24(p. 3)] Canadian privacy law is rapidly evolving and currently consists of a patchwork of statutory and common law (court-made law) legal frameworks that leaves many gaps in coverage. Laws may be federal, provincial or territorial, or municipal and may apply to the public sector or private actors.

Some privacy laws apply specifically to personal health information. *Personal health information* is generally defined as including health-related information about identifiable individuals. Most provinces and territories have specific legislation that applies to personal health information (see Table 10.1). Health privacy legislation refers to people who keep health information as custodians or trustees, and the legislation may apply to health care providers including, but not limited to, members of regulated health professions as well as institutions or organizations that provide health services, such as health authorities, hospitals, long-term care facilities, pharmacies, laboratories, and ambulance services.[25(p. 459)] Most statutes protect custodians or trustees from liability for actions under the legislation if they have acted reasonably and in good faith.[26]

Table 10.1. Privacy Legislation That Applies to Health Care Providers in Canadian Jurisdictions

Jurisdiction	Health information laws	Privacy protection laws
Federal	N/A	*Privacy Act*, RSC 1985, c P-21 *Personal Information Protection and Electronic Documents Act*, SC 2000, c 5
Alberta	*Health Information Act*, RSA 2000, c H-5	*Freedom of Information and Protection of Privacy Act*, RSA 2000, c F-25 *Personal Information Protection Act*, SA 2003, c P-6.5
British Columbia	*E-Health (Personal Health Information Access and Protection of Privacy) Act*, SBC 2008, c 38	*Freedom of Information and Protection of Privacy Act*, RSBC 1996, c 165 *Personal Information Protection Act*, SBC 2003, c 643
Manitoba	*The Personal Health Information Act*, CCSM c P33.5	*Freedom of Information and Protection of Privacy Act*, CCSM c F175
New Brunswick	*Personal Health Information Privacy and Access Act*, SNB 2009, c P-7.05	*Right to Information and Protection of Privacy Act*, SNB 2009, c R-10.6
Newfoundland and Labrador	*Personal Health Information Act*, SNL 2008, c P-7.01	*Access to Information and Protection of Privacy Act*, 2015, SNL 2015, c A-1.2 *Privacy Act*, RSNL 1990, c P-22
Northwest Territories	*Health Information Act*, SNWT 2014, c 2	*Access to Information and Protection of Privacy Act*, SNWT 1994, c 20
Nova Scotia	*Personal Health Information Act*, SNS 2010, c 41	*Freedom of Information and Protection of Privacy Act*, SNS 1993, c 5 *Part XX of the Municipal Government Act*, SNS 1998, c 18 *Personal Information International Disclosure Protection Act*, SNS 2006, c 3
Nunavut	No health-specific legislation	*Access to Information and Protection of Privacy Act*, CSNu 1996, c A-20
Ontario	*Personal Health Information Protection Act*, 2004, SO 2004, c 3, Sched A	*Freedom of Information and Protection of Privacy Act*, RSO 1990, c F.31 *Municipal Freedom of Information and Protection of Privacy Act*, RSO 1990, c M.56

(*Continued*)

Table 10.1. (Continued)

Jurisdiction	Health information laws	Privacy protection laws
Prince Edward Island	*Health Information Act*, SPEI 2014, c. 31	*Freedom of Information and Protection of Privacy Act*, RSPEI 1998, c F-15.01
Québec	*Act respecting the sharing of certain health information*, CQLR c P-9.0001 *An Act to amend the Act respecting health services and social services*, CQLR c S-4.2 *Health Insurance Act*, CQLR c A-29 *Act respecting the Régie de l'assurance maladie du Québec*, CQLR c R-5	*Act respecting access to documents held by public bodies and the Protection of personal information*, CQLR c A-2.1 *Act respecting the protection of personal information in the private sector*, CQLR c P-39.1
Saskatchewan	*Health Information Protection Act*, SS 1999, c H-0.021	*The Freedom of Information and Protection of Privacy Act*, SS 1990–91, c F-22.01 *The Local Authority Freedom of Information and Protection of Privacy Act*, SS 1990–91, c L-27.1
Yukon	*Health Information Privacy and Management Act*, SY 2013, c 16	*Access to Information and Protection of Privacy Act*, RSY 2002, c 1

Source: List of statutes was retrieved from Office of the Privacy Commissioner of Canada. Summary of privacy laws in Canada [Internet]. Ottawa: The Office; 2018. Available from: https://www.priv.gc.ca/en/privacy-topics/privacy-laws-in-canada/02_05_d_15/; see also section 5A:1 of McIsaac B, Klein K, Brown S. Law of privacy in Canada (loose-leaf updated 2022, release 2022–6). Toronto: Thomson Reuters; 2000.

N/A = not applicable.

Other legislation may apply to information or bodies that collect health information but fall outside the scope of health information legislation or where no health-specific legislation is in place.[27(p. 454)] One of those pieces of legislation is the *Personal Information Protection and Electronic Documents Act* (*PIPEDA*), a federal law that applies to personal information, including personal health information that is collected, used, or disclosed during commercial activities.[28]

Statutes, regulations, and codes of conduct applying to health professionals and institutions often supplement the relevant provisions of health information statutes regarding health records, and regulated professionals can face professional discipline for breaching those standards.[29(p. 457)]

Outside of the health care setting, other pieces of privacy legislation apply to the private and public sectors (see Table 10.1). Different levels of government are subject to different pieces of privacy legislation.[30] Each piece of privacy legislation governs the collection, use, and disclosure of personal information. The common law in some provinces also applies to protect the privacy of personal information (see the "Remedies for Breach of Privacy" section).

Disclosure of HIV Status

A person's HIV status is their personal health information, and it is the person's choice whether and in what circumstances to share it. Employers, housing providers, schools, childcare centres, health care providers, and other service providers are almost never entitled to know a person's HIV status. Such entities often mistakenly believe they are entitled to this information, but this misconception is typically based on unfounded and erroneous fears about the risk of HIV transmission.

In most workplace settings (with rare exceptions outlined next), there are no permissible questions about HIV on employment application forms, and it is unlikely that HIV testing or protective measures specific to HIV would be justifiable because very few jobs pose a real risk of HIV transmission.[31(p. 8)] Asking unnecessary questions about HIV or excluding someone from employment on the basis of their HIV-positive status would likely constitute discrimination. There is no obligation to share one's HIV status with an employer, colleagues, or clients.

There are rare circumstances in which a person is legally required to disclose their HIV status in the context of their employment. Under the criminal law, people living with HIV are required to disclose their status to their sexual partner before sexual activity that carries a realistic possibility of transmission (see the "How HIV Is Criminalized in Canada" section).[32] This law also applies to sex workers in the course of their work. Health care providers living with HIV who perform exposure-prone procedures (invasive procedures where there is a possibility of direct contact between the skin of the health care worker and a sharp instrument or sharp tissue inside a body cavity or anatomical space) may be required to disclose their status to their professional regulator, which can take steps to minimize any risk of transmission to patients.[33] This requirement varies across professions and jurisdictions; anyone who may fall into this category should seek legal advice before disclosing their HIV-positive status. Individuals may choose to disclose the fact that they have a chronic illness or disability to their employer to request accommodations in the workplace (see the "Supporting People Living with HIV in Requesting Accommodations" section).

Another situation in which a person may be required to disclose their status is in the rare case of mandatory post-exposure testing for HIV and other sexually transmitted and blood-borne infections (STBBIs). Post-exposure testing involves allowing a person (usually first responders and health care providers) exposed to the bodily fluids of another to apply to a court or tribunal for an order requiring the source individual to undergo testing for HIV and other STBBIs.[34] Alberta, British Columbia, Nova Scotia, Ontario, Manitoba, and Saskatchewan have implemented legislation allowing for mandatory testing of source individuals without consent. The result of the testing is generally disclosed only to the exposed individual or their physician.[35] Someone may also choose to voluntarily disclose their status when they know another person may have been exposed to their bodily fluids in a manner that could transmit HIV. Disclosing this information could help the exposed person decide whether to take post-exposure prophylaxis (PEP) to prevent transmission, which must be started within 72 hours of the potential exposure.[36]

Some people living with HIV choose to be public about their status or choose to share their status with select people. They may find that sharing their status alleviates the stress that comes with trying to keep it secret. This is an individual choice, and individuals should not be pressured to share their HIV-positive status if they do not want to. Once someone has disclosed their status, there is no going back, and, in the Internet age, they lose control over how that information may spread. Levels of stigma and accompanying discrimination vary across communities and life circumstances; the individual is best placed to assess the potential consequences of disclosure. AIDS service organizations can often assist people living with HIV in exploring their options for disclosure.[37]

Health Care Providers' Duty of Confidentiality and Exceptions

A health care provider cannot disclose a patient's HIV status without consent, aside from very limited exceptions discussed later. Respecting a patient's privacy requires health care providers to respect their patient's right to decide for themselves when and how their personal information will be shared, used, or disclosed. This includes not just their HIV status or the presence of other medical conditions, but any information the provider may have about their drug use, sexual activity, sexual orientation, or gender identity.[38] There is also no legal obligation for a person to tell their health care provider that they are living with HIV (although sharing this information may well be helpful to get the best care possible). Health care providers should be using universal precautions at all times.[39]

Health care providers may share a patient's personal health information with others in the patient's circle of care for the purpose of providing care to that individual. This is the default even if the person does not explicitly consent to disclosure of that information (i.e., consent is implied). In some provinces, including Ontario, British Columbia, Quebec, and Newfoundland and Labrador, the statute that governs personal health information allows patients to withdraw that implied consent when they do not want to share certain information with another health care provider.[40]

In Ontario, this limit on implied consent is called the *lock box*. For example, in Ontario a patient can activate the lock box by requesting that their family doctor not share their HIV status with a psychiatrist to whom they are being referred. The family doctor must tell the psychiatrist that there is information important to the patient's care that has not been included in the shared records. The psychiatrist can then discuss the missing information directly with the patient.[41]

Hospitals may have different processes in place to prevent all members of the medical team from accessing certain information.[42] Blocking access to certain health information becomes more difficult in jurisdictions with electronic health records, although British Columbia's *E-Health (Personal Health Information Access and Protection of Privacy) Act* allows individuals to make disclosure directives that limit otherwise permissible collection, use, and disclosure of personal health information.[43] Individuals can seek information about how to protect their personal health information by speaking to the privacy officer at their health care facility or by contacting the provincial privacy commissioner.[44]

There are exceptions to the rule that a patient's personal health information cannot be disclosed without consent. A provider can make two types of reports without their patient's express or implied consent: mandatory and permissive. Mandatory reports are legally required and considered necessary in the public interest. Examples include reporting child abuse or neglect or reporting impaired driving ability because of a medical condition. Permissive reports are rooted in professional responsibility, ethics, and law. Although they may be legally permitted in certain circumstances, the decision to make a permissive report is at the health care provider's discretion.[45] An example is disclosure to prevent harm to a third party, discussed further later. Provincial regulatory bodies or professional insurers may provide further guidance about mandatory and permissive disclosures in a given province or territory. At the beginning of the service relationship, patients should be informed about the provider's duty of confidentiality and its limits.[46]

Disclosure may be mandatory to comply with a warrant, subpoena, or court order. For more on this topic in the context of HIV criminalization, see the "Effect on Patient–Provider Relationships" section.

Public health laws (outside of Quebec) may permit or require certain health care providers to report known or suspected cases of specified communicable medical conditions, along with the patient's name and contact information, to public health authorities. Other types of disclosure may also be required or permitted for purposes outlined in public health statutes, including when there may be a risk to third parties.[47] Providers should inform patients in advance that this type of disclosure may be required when applicable (e.g., before nominal HIV testing). See the "HIV Testing, Reporting, and Contact Tracing" section for more information.

There is no recognized duty under Canadian common law that requires a health care provider to warn a third party (e.g., the sexual partner of a person living with HIV) of the risk of HIV infection, and no known cases in which a health care provider has been held liable for failing to do so.[48] However, all provinces have legislation that permits physicians to disclose confidential information without a patient's consent if there are reasonable grounds to believe this will avoid or minimize danger to another person.[49(p. 3)] A Supreme Court of Canada case called *Smith v Jones* sets out guiding principles for a public safety exception to determine when a service provider with a duty of confidentiality has the discretion (not an obligation) to disclose confidential information about a patient-client to prevent harm to another person:

- There is a clear risk of harm to an identifiable person or group of persons.
- There is a risk of serious bodily harm or death (i.e., the intended victim is in danger of being killed or of suffering serious bodily harm).
- The danger is imminent (i.e., a sense of urgency).[50]

If the professional determines they will disclose confidential information without the patient's consent, they should discuss the disclosure with the patient in advance when practicable, and the common law (court-made law) requires that they disclose as little information as possible to the third party to avoid or minimize the danger.[51] Before disclosing, consider that a professional or service provider can be sued by a patient-client for breaching confidentiality. It is also possible to be sued for failing to warn a third party if some harm comes to them, although, again, there are no known Canadian cases in the context of HIV disclosure.

If a health care provider is considering exercising their discretion to disclose a patient's HIV status to a third party (including a sexual partner or police), they must consider each step of the preceding legal test. First, they must be reasonably certain that their client is engaging in behaviour that carries a high risk of transmission, not just assume this to be the case. Second, they should consider that there may be no risk of serious bodily harm or death when the risk of transmission is low or negligible, for example if the person has a low or undetectable viral load, uses condoms, or engages only in low-risk or occasional sexual activity.[52] If the provider chooses to exercise discretion to disclose without consent, it is not necessary to report a perceived risk of HIV transmission directly to a sexual partner or police. Reporting to public health authorities is another option to consider (see the "Public Health Orders" section). This decision must be carefully considered and documented, taking into account both confidentiality concerns and the impact of the decision on the patient and the health care provider or organization. It is best to have an organizational policy to guide decisions in these difficult situations.[53]

Test Yourself: Disclosing to Prevent Harm to Another Person

Questions

- If I determine that my patient poses a clear, imminent risk of serious bodily harm to a particular person, I legally must disclose to the authorities without the patient's consent. True or false?
- My patient living with HIV has an undetectable viral load. I know they are having unprotected sex with their partner, and their partner does not know the patient's HIV status. It may be acceptable to breach confidentiality to tell the patient's partner about the risk of getting HIV. True or false?
- My patient living with HIV is a medical administrator. Her prospective employer has asked me to complete a medical fitness form. I have a legal obligation to share the patient's HIV status without her consent to protect others. True or false?

Answers

- False. The law may permit you to disclose to an authority to prevent harm to a third party in these circumstances, but you are not required to do so. If you decide to disclose, you may do so with or without the patient's consent.
- False. People with an undetectable viral load cannot transmit HIV through sexual activity. It would not be acceptable to breach confidentiality here.
- False. All health care personnel should take universal precautions to prevent transmission of communicable medical conditions. HIV is not relevant to the patient's fitness to do her job. Disclosing her HIV status to her prospective employer would be an illegal breach of privacy.

Remedies for Breach of Privacy

Unauthorized disclosure of a person's HIV status is unfortunately all too common. For example, sexual partners, friends, or family members may intentionally disclose a person's HIV-positive status to others without the person's consent, or a service provider may discuss sensitive health information where it can be overheard. The type of legal recourse available to an individual for the breach of their health-related privacy depends on where they live and who breached their privacy.

In some provinces it is possible for a person whose privacy has been breached to sue the person or organization responsible. Ontario and Nova Scotia have recognized a common law privacy tort, or legal claim, called intrusion upon seclusion that involves recklessly or intentionally intruding on a person's private affairs without legal justification in a highly offensive way.[54] Ontario,[55] Nova Scotia,[56] and Alberta[57] recognize the tort of public disclosure of embarrassing or private facts, which involves publication of an aspect of an individual's private life in a highly offensive way to which the person did not consent and that was not of legitimate concern to the public.[58] British Columbia, Saskatchewan, Newfoundland and Labrador, and Manitoba each have a tort created by a statute for breach of privacy.[59] The result of a successful lawsuit is monetary damages, and the amounts are generally small for breaches of privacy, compared with those for other types of lawsuits. There are strict time limits for starting a lawsuit, so it is important for individuals to seek legal advice soon after the breach occurs.

Some privacy breaches are also discriminatory. For example, a nurse disclosing a person's HIV status to the person's family member may cause more harm than disclosing other health information because of the stigmatized nature of HIV, or a person's housing provider or employer may choose to disclose a person's HIV status without their consent on the basis of myths or stereotypes about HIV transmission. Both of these acts would likely violate human rights legislation. In each case, the person living with HIV could bring a human rights complaint against the person or organization that breached their privacy. There are strict time limits for starting a human rights complaint. See the "Remedies for Discrimination" section for more on human rights complaints.

If the breach involved a violation by a health care provider; health facility; or other organization, business, or government agency covered by privacy legislation, the individual whose privacy was breached can make a complaint to a privacy commissioner or ombudsperson who is responsible for investigating complaints and encouraging compliance with privacy legislation.[60] There are provincial entities and a federal entity.[61] Individuals who want to make a complaint should check with the relevant privacy commissioner or ombudsperson before making a formal complaint to make sure they are directing it to the correct entity. Privacy commissioners can make recommendations to prevent future privacy breaches (which may or may not be binding), and they can sometimes impose fines (paid to the government), but they normally cannot award compensation to the individual who suffered the privacy breach. There may be a deadline to file such a complaint.

If the privacy breach was committed by a registered professional, a person can also make a complaint to the professional regulator (e.g., the College of Physicians and Surgeons, College of Nurses, or Law Society). Professional regulators cannot award compensation, but they can, for example, discipline the professional or require them to undergo training to prevent future breaches. There may also be time limits for making a complaint to a professional regulator.

A person should seek legal advice before pursuing any of these actions because taking one route could compromise their ability to later pursue another route.

Case Study: Privacy of Health Information

Roberto is a nurse at a family practice. He sees on a medical form that his patient, Ben, is living with HIV. Roberto is surprised and mentions it to a medical student who is not involved in Ben's care. The medical student sees Ben kiss a friend on the cheek when he leaves the clinic. The medical student is concerned that Ben might have transmitted HIV and discloses Ben's HIV status to the friend.

Questions

- What went wrong here in terms of patient privacy?
- What legal options does Ben have?

Consider

- Roberto was not legally permitted to disclose Ben's health information without consent under relevant legislation or the common law. His professional duties of confidentiality may also apply.
- Implied consent to disclosure only applies within the circle of care.
- The medical student disclosed private health information without consent.
- The medical student has a misunderstanding of how HIV is transmitted and made an inappropriate disclosure based on myths and stigma.
- Ben could make a complaint to the privacy commissioner, sue the clinic in court, bring a human rights complaint, or make a complaint to the College of Nurses.

Criminal Law and HIV Non-Disclosure

How HIV Is Criminalized in Canada

HIV criminalization refers to "the unjust application of the criminal law to people living with HIV based solely on their HIV status."[62] This can include both HIV-specific laws and general criminal laws used to prosecute people living with HIV for unintentional HIV transmission, potential exposure, or non-disclosure of their HIV status.[63] There is no criminal statute in Canada that explicitly imposes an obligation to disclose HIV-positive status before sex. Instead, the courts have established an obligation under the criminal law of (aggravated) sexual assault to disclose in some circumstances. Health records and the testimony of health care providers can play a key role in criminal prosecutions for HIV non-disclosure, so it is important that health care providers understand the high stakes for people living with HIV and the problems with criminalization.

People in Canada who face criminal charges related to HIV non-disclosure are typically charged with aggravated sexual assault, based on the idea that not disclosing one's HIV-positive status when there is a realistic possibility of HIV transmission is a fraud that makes their partner's consent to sex invalid.[64] The "aggravated" portion of the charge is added because the courts have considered that exposing a person to the possibility of acquiring HIV endangers their life. Aggravated sexual assault is the most serious sexual offence in the *Criminal Code*, carrying a maximum penalty of life imprisonment and other consequences described later. The law criminalises exposure; no transmission needs to have occurred for a person to be convicted of aggravated sexual assault.[65(p. 11)]

In 1998, the Supreme Court of Canada ruled in a case called *R v Cuerrier* that people living with HIV have an obligation to disclose their status to a sexual partner before sexual activity that poses a "significant risk of serious bodily harm."[66] In 2012, in a case called *R v Mabior*, the court added that such a risk exists when there is a "realistic possibility of transmission of HIV."[67] Based on their interpretation of the evidence before them in 2012, they decided that there is no realistic possibility of HIV transmission when having vaginal sex if a condom is used and the HIV-positive partner has a low viral load (defined as less than 1,500 copies per millilitre of blood).[68] The court concluded that when there is no realistic possibility of transmission, there is no duty to disclose. This decision was widely criticized for being unfair and at odds with the scientific evidence, given that using a condom properly (when it does not break) or having a low-enough viral load alone eliminates the risk of HIV transmission. This standard has led to convictions even in cases in which the risk of transmission was negligible or non-existent.

Although the majority of criminal cases involve non-disclosure to sexual partners, there have also been several cases in which criminal charges have been laid for alleged spitting, biting, and other non-sexual exposures to bodily fluids despite the lack of evidence for any risk of transmission in those circumstances.[69] There is also one known case in which a woman living with HIV pleaded guilty to criminal charges after her baby contracted HIV. She was charged for not taking measures during her pregnancy to reduce the risk of transmission and subsequently breastfeeding her baby.[70] At this time, there are no known prosecutions based on allegations of sharing drug consumption equipment.[71]

Harms of HIV Criminalization

Canada has the dubious distinction of having one of the highest rates of HIV non-disclosure prosecutions in the world. Since 1989, there have been at least 224 documented prosecutions for HIV non-disclosure in Canada.[72] A person can be convicted for not disclosing even if they had no intent to cause harm, HIV was not in fact transmitted, and there was little or no risk of transmission.

The harms of criminalization for those who face prosecution and conviction are severe.[73] A conviction for aggravated sexual assault carries a maximum penalty of life imprisonment, a possible designation as a sex offender, and almost certain deportation for non-citizens. This is despite the fact that charges relate to otherwise consensual sex. Even in circumstances in which charges are ultimately not pursued or there are acquittals, police forces may issue press releases containing the name, photo, and health information of the accused person. Such disclosures can and do have drastic consequences, ranging from loss of family, friends, employment and housing to violence.[74(p. 8)]

Criminalization also causes broader harms. No other medical condition has been criminalized to this extent. Not only does criminalization exacerbate the already burdensome stigma facing people living with HIV, but it is also at odds with public health objectives. It hinders HIV prevention efforts and hampers care, treatment, and support for those living with HIV by providing disincentives for testing and deterring honest and open conversations with health care and other providers, including public health authorities, for legitimate fears that such conversations will be used in court.[75(p. 8)]

Advocates argue that "HIV criminalization serves as a proxy for discrimination based on class, ethnicity, gender identity, migrant status, race, sex, sexual orientation, and other markers of social vulnerability" and that "the most aggressive push to criminalize people living with HIV tends to occur at the intersection of several stigmatized identities."[76(p. S395)] In Canada, Black men and Indigenous women are particularly overrepresented in prosecutions for HIV non-disclosure in comparison with the proportion of Black and Indigenous people living with HIV.[77(p. 11)] Black and Indigenous people also have higher rates of conviction and are more likely to receive prison sentences for HIV non-disclosure than their white counterparts charged with similar offences. This is a reflection of the systemic racism inherent in the Canadian criminal legal system.[78] GBMSM represent the largest proportion of people living with HIV in Canada and are therefore also disproportionately affected by the risk of HIV-related criminal prosecution in general.[79]

Women living with HIV who are unstably housed, engage in sex work, or were recently incarcerated tend to be least able to access care and treatment to achieve a low or suppressed viral load and are therefore most at risk of criminal liability for HIV non-disclosure.[80] Women living with HIV may stay in abusive relationships and be deterred from reporting gender-based violence for fear of facing criminal charges at the hands of partners seeking retribution.[81] Women may not be able to negotiate condom use in violent relationships, opening them up to either a risk of violence for insisting on condom use or a risk of aggravated sexual assault charges if they do not.[82] Even after disclosing, sexual assault law may be weaponized against women living with HIV. Many women fear that their partners may threaten or actually make a police complaint for HIV non-disclosure as a form of control and intimidation, even if they disclosed before sex.[83] Some women living with HIV who experience sexual violence are deeply concerned about reporting it to police for fear that they will be transformed into an accused person and themselves charged with aggravated sexual assault. Moreover, prosecuting HIV non-disclosure as aggravated sexual assault undermines important principles of sexual assault law, which is harmful to anyone at risk of sexual assault.[84]

Recent Developments

When taking HIV medications (antiretroviral therapy) as prescribed and engaged in care, many people lower their viral load (the amount of HIV virus that can be detected in a person's blood) to a level at which there are fewer than 200 copies per millilitre of blood. This is called a suppressed viral load.[85] HIV treatment that keeps a person's viral load suppressed prevents sexual transmission of HIV, even in circumstances involving sex without a condom. Large international studies have demonstrated that when a person taking antiretroviral therapy maintains a suppressed viral load, they do not transmit HIV to their sexual partners.[86] This consensus has been promoted with the slogan "Undetectable = Untransmittable" (U=U).[87] The term *undetectable* currently refers to viral loads of less than 20 copies per millilitre, which cannot be detected with today's standard blood tests. Although the term *undetectable* is used in the U=U slogan, it is more accurate to say that a suppressed viral load of less than 200 copies per millilitre prevents sexual transmission. Legal directives refer to a suppressed viral load. By contrast, the term undetectable is mostly used in the medical context.

Since the *R v Mabior* decision in 2012, the law has been evolving towards the recognition that there is no "realistic possibility of HIV transmission" and hence no duty to disclose when a person has a suppressed viral load, even when no condom is used. The law has evolved through court cases as well as prosecutorial policy, as described later. Health care providers have been instrumental in helping the law catch up to the science of HIV transmission through expert consensus statements.[88]

However, in comparison with viral load, the law in relation to condom use has not evolved to the same extent. There are conflicting court decisions about whether using only a condom, without having a suppressed or low viral load, is enough to prevent a realistic possibility of transmission. Nova Scotia courts have accepted that a person should not be convicted for HIV non-disclosure if they used a condom (regardless of their viral load).[89] But Ontario's Court of Appeal came to the opposite conclusion: it upheld the conviction of a man living with HIV who had used condoms but did not have a suppressed or low viral load (even though he was not accused of using condoms incorrectly or of transmitting HIV).[90] Consequently, some people living with HIV in Canada are still at risk of non-disclosure prosecutions when they use condoms.[91]

Thanks to tireless work by HIV advocates, the prosecution of HIV non-disclosure has been limited by instructions to prosecutors in some provinces and territories. These instructions do not change the law itself as decided by the Supreme Court of Canada, but they can restrict prosecutors' ability to prosecute cases of HIV non-disclosure – or at least influence whether and when they choose to prosecute. This has resulted in a decreasing number of HIV non-disclosure prosecutions in recent years.[92] Additional efforts by advocates to reform HIV criminalization are ongoing, most recently with an effort to remove HIV non-disclosure from the realm of sexual assault law and to limit prosecutions to circumstances involving intentional and actual transmission.[93] Health care providers can get involved in law reform efforts through organizations such as the HIV & AIDS Legal Clinic Ontario (HALCO), the HIV Legal Network and the Canadian Coalition to Reform HIV Criminalization.[94]

In Ontario,[95(p. 131)] Quebec, Alberta, and British Columbia,[96] a person living with HIV who is on antiretroviral therapy and maintains a viral load of less than 200 copies per millilitre for at least four to six months (or for at least six months, in the case of Ontario) should not be prosecuted for HIV non-disclosure. This is the case for anal, vaginal, or oral sex and regardless of whether a condom was used. In British Columbia, the correct use of a condom during a single act of vaginal or anal sex, where HIV was not transmitted, is a factor that may weigh against prosecution. No specific directives for prosecutors exist in any other province.[97]

A 2018 directive to federal prosecutors from the Attorney General of Canada that applies to the Northwest Territories, Yukon, and Nunavut states that a person living with HIV will not be prosecuted if they maintained a viral load of less than 200 copies per millilitre and should generally not be prosecuted if they were taking treatment as prescribed, a condom was used, or they and their partners only had oral sex. The federal directive also calls for prosecutions to be carried out using non-sexual criminal offences where appropriate, and it requires consideration of whether public health authorities have provided services to the person in question.[98]

Even in situations in which prosecutions should no longer take place, individuals can still report allegations of non-disclosure to police, and the accused person can be caught up in a criminal investigation. A person accused of non-disclosure should always get legal advice from a criminal lawyer before speaking with police or anyone else, including a health care or other service provider. A provider's notes can be used against an accused person, as further explained later. The HIV & AIDS Legal Clinic Ontario (HALCO) or the HIV Legal Network can provide advice or referrals to people living with HIV who may be facing HIV criminalization.[99]

Effect on Provider–Patient Relationships

Police and courts can require the disclosure of clinical notes and records as part of a criminal investigation or prosecution by providing a warrant or subpoena to a health care provider or organization.[100] Health care and other service providers can also be called to testify against a patient or client accused of HIV non-disclosure. Professional duties of confidentiality usually do not apply to protect the patient–client's privacy in the context of a criminal trial. As a result, some organizations opt to minimize note-taking on discussions of HIV non-disclosure and sexual practices, to the extent that their duties as regulated professionals permit.[101(p. 11)] Patients should receive legal advice from a criminal lawyer before discussing the details of sexual activity with their health care or service provider or any other person who is not a lawyer when they may be at risk of criminal charges.

There is no obligation under the criminal law to report a suspected crime to police or to provide information about a patient to the police absent a search warrant requiring that information. There is also no legal obligation to advise a patient's sexual partner about the option to press charges against a patient who may have exposed them to HIV. It is not a health care provider's role to enforce the criminal law.

Public Health Law

HIV Testing, Reporting, and Contact Tracing

HIV testing is an important first step in maintaining the health of people living with HIV and preventing transmission, two goals that fall within the mandate of public health authorities. In Canada, 10 per cent of people living with HIV are unaware of their HIV status.[102] The Public Health Agency of Canada's (PHAC's) current approach to HIV testing promotes adherence to the three Cs: confidentiality, counselling (pre- and post-test), and informed consent. It adopts the following definition of *informed consent*: "Informed consent means that the client understands what is involved in the test procedures (advantages and disadvantages of being tested and of refusing to be tested), is prepared for a potential positive result, and provides permission to be tested."[103]

Provinces and territories have jurisdiction over the implementation of HIV testing, and approaches vary. Testing can be nominal, non-nominal, or anonymous.[104] Anonymous testing provides the best protection for the confidentiality of the person being tested. Anonymous testing usually takes place in a specialized clinic setting that provides enhanced pre- and post-test counselling. A positive anonymous test is reported to public health, but the result is not linked with the identity of the person being tested because the person does not provide their name and is identified only with a code.[105] Although the result of an anonymous test is not included in a person's health record, in some provinces an anonymous test must be followed by a confirmatory nominal test to access care.[106]

Nominal testing is the most common mode of testing in Canada. It links the identity of the person being tested, as well as their demographic information, contact information, and HIV risk factors, to their test result. Test results are recorded in a person's medical records and, if positive, are reported, along with the person's name and contact information, to the local public health authority and kept in a database (in all provinces except Quebec, where the name of the person testing positive is not reported).[107]

STI diagnoses, including HIV and AIDS, are typically subject to mandatory reporting set out in each province's or territory's public health legislation. Certain professionals, including physicians, nurses, lab technicians, hospital administrators, and others, often have a duty to report known or suspected cases of certain reportable medical conditions to local public health authorities.[108] After a person is diagnosed with HIV or another STI, public health unit staff will typically contact them to provide counselling and request the names of their sexual and needle-sharing partners. Health unit staff then use this information to carry out partner notification, which is mandatory in some provinces and permissible in others.[109] Although the public health unit should not disclose the name of the diagnosed person to their partners, partners might determine the identity of the diagnosed person. The diagnosed person, or their health care provider, are sometimes permitted to notify partners themselves.

Public health action and criminalization of HIV can interact in several ways. Partner notification can sometimes be the catalyst for individuals initiating complaints to police about non-disclosure. Records from public health counselling and contact tracing can be (and have been) used in police investigations and prosecutions.[110]

Public Health Orders

There are rare instances in which a person living with HIV is not compliant with public health measures to reduce transmission. Public health units may become aware of non-compliance through third-party or physician reports, including reporting of positive test results for other STIs. A physician or other health care provider may choose to contact public health about a patient when they believe the patient's behaviour is putting sexual or needle-sharing partners at risk of HIV and their own counselling and support efforts have failed. See the "Health Care Providers' Duty of Confidentiality and Exceptions" section for more on how to approach the decision to make a permitted report to public health.[111] In these situations, the medical officer of health (or equivalent head of public health) is empowered to make orders, sometimes called certificates, to minimize the risk of transmission. However, before using order-making powers, public health units should engage in a graduated response that supplements gaps in counselling, education, and care.[112]

Public health orders can require that a person diagnosed with HIV take or refrain from taking certain actions to protect public health, reduce the transmission of a communicable medical condition, or both. For example, typical orders may include terms requiring the individual to always disclose their HIV status before penetrative sexual activities (even when not required to do so under the criminal law), to always wear a condom, and to remain under the care of a physician.[113] Orders in Ontario are typically issued without a time limit. These orders significantly infringe on the liberty of people living with HIV and can undermine trust in public health authorities. For this reason, it is important to consider and exhaust less coercive options before choosing to report a patient to public health.

Most public health authorities in Ontario have changed their practice to reflect the science of U=U.[114(p. 13)] It would be unusual for a public health unit to issue orders against persons who have maintained a suppressed viral load (less than 200 copies per millilitre) for at least six months. It is hoped that other public health authorities will heed guidance from PHAC on suppressed viral load and adapt their practices as well.[115]

Orders can be enforced using fines or court orders or by any peace officer, depending on the jurisdiction.[116] Breach of a court order can result in the person being found in contempt of court, which raises the possibility of imprisonment.[117] The person against whom the order has been issued typically has appeal rights, but the time for initiating an appeal can be very short, so timely legal advice is imperative.[118]

Case Study: Patient Poses a Clear Risk of Transmission to Others

You recently diagnosed Marie, aged 20 years, with HIV. She has a history of anxiety and has had a difficult time accepting her diagnosis. She has not yet started antiretroviral therapy because she is concerned about the side effects, and her viral load is high. She has one sexual partner and has not yet disclosed her HIV diagnosis to him. Marie has told you it is difficult for her to ask her partner to use a condom for vaginal sex, and you suspect the relationship may be abusive.

Questions

- What are your options to address this situation?
- What are the advantages and disadvantages of each approach?

Options

Options could include

- referring Marie to a legal clinic or other legal services for advice (and cautioning her against sharing details of her sexual activity with anyone until she has spoken to a lawyer);

- referring Marie to a local AIDS service organization or services for women experiencing intimate partner violence for support to ensure she has a safety plan if she is experiencing violence;
- counselling Marie about the risk of transmission and how condoms and antiretroviral therapy can reduce the risk;
- counselling Marie regarding her concerns regarding the side effects of antiretroviral therapy;
- making an anonymous report to the local public health unit naming the partner (if known) as a person who should seek HIV testing and alerting public health to the risk of intimate partner violence; or
- reporting Marie by name to the local public health unit to prevent an imminent risk of serious bodily harm to her partner, with or without her consent, and alerting public health to the risk of intimate partner violence.

In any scenario in which you decide a report to public health authorities is necessary, advise Marie in advance that you intend to report and provide her an opportunity to seek legal advice before making your report.

Note that if Marie's partner is also your patient, your obligation may change. Seek advice yourself before taking any action.

Access to Medications

Consistent adherence to antiretroviral medication starting as soon as possible after diagnosis and continuing throughout the lifetime helps people living with HIV to maintain their health and prevent onward transmission. As a result of Canada's piecemeal approach to prescription medication coverage, people living with HIV face many structural barriers in maintaining consistent, affordable access to medication. HIV medications can be extremely expensive – $15,000 per year on average for a single-tablet first-line treatment[119] – and inadequate drug coverage may affect antiretroviral adherence and viral suppression.[120] Helping people living with HIV to access stable medication coverage is essential in helping them maintain their health. Of course, access to health care is also essential for maintaining the health of people living with HIV. See chapter 7 for more information on barriers to accessing health care based on immigration status.

The main sources of coverage for antiretroviral medications are provincial or territorial or federal public insurance (see Table 10.2), private insurance, and compassionate access programs through pharmaceutical companies.

The federal government provides drug coverage programs for First Nations and Inuit peoples (but not for Métis peoples), refugees and refugee claimants, federal inmates, Canadian military personnel, veterans, and some federal public service employees.[121] Canada's national pharmacare plan is set to provide coverage for certain diabetes treatments and contraception in provinces that reach agreements with the federal government, but antiretrovirals are not covered under the plan at this time.[122]

Federal programs are portable when individuals move across Canada. Each provincial and territorial government provides public drug coverage for antiretrovirals and other drugs with a patchwork of coverage that depends on immigration status, income, age, receipt of social assistance, drug costs, and the presence of private insurance.[123] Provincial and territorial programs are not portable and are generally only available to residents of that province, creating the potential for gaps in coverage when a person moves across the country. Many require out-of-pocket payments in the form of premiums, deductibles, or co-payments. Most antiretroviral drugs are covered under most provincial and territorial formularies, but there may be conditions or restrictions on coverage for certain treatments (e.g., second-line treatments if a person has not yet tried first-line treatments).[124] People with precarious or no immigration status may have difficulty accessing public drug programs in certain provinces or territories.

Private group insurance (which covers a group of people under a single plan) is often offered through employers and post-secondary institutions, and it may include disability and life insurance in addition to medication and other health care coverage. It is often possible to join a group insurance plan without providing any health information, making these plans more accessible to people with a pre-existing condition such as HIV. Private individual insurance that covers prescription medication is available for purchase for those who do not have access to a group plan. When applying to purchase individual insurance or additional insurance coverage under a group plan, an applicant may be asked to give detailed health information or have an HIV test. If an insurance company finds out that an applicant did not provide accurate information, the insurance policy will not be legally valid.

Private insurance may have an annual or lifetime spending cap, limits on the type of prescriptions covered, or other types of restrictions.

Table 10.2. Publicly Funded Drug Plans in Canada That Cover Antiretroviral Medication

Program	Eligibility	Notes
Federal		
Non-Insured Health Benefits Program (NIHB)	Registered First Nations persons, Inuk recognized by an Inuit land claim organization, or child younger than age two whose parent is NIHB-eligible.	Fully subsidizes the cost of antiretrovirals for eligible patients regardless of their age or income.
Interim Federal Health Program	Resettled refugees, protected persons, refugee claimants, victims of human trafficking, detainees	Fully subsidizes the cost of antiretrovirals for eligible patients regardless of their age or income.
Veteran Affairs Canada Prescription Drug Program	Clients must have a Veteran Affairs Canada Health Care Identification Card on which an A, B, or both are indicated under the heading "Program Number 10."	Fully subsidizes the cost of antiretrovirals for eligible patients regardless of their age or income. Group A clients may only use their card to obtain benefits directly related to the treatment of their Veterans Affairs Canada pensioned medical condition. Group B clients are eligible for approved benefits, provided that they have a clearly demonstrated health need and the benefits are not available to them under a provincial health plan.
Correctional Service Canada, Health Services	Federal inmates	Places restrictions on the prescriber authorizing the regimen. Assigns designated pharmacies to dispense medication. Fully subsidizes the cost of antiretrovirals for eligible patients regardless of their age or income.
Canadian Forces Drug Benefit Plan	Canadian Armed Forces personnel, authorized visiting military forces, foreign military exchange personnel and their dependents	Fully subsidizes the cost of antiretrovirals for eligible patients regardless of their age or income.

(*Continued*)

Table 10.2. (Continued)

Program	Eligibility	Notes
Alberta		
Alberta Health Care Insurance Plan, Specialized High Cost Drug Program (AHCIP)	Alberta residents registered for AHCIP	Provides antiretrovirals at no cost to residents. Does not provide universal coverage of prescriptions not related to HIV. Places restrictions on the prescriber authorizing the regimen.
British Columbia		
British Columbia Centre for Excellence HIV Drug Treatment Program	HIV-positive residents with Medical Services Plan coverage and residents with coverage from another jurisdiction awaiting BC medical coverage	Provides antiretrovirals at no cost to residents. Does not provide universal coverage of prescriptions not related to HIV. Places restrictions on the prescriber authorizing the regimen.
Manitoba		
Pharmacare Program	Registered Manitoba residents	No limit to the annual income-based deductible collected. Seniors incur the same out-of-pocket expenses as non-senior counterparts with the same income.
HIV ART Medication Program	Manitoba residents with significant financial barriers to treatment who have no other drug insurance.	No deductible. Coverage is temporary until recipients can access other coverage.
Employment and Income Assistance Program – Prescription Drugs	Persons living in Manitoba and in financial need	Provides benefits to help eligible recipients with the cost of prescription drugs or health-related equipment not provided for by other programs.
New Brunswick		
Prescription Drug Program, HIV/AIDS Plan	Registered New Brunswick residents not receiving private insurance for the drugs they require	Provides antiretrovirals at no cost to residents. Does not provide universal coverage of prescriptions not related to HIV. Patients not eligible for free antiretrovirals if they receive any benefits from a private plan. Places restrictions on the prescriber authorizing the regimen. Co-payment and registration fees required.

Table 10.2. (Continued)

Program	Eligibility	Notes
Newfoundland and Labrador		
Foundation Plan	Residents who qualify for income support benefits	Provides 100% coverage of eligible prescription drugs.
Access Plan and Assurance Plan	For low and middle-income individuals and families Based on income	Covers 20%–70% of total prescription cost, depending on income. Co-payment and deductible may be required depending on level of household income.
65Plus Plan	Residents age ≥65 years who receive Old Age Security benefits and Guaranteed Income Supplement	Copayment is a maximum $6 dispensing fee. No limit to the annual income-based deductible collected. No assistance available for residents with a net annual household income ≥ $150,000. Seniors incur the same out-of-pocket expenses as non-senior counterparts with the same income.
Northwest Territories		
Extended Health Benefits for Specified Disease Conditions Program	Non-Indigenous registered Northwest Territories residents under the care of an MD or nurse practitioner	Universal coverage of antiretrovirals for all of residents living with HIV
Métis Health Benefits Program	For registered Métis who are residents of Northwest Territories	Universal coverage of antiretrovirals for all of residents living with HIV.
Extended Health Benefits for Seniors Program	For non-Indigenous and non-Métis registered residents of Northwest Territories who are age ≥ 60 years under the care of an MD or NP	Coordination of private insurance benefits allowed. Universal coverage of antiretrovirals for all residents living with HIV
Nova Scotia		
Nova Scotia Family Pharmacare Program	Registered residents of Nova Scotia	Coordination of private insurance benefits is required. Places restrictions on the prescriber authorizing the regimen. Seniors incur same out-of-pocket expenses as non-senior counterparts with the same income.

(Continued)

Table 10.2. (Continued)

Program	Eligibility	Notes
Nunavut		
Extended Health Benefits Program	Non-Indigenous registered Nunavut residents with a specified condition Non-Indigenous residents aged $\geq$ 65 years Registered residents who are not fully covered by third-party insurance	Universal coverage of antiretrovirals for all residents living with HIV
Ontario		
Ontario Drug Benefit Program	Residents of long-term care facilities Ontario residents enrolled in the Health atHome home care program People enrolled in Ontario Works for income support People enrolled in the Ontario Disability Support Program for income support and other services Registered residents aged $\geq$ 65 years	Seniors pay a deductible but a waiver is available for low-income seniors.
Trillium Drug Program	Registered Ontario residents enrolled in the Trillium Drug Program who have high drug costs relative to their income Patients can register in the Trillium Drug Program if they • do not have private insurance coverage or their private insurance does not cover 100% of their prescription drug costs; • have valid Ontario Health Insurance and are a resident of Ontario; or • are not eligible for drug coverage as another category of recipient under the Ontario Drug Benefit Program	Recipients pay a deductible equal to 4% of their annual net household income.
OHIP+	Ontario residents aged 24 years and younger who have an OHIP card and do not have private insurance.	No coverage available for those with private insurance even if private insurance does not cover the prescribed drug.

Table 10.2. (Continued)

Program	Eligibility	Notes
Prince Edward Island		
Health PEI: HIV Drug Program	Registered HIV-positive residents of Prince Edward Island	Does not provide universal coverage of prescriptions not related to HIV. Provides universal coverage of antiretrovirals for all residents living with HIV.
Quebec		
Régie de l'assurance maladie du Québec	Recipients of Social Assistance and Social Solidarity Program Single adults, aged 18–25 years, living with parents and full-time students in an educational institution at the secondary, college, or university level Registered Quebec residents aged ≥ 65 years Registered residents of Quebec without private insurance	Collects a yearly income-based premium of $0–$710 from non-insured people whether they purchased drugs or not. Some low-income groups, children, and persons with disabilities can access the program at no cost.
Saskatchewan[a]		
Saskatchewan Drug Plan, Exceptional Drug Status Program	Registered Saskatchewan residents living with HIV, regardless of age or income.	Places restrictions on the prescriber authorizing the regimen. Provides universal coverage of antiretrovirals for all residents living with HIV.
Seniors' Drug Plan	Aged ≥ 65 years with net income of ≤ $75,918	No deductible, but co-payment is required.
Supplementary Health Program	Government wards Inmates of provincial correctional institutions Residents of special care facilities who are eligible for the Senior's Income Plan Those enrolled in the following income support programs: • Saskatchewan Assured Income for Disability • Provincial Training Allowance • Saskatchewan Income Support	Co-payment and coverage depends on which sub-plan a person qualifies for.

(Continued)

Table 10.2. (Continued)

Program	Eligibility	Notes
Yukon		
Chronic Disease and Disability Benefits Program	Registered Yukon residents	Places restrictions on the prescriber authorizing the regimen. Annual deductible may be waived on the basis of income. Coordination with private insurance is required.
Pharmacare and Extended Health Benefits Program	Registered residents aged $\geq$ 65 years or aged > 60 years and married to a Yukon resident who is aged $\geq$ 65 years	Places restrictions on the prescriber authorizing the regimen.

Source: Data were retrieved from Yoong D, Bayoumi AM, Robinson L, et al. Public prescription drug plan coverage for antiretrovirals and the potential cost to people living with HIV in Canada: a descriptive study. CMAJ. 2018;6(4): E551–E560https://doi.org/10.9778/cmajo.20180058; Public Health Agency of Canada (PHAC). HIV antiretroviral medication coverage in Canada [Internet]. Ottawa: PHAC; 2023. Available from: https://www.canada.ca/content/dam/phac-aspc/documents/services/publications/diseases-conditions/summary-hiv-antiretroviral-medication-coverage/phac-drugcoveragedoc.pdf.

Note: ART = antiretroviral therapy; OHIP = Ontario Health Insurance Plan.
[a] These plans are part of the general Saskatchewan Drug Plan.

Private plans may provide partial coverage or require plan members to pay a deductible, premium, or co-payment. People living with HIV often face medication disruptions when they lose a job and the health benefits associated with it. It is important for any person living with HIV who has left or plans to leave their employment or has otherwise lost their private insurance coverage to get legal or other advice about their entitlement to benefits and to plan with their primary care provider to maintain access to medications.

Compassionate supply through pharmaceutical companies is an option to avoid treatment interruptions or initiate treatment for those without coverage.[125] Each pharmaceutical company has a different process for accessing compassionate medication coverage, and the access is usually time-limited. Patients must access these programs through their prescriber.

Local AIDS service organizations will often be familiar with options for emergency medication and sources of drug coverage. Local services can be found through the Where To? website operated by CATIE, Canada's source for HIV and hepatitis C information.[126]

Immigration and Refugee Law

People living with HIV are allowed to travel to Canada. They are also allowed to apply to remain in Canada as temporary or permanent residents and to make claims for refugee protection. However, HIV status is a factor that immigration and refugee decision makers may consider when deciding whether a person can stay in Canada for an extended period or permanently.[127]

The effect of HIV status on an individual's ability to remain in Canada will vary depending on the type of immigration application being submitted. For some immigration applicants and refugee claimants, considerations such as HIV-related stigma and discrimination and limited access to HIV-related medical care in their countries of origin may support a refugee claim or an application for permanent residence from within Canada on humanitarian and compassionate grounds. Other immigration applicants face potential barriers to temporary or permanent residence in Canada because of the estimated cost of their medical care. This is known as medical inadmissibility due to excessive demand on health or social services and is discussed in more detail in the following section.

Medical Inadmissibility

A foreign national who applies for temporary or permanent residence may be inadmissible to Canada if they have a health condition that

- is likely to be a danger to public health;[128]
- is likely to be a danger to public safety;[129] or
- might reasonably be expected to cause excessive demand on health or social services.[130]

Canadian immigration authorities do not consider HIV to be a danger to public health or public safety.[131] However, persons living with HIV may be medically inadmissible for excessive demand on health or social services. An applicant is considered to place an excessive demand on health or social services when

- the cost of the health or social services for an applicant is expected to exceed the annual average per capita costs of these services for Canadians[132] and
- the health or social services needed to treat their health condition would negatively affect wait times for services in Canada.[133]

To assess an applicant's medical admissibility, Immigration, Refugees and Citizenship Canada (IRCC) looks at cost of the estimated health care and social services an applicant is expected to use over the five years after their Immigration Medical Exam (IME).[134] When there is evidence that significant costs are likely to be incurred after five years, a decision-maker may look at estimated health and social services costs over 10 consecutive years.[135]

In June 2018, IRCC enacted a temporary policy that significantly increased the excessive demand threshold cost amount. The June 2018 policy allows immigration officers to exempt individuals from the excessive demand threshold if their health care costs are less than three times the average Canadian per capita health and social services costs over five consecutive years.[136] In 2025, the cost threshold under the temporary public policy is $27,162 per year, or $135,810 over five years.[137] The IRCC website provides detailed information on how it calculates medical and social service costs.

Until the June 2018 temporary public policy, most people living with HIV were inadmissible for excessive demand because of the high cost of antiretroviral medications. Now, health care costs for many people living with HIV fall under the new threshold. However, the cost of medical care for some people living with HIV continues to exceed the present threshold, especially when applicants are receiving treatment for other illnesses or have other co-morbidities.

When IRCC believes an applicant is likely inadmissible to Canada because of excessive demand, they will send the applicant a procedural fairness letter. This letter informs the applicant of the health and social services that IRCC believes the applicant will require. The applicant has 60 days to provide additional information and documentation to address and try to convince IRCC to overturn the finding of medical inadmissibility.[138]

A person living with HIV may be able to satisfy an immigration or visa officer that they will not cause an excessive demand on health or social services if they can demonstrate that the cost of their care will be less than the amount calculated by IRCC or that they have a viable mitigation plan.[139] An applicant who can demonstrate that the cost of their required medical care is under the excessive demand threshold or that they have private medical insurance in Canada that will cover the cost of their HIV medications may be able to overcome a finding of medical inadmissibility.

Applicants who are found to be medically inadmissible will usually be denied the visa for which they have applied. Applicants for permanent residence may be able to request an exemption from the medical admissibility requirements on humanitarian and compassionate grounds. Applicants may also be able to obtain a Temporary Resident Permit (TRP) in exceptional circumstances.[140]

An applicant who has been found to be medically inadmissible is not banned from entering Canada under different circumstances (i.e., someone who has been refused a permanent resident visa because they have been found to be medically inadmissible may be able to enter Canada as a visitor). Applicants who have been found to be medically inadmissible may also be able to obtain a TRP in exceptional circumstances.[141]

Tips for Primary Care Providers to Support Patients Facing Potential Medical Inadmissibility

- Advise your patient to consult with or retain immigration counsel who has experience with medical inadmissibility cases.
- Review the breakdown of services and associated costs as well as the prognosis outlined by the immigration medical officer that can be found in the procedural fairness letter to ensure that it accurately reflects your patient's medical condition and care.
- If your patient's medications are very expensive, consider whether there are less expensive substitutes.
- You may be asked to write a letter to support your patient's response to the procedural fairness letter. See the general tips on writing letters of support in the text box in the "HIV Status and Applications for Permanent Residence from Within Canada on Humanitarian and Compassionate Grounds" section.

Applicants may challenge a final decision of medical inadmissibility before either the Immigration Appeal Division or the Federal Court, depending on the type of application that was submitted.[142] The timelines for challenging immigration decisions are short – 15, 30, or 60 days, depending on the situation.[143] Applicants who want to challenge a finding of medical inadmissibility should contact a lawyer who specializes in immigration law as soon as possible. Paralegals or registered immigration consultants may also be able to assist in some circumstances.

Certain categories of foreign nationals cannot be inadmissible for excessive demand on health or social services:

- sponsored members of the family class, including spouses, common-law partners, and dependent children, and
- *Convention* refugees and protected persons and their dependants, including government-assisted and privately sponsored refugees.[144]

Most applicants for temporary residence will not be subject to the excessive demand provisions because they will not be eligible for government-funded health or social services in Canada. Applicants for temporary residence who may become eligible for publicly funded health and social services while in Canada, such as some international students and foreign workers, will be assessed to determine whether they are medically inadmissible for excessive demand.

The eligibility of international students and foreign workers for publicly funded health and social services varies from one province or territory to another. Applicants living with HIV should check whether they are eligible for publicly funded health and social services, including drug coverage, in the province or territory where they intend to work or study. They should also check whether any health insurance provided by their employer or educational institution covers HIV-related medical care and, if so, the extent of the coverage.

The Immigration Medical Examination

Everyone aged 15 years and older who is required to complete an IME is also required to undergo an HIV test as part of the IME.[145] Panel physicians may also request HIV testing for an individual younger than age 15 in some circumstances.[146] Although IRCC requires physicians who are authorized to conduct the IME to provide pre- and post-HIV test counselling, anecdotal evidence suggests that this does not always occur.

After the IME is complete, the panel physician's office sends the results to IRCC for assessment by an immigration medical officer.

If an applicant tests positive for HIV in an IME that is conducted in Canada, the panel physician will notify the applicable public health authorities.[147] They will advise the applicant of any obligations to notify sexual partners. When an IME is conducted outside of Canada, the applicant's HIV status may be shared with local public health authorities or third parties (such as sexual partners) when local law requires it.[148] The applicant's HIV status will be shared with the provincial or territorial public health authorities where the applicant intends to settle only if the applicant's immigration application is successful. The public health agency may contact the applicant after they arrive in Canada.[149]

Partner Notification in Immigration and Refugee Cases

IRCC previously had an automatic partner notification policy for HIV-positive applicants. The automatic partner notification policy required HIV-positive applicants to voluntarily disclose their HIV status to their spouse or common-law partner living in Canada within a specified period or to withdraw their application. If an applicant did neither, an immigration officer would send a formal notification letter to the partner living in Canada. IRCC discontinued this policy as of 7 July 2023.[150] Applicants who test positive for HIV in the sponsored family class and dependant refugee class are now subject to generally the same procedural process as all other applicants who test positive for HIV, as described earlier.

Family Sponsorship for Sponsors Receiving Disability Support

Some people living with HIV in Canada receive government financial assistance for people living with disabilities through programs such as the Ontario Disability Support Program or British Columbia's Employment and Assistance Program for Persons with Disability. Canada's immigration law excludes people on social assistance for reasons other than disability from sponsoring their family members.[151] Individuals who receive financial support for reasons related to disability are eligible to apply to sponsor members of the family class – their spouse or common-law partner or conjugal partner, dependent children, or both.[152] However, some difficulties may arise during and after the sponsorship application if the sponsor is receiving financial support for reasons related to disability. As a result, all parties should be referred to a legal professional for advice before initiating an application.

Minimum income requirements must be met to sponsor other family members (family members who are not part of the family class), such as parents and grandparents.[153] Family members who are not part of the family class are also subject to Canada's excessive demand provisions.

More detailed information about family sponsorship while receiving social assistance can be found in chapter 7.

HIV Status and Claims for Refugee Protection

A *Convention* refugee is a person who is living outside of their country and not able or willing to return because they have good reason to fear being persecuted for their race, religion, nationality, political opinion, or membership in a particular social group.[154] A person in need of protection is a person in Canada who would likely face a risk of torture, a risk to their life, or a risk of cruel and unusual treatment or punishment if they had to return to their country.[155] In Canada, people who have been determined to be *Convention* refugees or persons in need of protection may be referred to as *protected persons*.

Persecution because of HIV status can be the basis of a claim for refugee protection or part of the overall risk profile of a claimant, especially when it intersects with gender, gender identity, gender expression, sexual orientation, political opinion, drug use (disability), or other grounds of persecution. HIV status may also be relevant to other aspects of the analysis of whether someone is a *Convention* refugee or a person in need of protection. For example, a refugee claimant living with HIV does not have a viable internal flight alternative in a location where HIV-related medical care is not available.[156]

That HIV-related medical care is not equivalent to what someone may receive in Canada or is not available at all is not relevant to the determination of *Convention* refugee or protected person status unless medical care is not being provided for a discriminatory reason.[157] This factor may be considered as part of an application for permanent residence from within Canada on humanitarian and compassionate grounds.[158]

Refugee claimants and others seeking Canada's protection should be encouraged to include their HIV status in their claim and to seek advice from counsel who has experience with these types of cases. In some jurisdictions, a paralegal or registered immigration consultant may be able to represent a claimant at a refugee hearing.

HIV Status and Applications for Permanent Residence from within Canada on Humanitarian and Compassionate Grounds

As discussed in chapter 7, applications for permanent residence from within Canada on humanitarian and compassionate factors (H&C applications) can be based on much broader considerations than a claim for refugee protection. Applicants can put forward any reason that they should be allowed to remain in Canada, including access to HIV-related medical care and HIV-related stigma and discrimination that may not meet the legal test of being persecutory for the purposes of a claim for refugee protection.

Although H&C applications allow decision-makers to consider a wider range of factors than a claim for refugee protection, there are significant downsides to making an H&C application as opposed to a refugee claim. H&C applicants do not have a right to remain in Canada while their application is considered and are generally not eligible for a work permit or provincial or territorial health insurance coverage. It is very important that individuals get advice about their options from an experienced immigration lawyer.

Tips for Writing Letters of Support for Immigration Applicants and Refugee Claimants Living with HIV

- Communicate with counsel to ensure that you understand the reason you are providing the letter and what specific information counsel requires.
- Letters should be on letterhead, signed, and dated.
- Briefly outline your relevant qualifications and experience and how long you have been treating the patient.
- Use professional, neutral language. Avoid language that may be seen as advocacy for your patient.
- Use plain language when possible, because the audience for your letter will primarily be people without medical training.
- Avoid discussions of access to medical care or HIV-related stigma or discrimination in the patient's country of origin unless you have direct experience with and knowledge of these topics, such as experience providing medical care in that country.

See chapter 7 for more information about H&C applications.

Travelling Outside of Canada

People living with HIV can travel to many countries. However, some countries restrict entry for people living with HIV. These restrictions may apply only to individuals who are applying for work or residence permits or may restrict all people living with HIV from entering the country for any reason. Enforcement of HIV-related entry restrictions may vary.

It is recommended that people living with HIV check for any HIV-related travel restrictions before making travel plans. Information about

HIV-related entry restrictions can be found online or by checking with the consulate of the destination country.[159]

Bringing HIV Medications into Canada

As a general rule, citizens and permanent residents of Canada may not bring prescription medications into Canada. This includes carrying medications across the border or having medications delivered by mail or by courier.[160]

Newly landed immigrants, refugees, and temporary residents may bring a personal supply of prescription medications with them into Canada. Health Canada defines a personal supply as a 90-day supply of medication or a single course of treatment, whichever is less.[161] Temporary residents of Canada staying for longer than three months may obtain an additional 90-day supply of their prescription medications for their own personal use by mail or courier every three months.[162] International students and other temporary residents from countries that provide free or low-cost HIV medications may prefer to have medications shipped from their country of citizenship.

Any medications brought into Canada for personal use must be in the package dispensed by the hospital or pharmacy, be in the original retail package, or have the original label attached to it that states what the medication is and what it contains.[163] Temporary residents who are having medications mailed or couriered to them should be prepared to provide a copy of their passport and proof of their temporary resident status, such as a copy of their visitor visa or visitor record, work permit, or study permit.[164]

Conclusion

There is much good news for people living with HIV in Canada. People who have access to sustained treatment and care now have more or less the same life expectancy as those who are HIV-negative. Because of advances in treatment, HIV has now become a manageable chronic condition. That ought to be celebrated. However, the legal problems that often accompany an HIV diagnosis remain. Many people face significant institutional, social, and economic barriers to accessing health care and life-saving medications. These barriers are not evenly distributed; key affected populations, including men who have sex with men, Indigenous Peoples, Black persons, migrants, and people who use drugs, are particularly affected by the stigma, discrimination, and criminalization that can accompany an HIV diagnosis. From being denied services to being refused accommodation in the workplace, human rights concerns are widespread. Privacy is a constant worry for many, whether it is related to institutional actors, service providers, or neighbours, and legal recourse may be difficult to obtain. Canada remains a world leader in prosecuting people living with HIV, with upwards of 220 such prosecutions. Public health orders can infringe on the liberty of people living with HIV. Vital access to medication remains challenging because of Canada's patchwork of medication coverage. Immigrants and refugees living with HIV and their families face unique challenges in Canada's immigration system.

Access to legal information and services at an early stage can help people living with HIV resolve problems before they become crises. Identifying and resolving legal issues early can also reduce stress that can negatively affect the immune system and adherence to medications, thus directly affecting health outcomes. People living with HIV are experts on their own lives and can identify the problems most affecting their well-being. This chapter has aimed to equip health care providers with the knowledge to support people living with HIV to take action on those problems.

Acknowledgment

The authors express their deep gratitude to the lived experience advisors who provided invaluable feedback on the development of this chapter: Pat Brown, Muluba Habanyama and Trevor Stratton. The authors thank Jonathan Glenn Betteridge, former staff lawyer at the HIV & AIDS Legal Clinic Ontario (HALCO); Léo Bourgeois, summer law student at HALCO; Avineet Cheema, former staff lawyer at HALCO; Alexandra Veall, staff lawyer at HALCO; and Glen Stratton, workplace lawyer, for their contributions to this chapter.

NOTES

1 We use the term *person* or *people living with HIV* throughout this chapter, rather than *patients, HIV- or AIDS-infected persons*, or other terms that centre the medical side of HIV and AIDS. The Denver Principles, the seminal statement created by people living with HIV/AIDS in 1983, puts it this way: "We condemn attempts to label us as 'victims,' a term which implies defeat, and we are only occasionally 'patients,' a term which implies passivity, helplessness, and dependence upon the care of others. We are 'People With AIDS'" (Joint United Nations Programme on HIV/AIDS.

The Denver principles: 1983 [Internet]. Geneva: Joint United Nations Programme on HIV/AIDS; 2007 [cited 2022 July 19]. https://data.unaids .org/pub/externaldocument/2007/gipa1983denverprinciples_en.pdf). As a result, we use the term *patient* only when it reflects the legal language of a law. We also refer to HIV, the virus that causes AIDS, throughout this chapter rather than HIV/AIDS. Given advances in treatment, progression to AIDS is now relatively rare among people living with HIV in North America who have access to medical care.

2 World Health Organization. Summary report: World Conference on Social Determinants of Health. Geneva: World Health Organization; 2013.

3 Nobleman R. Addressing access to justice as a social determinant of health. Health Law J. 2014; 49(21):52. *Access to justice* can be defined as access to legal services, courts, and tribunals, but it also encompasses access to legal information, effective and affordable means of resolving legal disputes, and laws and policies that help people avoid legal problems in the first place.

4 Public Health Agency of Canada (PHAC). HIV in Canada: 2022 surveillance highlights [Internet]. Ottawa: PHAC; 2022. Available from: https://www.canada.ca/en/public-health/services/publications /diseases-conditions/hiv-2022-surveillance-highlights.html.

5 Centers for Disease Control and Prevention. Revised guidelines for HIV counselling, testing, and referral and revised recommendations for HIV screening of pregnant women. MMWR Recomm Rep. 2001;50(1):37.

6 Public Health Agency of Canada (PHAC). Estimates of HIV incidence, prevalence and Canada's progress on meeting the 90-90-90 HIV targets [Internet]. Ottawa: PHAC; 2021. Available from: https://www.canada.ca /en/public-health/services/publications/diseases-conditions/summary -estimates-hiv-incidence-prevalence-canadas-progress-90-90-90.html#s11.

7 Joint United Nations Programme on HIV/AIDS (UNAIDS). The Denver principles: 1983 [Internet]. Geneva: UNAIDS; 2007 [cited 2022 July 19]. Available from: https://data.unaids.org/pub/externaldocument/2007 /gipa1983denverprinciples_en.pdf; Joint United Nations Programme on HIV/AIDS (UNAIDS). UNAIDS policy brief: the greater involvement of people living with HIV [Internet]. Geneva: UNAIDS; 2007. Available from: https://www.unaids.org/sites/default/files/media_asset/jc1299 -policybrief-gipa_en_0.pdf. For a Canadian example, see Ontario AIDS Network (OAN). The Ontario accord [Internet]. Toronto: OAN; n.d. [cited 2022 July 19]. Available from: https://oan.red/ontario-accord/.

8 For more information about HIV and the law in Canada, see HIV Legal Network, https://www.hivlegalnetwork.ca. For information and advice about HIV and the law in Ontario, see HIV & AIDS Legal Clinic Ontario (HALCO), https://www.halco.org or call 416-340-7790 or

1-888-705-8889. For information and advice about HIV and the law in Quebec, see Coalition des organismes communautaires québécois de lutte contre le sida (COCQ-Sida), www.cocqsida.com (in French only) or call 514-844-2477 or 1-866-535-0481.

9 McCullagh J. A guide for service providers [Internet]. Toronto: Canada's source for HIV and hepatitis C Information; 2019. Available from: https://www.catie.ca/sites/default/files/2021-10/catie-uuguide-en2.pdf.

10 Pp. 45–58 and 66–72 of EKOS Research Associates. 2012 HIV/AIDS Attitudinal Tracking Survey: final report [Internet]. Ottawa: EKOS Research Associates; 2012. Available from: https://www.catie.ca/sites/default/files/2012-HIV-AIDS-attitudinal-tracking-survey-final-report.pdf; pp. 41–45 of EKOS Research Associates. Canadians' awareness, knowledge and attitudes related to sexually transmitted and blood-borne infections: 2018 findings report [Internet]. Ottawa: EKOS Research Associates; 2018. Available from: https://epe.lac-bac.gc.ca/100/200/301/pwgsc-tpsgc/por-ef/public_health_agency_canada/2018/056-17-e/report.pdf.

11 Ontario Human Rights Commission. Policy on ableism and discrimination based on disability [Internet]. Toronto: The Commission; 2016. Available from: https://www3.ohrc.on.ca/sites/default/files/Policy%20on%20ableism%20and%20discrimination%20based%20on%20disability_accessible_2016.pdf.

12 See, for example, *Quebec (Commission des droits de la personne et des droits de la jeunesse) v Montréal (City)*, [2000] 1 SCR 665, at para 48, 2000 SCC 27 (CanLII).

13 Ontario Human Rights Commission. Policy on ableism and discrimination based on disability [Internet]. Toronto: The Commission; 2016. Available from: https://www3.ohrc.on.ca/sites/default/files/Policy%20on%20ableism%20and%20discrimination%20based%20on%20disability_accessible_2016.pdf.

14 *Frank v AJR Enterprises Ltd. (c.o.b. "Nelson Place Hotel")*, (1993), 23 CHRR D/228 (BCCHR).

15 Ontario Human Rights Commission. Policy on ableism and discrimination based on disability [Internet]. Toronto: The Commission; 2016. Available from: https://www3.ohrc.on.ca/sites/default/files/Policy%20on%20ableism%20and%20discrimination%20based%20on%20disability_accessible_2016.pdf.

16 *Hydro-Québec v Syndicat des employé-e-s de techniques professionnelles et de bureau d'Hydro-Québec, section locale 2000 (SCFP-FTQ)*, 2008 SCC 43 (CanLII), at para 14.

17 See chapter 2 for more information on the features of undue hardship.

18 See, for example, *Human Rights Code*, RSO 1990, c H.19, s 11(2).

19 See, for example, Ontario Human Rights Commission. Policy on ableism and discrimination based on disability [Internet]. Toronto: Ontario Human

Rights Commission; 2016 [cited 27 December 2024], at section 10: Other limits on the duty to accommodate. Available from: https://www3.ohrc .on.ca/en/policy-ableism-and-discrimination-based-disability.

20 For example, it may be relevant to know a patient's CD4 count and viral load before major surgery. Their HIV status alone is usually insufficient information on which to base a decision about eligibility for a given service or procedure.

21 Ontario Human Rights Commission. Policy position on medical documentation to be provided when a disability-related accommodation request is made [Internet]. Toronto: Ontario Human Rights Commission; n.d. [cited 2022 July 20]. Available from: https://www.ohrc.on.ca /en/ohrc-policy-position-medical-documentation-be-provided-when -disability-related-accommodation-request.

22 *Saskatchewan Human Rights Code*, SS 1979, c S-24.1, ss 31.3–31.4; *Human Rights Code*, RSO 1990, c H19, 2.45.2; *Human Rights Code*, RSBC 1996, c 210, s 37.

23 See, for example, Saskatchewan Human Rights Commission. A restorative approach [Internet]. Saskatoon (SK): Saskatchewan Human Rights Commission; n.d. Available from: https://saskatchewanhumanrights.ca /education-resources/information-sheets/restorative-approach/.

24 Canadian HIV/AIDS Legal Network, Canadian Public Health Association. Reducing stigma and discrimination through the protection of privacy and confidentiality [Internet]. Ottawa: Canadian Public Health Association; 2017. Available from: https://www.cpha.ca/reducing-stigma-and -discrimination-through-protection-privacy-and-confidentiality.

25 Von Tigerstrom B. Information & privacy law in Canada. Toronto: Irwin Law; 2020.

26 *Health Information Act*, RSA 2000, c H-5, s 105; *Personal Health Information Act*, CCSM c P33.5, s 62; *Personal Health Information Protection Act*, 2004, SO 2004, c 3, Sched A, s 71(1); *Health Information Privacy and Management Act*, SY 2013, c 16, s 119.

27 Von Tigerstrom B. Information & privacy law in Canada. Toronto: Irwin Law; 2020.

28 *Personal Information Protection and Electronic Documents Act* (PIPEDA), SC 2000, c 5, s 30. *PIPEDA* does not apply where and to the extent that provincial legislation that is substantially similar applies. Health information statutes in Ontario, New Brunswick, Newfoundland and Labrador, and Nova Scotia are considered to be substantially similar. *PIPEDA* can still apply to PHI when it overlaps with health information legislation, except in Quebec, Alberta, and British Columbia, where general private sector privacy legislation has been deemed substantially similar and applies instead; see p. 455 of Von Tigerstrom B. Information & privacy law in Canada. Toronto: Irwin Law; 2020.

29 Von Tigerstrom B. Information & privacy law in Canada. Toronto: Irwin Law; 2020. See, for example, Canadian Medical Association. Principles for the protection of patient privacy. Ottawa: The Association; 2017. Available from: https://www.cma.ca/sites/default/files/2018-11/PD18-02.pdf.

30 For example, *Privacy Act*, RSC 1985, c P-21; *Freedom of Information and Protection of Privacy Act*, RSO 1990, c F.31; *Municipal Freedom of Information and Protection of Privacy Act*, RSO 1990, c M.56.

31 Ontario Human Rights Commission. Human rights at work 2008 – third edition [Internet]. Toronto: Carswell; 2008. Available from: https://www .ohrc.on.ca/en/iv-human-rights-issues-all-stages-employment/4 -designing-application-forms.

32 *R v Mabior*, 2012 SCC 47.

33 HIV Legal Network. Know your rights 1: disclosure at work [Internet]. Toronto: The Network; 2013. Available from: https://www.hivlegalnetwork .ca/site/know-your-rights-1-disclosure-at-work/?lang=en.

34 See, for example, *Mandatory Blood Testing Act*, 2006, SO 2006, c 26.

35 See, for example, Renke W. Appendix N: Uniform Mandatory Testing and Disclosure Act [Internet]. Nepean (ON): Uniform Law Conference of Canada; n.d. Available from: https://www.ulcc-chlc.ca/ULCC/media /EN-Annual-Meeting-2004/Uniform-Mandatory-Testing-and-Disclosure -Act-(2004)-Adopted_1.pdf.

36 PEP helps prevent the transmission of HIV to an HIV-negative person who may recently have been exposed to the virus. It must be started as soon as possible after exposure, within 72 hours at most, and taken for 28 days. For more information about PEP, see Arkell C. Post exposure prophylaxis (PEP) [Internet]. Toronto: Canada's source for HIV and hepatitis C information; 2019. Available from: https://www.catie.ca/post-exposure -prophylaxis-pep.

37 Local AIDS service organisations can be located on the Where To? website: https://whereto.catie.ca/.

38 Canadian HIV/AIDS Legal Network, Canadian Public Health Association. Reducing stigma and discrimination through the protection of privacy and confidentiality [Internet]. Ottawa: Canadian Public Health Association; 2017. Available from: https://www.cpha.ca/reducing-stigma-and -discrimination-through-protection-privacy-and-confidentiality.

39 See Part I(D) of Public Health Agency of Canada [PHAC]. Routine practices and additional precautions for preventing the transmission of infection in healthcare settings [Internet]. Ottawa: PHAC; 2017. Available from: https://www.canada.ca/en/public-health/services/publications /diseases-conditions/routine-practices-precautions-healthcare-associated -infections.html.

40 *Personal Health Information Protection Act*, 2004, SO 2004, c 3, Sch A, s 20(2).

41 *Personal Health Information Protection Act*, 2004, SO 2004, c 3, Sch A, s 20(3).

42 HIV Legal Network. Know your rights 6: privacy and health records [Internet]. Toronto: The Network; 2014. Available from: https://www .hivlegalnetwork.ca/site/know-your-rights-6-privacy-and-health -records/?lang=en.

43 *E-Health (Personal Health Information Access and Protection of Privacy) Act*, SBC 2008, c 38, ss 9–10.

44 HIV Legal Network. Know your rights 6: privacy and health records [Internet]. Toronto: The Network; 2014. Available from: https://www .hivlegalnetwork.ca/site/know-your-rights-6-privacy-and-health -records/?lang=en.

45 College of Physicians and Surgeons of Ontario. Reporting requirements [Internet]. Toronto: The College; 2000 [updated November 2024]. Available from: https://www.cpso.on.ca/Physicians/Policies-Guidance/Policies /Mandatory-and-Permissive-Reporting#offences.

46 For guidelines on counselling about HIV non-disclosure, see Canadian HIV/AIDS Legal Network. Counselling in the context of the criminalization of HIV non-disclosure [Internet]. In: HIV disclosure and the law: a resource kit for service providers. Toronto: The Network; 2017. Available from: https://www.hivlegalnetwork.ca/site/wp-content /uploads/2014/02/Chapter4.2-ENG.pdf.

47 For example, in British Columbia, if a physician believes that a patient poses a risk of HIV infection to another person, the physician may provide information about that person to the medical officer of health, in accordance with the regulations on communicable diseases made under the *Health Act*. In Nova Scotia, the applicable public health legislation requires a physician who is not satisfied that an HIV-positive patient has informed his or her partner of a risk of exposure to HIV to consult the medical officer.

48 Canadian HIV/AIDS Legal Network. Client confidentiality and record-keeping: preventing harm to others [Internet]. In: HIV disclosure and the law: a resource kit for service providers. Toronto: The Network; 2017. Available from: https://www.hivlegalnetwork.ca/site/wp-content /uploads/2014/02/Chapter5.3-ENG.pdf. Note that courts have ruled that some institutions and professionals with specific mandates – including hospitals, psychiatrists, social workers, and police – have a duty, in some specific circumstances, to take reasonable steps to protect someone they can identify as being at risk of harm, either by better controlling or supervising a patient or by warning specific people known to be at risk. This has not been applied to risk of HIV transmission in Canada.

49 Canadian HIV/AIDS Legal Network, Canadian Public Health Association. Reducing stigma and discrimination through the protection of privacy and confidentiality [Internet]. Ottawa: Canadian Public Health Association;

2017. Available from: https://www.cpha.ca/reducing-stigma-and -discrimination-through-protection-privacy-and-confidentiality.

50 *Smith v Jones*, 1999 CanLII 674 (SCC), [1999] 1 SCR 455.

51 *Smith v Jones*, 1999 CanLII 674 (SCC), [1999] 1 SCR 455.

52 For guidance in developing such policies, see Canadian HIV/AIDS Legal Network. Client confidentiality and record-keeping: preventing harm to others [Internet]. In: HIV disclosure and the law: a resource kit for service providers. Toronto: The Network; 2017. Available from: https://www .hivlegalnetwork.ca/site/wp-content/uploads/2014/02/Chapter5.3 -ENG.pdf.

53 For additional guidance see Canadian HIV/AIDS Legal Network. Client confidentiality and record-keeping: preventing harm to others [Internet]. In: HIV disclosure and the law: a resource kit for service providers. Toronto: The Network; 2017. Available from: https://www.hivlegalnetwork.ca/site /wp-content/uploads/2014/02/Chapter5.3-ENG.pdf.

54 *Jones v Tsige*, 2012 ONCA 32; *VonMaltzahn v Koppernaes*, 2018 NSSC 192; see also *Marson v Nova Scotia*, 2017 NSCA 17. Courts in Manitoba, Nova Scotia, Alberta, New Brunswick, and Newfoundland and Labrador, and the Federal Court have recognized intrusion upon seclusion as a potential legal claim, but none have decided cases recognizing the tort.

55 *Jane Doe 72511 v M.N*, 2018 ONSC 6607.

56 *Racki v Racki*, 2021 NSSC 46.

57 *ES v Shillington*, 2021 ABQB 739.

58 *Jane Doe 72511 v M.N*, 2018 ONSC 6607.

59 *Freedom of Information and Protection of Privacy Act*, RSBC 1996, c 165; *Freedom of Information and Protection of Privacy Act*, SS 1990–91, c F-22.01; *Freedom of Information and Protection of Privacy Act*, CCSM c F175; *Privacy Act*, RSNL 1990, c P-22.

60 See section 5A:1 of McIsaac B, Klein K, Brown S. Law of privacy in Canada (loose-leaf updated 2022, release 2022–6). Toronto: Thomson Reuters; 2000. The equivalent entity in Nova Scotia is the Review Officer; in New Brunswick, it is the Ombud; the Quebec law is enforced by the Commission d'accès à l'information, although the administration of the law is overseen by the Minister of Health and Social Services.

61 For a list of provincial and territorial privacy laws and oversight bodies, see Office of the Privacy Commissioner of Canada. Provincial and territorial privacy laws and oversight [Internet]. Ottawa: The Office; 2020 [modified 2024 Nov 28]. Available from: https://www.priv.gc.ca/en /about-the-opc/what-we-do/provincial-and-territorial-collaboration /provincial-and-territorial-privacy-laws-and-oversight/.

62 HIV Justice Worldwide. Frequently asked questions: what is HIV criminalisation? [Internet]. HIV Justice Worldwide; n.d. [accessed 2022

July 20]. Available from: https://www.hivjusticeworldwide.org/en
/frequently-asked-questions/.

63 HIV Justice Worldwide. Frequently asked questions: what is HIV
criminalisation? [Internet]. HIV Justice Worldwide; n.d. [accessed 2022
July 20]. Available from: https://www.hivjusticeworldwide.org/en
/frequently-asked-questions/.

64 This approach could also apply to other sexually transmitted infections
(STIs), but there have been only a handful of cases related to STIs other
than HIV.

65 A recent report found that the majority of HIV non-disclosure cases in
Canada (64 per cent) involved no transmission of HIV. See Hastings C,
Massoquoi N, Elliott R, et al. HIV criminalization in Canada: key trends
and patterns (1989–2020) [Internet]. Toronto: HIV Legal Network; 2022.
Available from: https://www.hivlegalnetwork.ca/site/hiv
-criminalization-in-canada-key-trends-and-patterns-1989-2020/?lang=en.

66 *R v Cuerrier*, [1998] 2 SCR 371.

67 *R v Mabior*, 2012 SCC 47.

68 Courts have applied the same standard to anal sex. Although the law on oral
sex is unclear, there have been very few prosecutions for oral sex alone in
Canada. The prosecutions that have taken place have established that oral sex
alone does not pose a sufficient risk of transmission to justify criminal liability.

69 *R v Bear*, 2011 MBQB 191; *R v Ratt*, 2012 SKPC 154.

70 *R v JI*, 2006 ONCJ 356. For more on breastfeeding and HIV in high-resource
settings, see Agwu A, Auerbach JD, Cameron B, et al. Expert consensus
statement on breastfeeding and HIV in the United States and Canada
[Internet]. The Well Project; 2020. Available from: https://www
.thewellproject.org/hiv-information/expert-consensus-statement
-breastfeeding-and-hiv-united-states-and-canada. See also Symington A,
Chingore-Munazvo N, Moroz S. When law and science part ways: the
criminalization of breastfeeding by women living with HIV. Ther Adv
Infect Dis. 2022;9:20499361221122481.

71 Chaisson A, Janmohamed K, Peck R, et al. Criminal law and public health.
In: Radbord J, editor. LGBTQ2+ law: practice issues and analysis. Toronto:
Emond Publishing; 2019. p. 496.

72 A recent report found that the majority of HIV non-disclosure cases
in Canada (64 per cent) involved no transmission of HIV: Hastings C,
Massoquoi N, Elliott R, et al. HIV criminalization in Canada: key trends
and patterns (1989–2020) [Internet]. Toronto: HIV Legal Network;
2022. Available from: https://www.hivlegalnetwork.ca/site/hiv
-criminalization-in-canada-key-trends-and-patterns-1989-2020/?lang=en.

73 See, for example, McClelland A. The criminalization of HIV in Canada:
experiences of people living with HIV [Internet]. Hamilton (ON): Positive

Health Network; 2019. Available from: https://aidsnetwork.ca/the
-criminalization-of-hiv-in-canada-experiences-of-people-living-with-hiv/;
Michaud L, Annamanthadoo I, Chu SKH, et al. Harms of sex offender
registries in Canada among people living with HIV [Internet]. Toronto:
HIV Legal Network; 2021. Available from: https://www.hivlegalnetwork
.ca/site/harms-of-sex-offender-registries-in-canada-among-people-living
-with-hiv/?lang=en.

74 Canadian HIV/AIDS Legal Network. The criminalization of HIV non-
disclosure in Canada: current status and the need for change [Internet].
Toronto: The Network; 2019. Available from: https://www
.hivlegalnetwork.ca/site/the-criminalization-of-hiv-non-disclosure-in
-canada-report/?lang=en.

75 Canadian HIV/AIDS Legal Network. The criminalization of HIV non-
disclosure in Canada: current status and the need for change [Internet].
Toronto: The Network; 2019. Available from: https://www
.hivlegalnetwork.ca/site/the-criminalization-of-hiv-non-disclosure
-in-canada-report/?lang=en; Bernard EJ, Symington A, Beaumont S.
Punishing vulnerability through HIV criminalization. Am J Public Health.
2022;112(S4):S395–S397. https://doi.org/10.2105/AJPH.2022.306713.

76 Bernard EJ, Symington A, Beaumont S. Punishing vulnerability through
HIV criminalization. Am J Public Health. 2022;112(S4):S395–S397. https://
doi.org/10.2105/AJPH.2022.306713.

77 See Hastings C, Massoquoi N, Elliott R, et al. HIV criminalization in
Canada: key trends and patterns (1989–2020) [Internet]. Toronto: HIV
Legal Network; 2022. Available from: https://www.hivlegalnetwork.ca
/site/hiv-criminalization-in-canada-key-trends-and-patterns-1989
-2020/?lang=en.

78 See, for example, *R v Morris*, 2021 ONCA 680.

79 See Hastings C, Massoquoi N, Elliott R, et al. HIV criminalization in
Canada: key trends and patterns (1989–2020) [Internet]. Toronto: HIV
Legal Network; 2022. Available from: https://www.hivlegalnetwork.ca
/site/hiv-criminalization-in-canada-key-trends-and-patterns-1989
-2020/?lang=en.

80 Krüsi A, Deering K, Ranville, F, et al.; SHAWNA Project Team.
Marginalized women living with HIV at increased risk of viral load
suppression failure: Implications for prosecutorial guidelines regarding
criminalization of HIV non-disclosure in Canada and globally. Abstract
TUAD0204. J Int AIDS Conf. 2018; 21(S6):e25148. https://doi.org/10.1002
/jia2.25148. Since *Mabior*, studies have established even more clearly that a
person living with HIV with a suppressed viral load cannot transmit HIV
through sex: see Barré-Sinoussi F, Abdool Karim SS, Albert J, et al. Expert
consensus statement on the science of HIV in the context of criminal law.

J Intern AIDS Soc. 2018;21(7):e25161. https://doi.org/10.1002%2Fjia2.25161.
Regarding updated prosecutorial guidelines across Canada, see also p. 8
of Canadian HIV/AIDS Legal Network. The criminalization of HIV non-
disclosure in Canada: current status and the need for change [Internet].
Toronto: The Network; 2019. Available from: https://www
.hivlegalnetwork.ca/site/the-criminalization-of-hiv-non-disclosure-in
-canada-report/?lang=en.

81 Krüsi A, Ranville F, Gurney L, et al. Positive sexuality: HIV disclosure,
gender, violence and the law – a qualitative study. PloS One. 2018;3(8):
e0202776. https://doi.org/10.1371/journal.pone.0202776.

82 Pp. 10–11 of Krüsi A, Ranville F, Gurney L, et al. Positive sexuality: HIV
disclosure, gender, violence and the law – a qualitative study. PloS One.
2018;3(8): e0202776. https://doi.org/10.1371/journal.pone.0202776; pp. 18–19
of House of Commons, Standing Committee on Justice and Human Rights,
The criminalization of HIV non-disclosure in Canada (June 2019), 42nd Parl, 1st
Sess. Available from: https://www.ourcommons.ca/Content
/Committee/421/JUST/Reports/RP10568820/justrp28/justrp28-e.pdf.

83 Krüsi A, Ranville F, Gurney L, et al. Positive sexuality: HIV disclosure,
gender, violence and the law – a qualitative study. PloS One. 2018;3(8):
e0202776. https://doi.org/10.1371/journal.pone.0202776.

84 Grant I. The complex legacy of *R. v. Cuerrier*: HIV nondisclosure prosecutions
and their impact on sexual assault law. Alberta Law Rev. 2020;58(1):45–81.
https://albertalawreview.com/index.php/ALR/article/view/2609/2569.

85 For the purpose of the criminal law in Canada, a low viral load has been
defined as a viral load of less than 1,500 copies per millilitre of blood,
and a suppressed viral load has been defined as a viral load of less than
200 copies per millilitre of blood. Prosecutorial directives now refer to a
suppressed viral load. By contrast, the term *undetectable* is mostly used
in the medical context. It refers to viral loads of less than 20 copies per
millilitre of blood.

86 Loutfy M, Tyndall M, Baril J-G, et al. Canadian consensus statement on
HIV and its transmission in the context of criminal law. Can J Infect Dis
Med Microbiol. 2014;25(3):135–40, https://doi.org/10.1155/2014/498459;
see also Barré-Sinoussi F, Abdool Karim SS, Albert J, et al. Expert
consensus statement on the science of HIV in the context of criminal law. J
Intern AIDS Soc. 2018;21(7):e25161. https://doi.org/10.1002%2Fjia2.25161.

87 Public Health Agency of Canada (PHAC). HIV factsheet: U = U for health
professionals [Internet]. Ottawa: PHAC; 2020. Available from: https://www
.canada.ca/en/public-health/services/publications/diseases-conditions
/hiv-factsheet-undetectable-untransmittable-health-professionals.html.

88 See, for example, Loutfy M, Tyndall M, Baril J-G, et al. Canadian
consensus statement on HIV and its transmission in the context of criminal

law. Can J Infect Dis Med Microbiol. 2014;25(3):135–40, https://doi
.org/10.1155/2014/498459; see also Barré-Sinoussi F, Abdool Karim SS,
Albert J, et al. Expert consensus statement on the science of HIV in the
context of criminal law. J Intern AIDS Soc. 2018;21(7):e25161. https://doi
.org/10.1002%2Fjia2.25161.

89 *R v Thompson*, [2018] NSCA 13.

90 *R v N.G*, [2020] ONCA 494.

91 HIV Legal Network. Overview of HIV criminalization in Canada 2022
    [Internet]. Toronto: The Network; 2022 [cited 2022 July 20]. Available from
    https://www.hivlegalnetwork.ca/site/overview-of-hiv-criminalization
    -in-canada-2022/?lang=en.

92 Hastings C, Massoquoi N, Elliott R, et al. HIV criminalization in Canada:
    key trends and patterns (1989–2020) [Internet]. Toronto: HIV Legal
    Network; 2022. Available from: https://www.hivlegalnetwork.ca/site/hiv
    -criminalization-in-canada-key-trends-and-patterns-1989-2020/?lang=en.

93 See Canadian Coalition to Reform HIV Criminalization. Change the
    code: reforming Canada's criminal code to limit HIV criminalization: a
    community consensus statement [Internet]. The Coalition; n.d. [cited 2022
    Sept 12]. Available from: http://www.hivcriminalization.ca/2022
    -consensus-statement/.

94 For the HIV & AIDS Legal Clinic Ontario (HALCO), see https://www
    .halco.org/; for the HIV Legal Network see https://www.hivlegalnetwork
    .ca; for the Canadian Coalition to Reform HIV Criminalization, see http://
    www.hivcriminalization.ca/.

95 Ministry of the Attorney General. Crown prosecution manual: sexual
    offences against adults [Internet]. Toronto: Queen's Printer for Ontario;
    2017. Available from: https://www.ontario.ca/document/crown
    -prosecution-manual/d-33-sexual-offences-against-adults.

96 BC Prosecution Service. Sexual transmission, or realistic possibility of
    transmission, of HIV [Internet]. In: Crown Counsel policy manual. Victoria
    (BC): The Service; 2019. Available from: https://www2.gov.bc.ca/assets
    /gov/law-crime-and-justice/criminal-justice/prosecution-service/crown
    -counsel-policy-manual/sex-2.pdf.

97 HIV Legal Network. Overview of HIV criminalization in Canada 2022
    [Internet]. Toronto: The Network; 2022 [cited 2022 July 20]. Available from
    https://www.hivlegalnetwork.ca/site/overview-of-hiv-criminalization
    -in-canada-2022/?lang=en.

98 *Director of Public Prosecutions Act*, (2018) C Gaz, 1, Vol. 152. Available from:
    https://gazette.gc.ca/rp-pr/p1/2018/2018-12-08/html/notice-avis-eng
    .html.

99 Contact the HIV & AIDS Legal Clinic Ontario through https://www.halco
    .org or the HIV Legal Network through https://www.hivlegalnetwork.ca.

100 For more detailed guidance, see Canadian HIV/AIDS Legal Network.
Client confidentiality and record-keeping. In: HIV disclosure and the
law: a resource kit for service providers [Internet]. Toronto: The Network;
2017. Available from: https://www.hivlegalnetwork.ca/site/wp
-content/uploads/2014/02/Chapter5.7-ENG.pdf.

101 For more detailed guidance, see Canadian HIV/AIDS Legal Network.
Client confidentiality and record-keeping. In: HIV disclosure and the
law: a resource kit for service providers [Internet]. Toronto: The Network;
2017. Available from: https://www.hivlegalnetwork.ca/site/wp
-content/uploads/2014/02/Chapter5.7-ENG.pdf; Canadian HIV/AIDS
Legal Network, Canadian Public Health Association. Reducing stigma
and discrimination through the protection of privacy and confidentiality
[Internet]. Toronto: The Network; 2017. Available from: https://www
.cpha.ca/reducing-stigma-and-discrimination-through-protection
-privacy-and-confidentiality.

102 Public Health Agency of Canada (PHAC). Estimates of HIV incidence,
prevalence and Canada's progress on meeting the 90-90-90 HIV targets
[Internet]. Ottawa: PHAC; 2021. Available from: https://www.canada
.ca/en/public-health/services/publications/diseases-conditions
/summary-estimates-hiv-incidence-prevalence-canadas-progress
-90-90-90.html#s11.

103 Joint United Nations Programme on HIV/AIDS (UNAIDS), World
Health Organization. Policy statement on voluntary HIV testing
[Internet]. Geneva: UNAIDS; 2004. Available from: https://data.unaids
.org/una-docs/hivtestingpolicy_en.pdf.

104 Harrigan M. The HIV testing process [Internet]. Canada's source for
HIV and hepatitis C Information; 2021 [updated 2021]. Available from:
https://www.catie.ca/the-hiv-testing-process; Public Health Agency of
Canada (PHAC). Human immunodeficiency virus – HIV screening and
testing guide [Internet]. Ottawa: PHAC; 2014. Available from: https://
www.canada.ca/en/public-health/services/hiv-aids/hiv-screening
-testing-guide.html#b.

105 Harrigan M. The HIV testing process [Internet]. Toronto: Canada's source
for HIV and hepatitis C Information; 2021 [updated 2021]. Available
from: https://www.catie.ca/the-hiv-testing-process.

106 Public Health Agency of Canada (PHAC). Human immunodeficiency
virus – HIV screening and testing guide [Internet]. Ottawa: PHAC; 2014.
Available from: https://www.canada.ca/en/public-health/services/hiv
-aids/hiv-screening-testing-guide.html#b. Ontario is an exception
because its *Health Protection and Promotion Act* regulations (*Reports*, RRO
1990, Reg 569, s. 5.1) allow for anonymous viral load testing using the
same code that was used for anonymous HIV testing.

107 Public Health Agency of Canada (PHAC). Human immunodeficiency
     virus – HIV screening and testing guide [Internet]. Ottawa: PHAC; 2014.
     Available from: https://www.canada.ca/en/public-health/services
     /hiv-aids/hiv-screening-testing-guide.html#b; regulation under the
     Public Health Act, CQLR c S-2.2, r 2.1, ss 11–13.

108 See e.g., *Public Health Act*, RSA 2000, c P-37, ss 22–23; *Public Health Act*,
     SBC 2008, c 28, ss 2–3; *Health Protection and Promotion Act*, RSO 1990,
     c H.7, ss 22 and 102.

109 For more information, see p. 470 of Chaisson A, et al. Criminal law
     and public health. In: Radbord J, editor. LGBTQ2+ law: practice issues
     and analysis. Toronto: Emond Publishing; 2019. British Columbia,
     Saskatchewan, Manitoba, Prince Edward Island, Nunavut, and the
     Northwest Territories require partner notification, and Alberta, Ontario,
     New Brunswick, Nova Scotia, and Yukon require it in their public
     health statutes. The remaining provinces' statutes are silent on partner
     notification. In Quebec, partner notification will only be done with the
     diagnosed person's consent barring exceptional circumstances involving
     an imminent threat of serious bodily harm or death.

110 For more information see pp. 540–1 of Chaisson A, et al. Criminal law
     and public health. In: Radbord J, editor. LGBTQ2+ law: practice issues
     and analysis. Toronto: Emond Publishing; 2019. The accused in *R v Aziga*,
     2006 CanLII 42798 (Ont Sup Ct) was successful in excluding some public
     health records from his criminal trial because his statements to public
     health were compulsory and not voluntary, such that admitting them
     would have breached his rights under the *Canadian Charter of Rights and
     Freedoms*.

111 For additional guidance, see Canadian HIV/AIDS Legal Network. Client
     confidentiality and record-keeping: preventing harm to others [Internet].
     In: HIV disclosure and the law: a resource kit for service providers.
     Toronto: The Network; 2017. Available from: https://www
     .hivlegalnetwork.ca/site/wp-content/uploads/2014/02/Chapter5.3
     -ENG.pdf.

112 See, for example, Council of Ontario Medical Officers of Health HIV
     Workgroup. Public health approach to HIV case management [Internet].
     Toronto: Association of Local Public Health Agencies; 2017. https://cdn.
     ymaws.com/www.alphaweb.org/resource/collection/822EC60D
     -0D03-413E-B590-AFE1AA8620A9/COMOH_Position_HIV_Case
     _Management_190417.pdf.

113 See, for example, *Health Protection and Promotion Act*, RSO 1990, c H.7, ss
     22; *Public Health Act*, SBC 2008, c 28, ss 27–29.

114 Council of Ontario Medical Officers of Health HIV Workgroup. Public
     health approach to HIV case management [Internet]. Toronto: Association

of Local Public Health Agencies; 2017. Available from: https://cdn
.ymaws.com/www.alphaweb.org/resource/collection/822EC60D
-0D03-413E-B590-AFE1AA8620A9/COMOH_Position_HIV_Case
_Management_190417.pdf.

115 Public Health Agency of Canada (PHAC). HIV factsheet: U = U for health
professionals [Internet]. Ottawa: PHAC; 2020. Available from: https://
www.canada.ca/en/public-health/services/publications
/diseases-conditions/hiv-factsheet-undetectable-untransmittable-health
-professionals.html.

116 See, for example, *Public Health Act*, RSA 2000, c P-37, s 39; *Health
Protection and Promotion Act*, RSO 1990, c H.7, s 102.

117 *Health Protection and Promotion Act*, RSO 1990, c H.7, s 102.

118 In Ontario, the individual has only 15 days under the *Health Protection
and Promotion Act* to start an appeal of a section 22 order to the Health
Services Appeal and Review Board. The HIV & AIDS Legal Clinic
Ontario (https://www.halco.org) can provide free legal advice to people
living with HIV facing such an order.

119 Yoong D, Bayoumi AM, Robinson L, et al. Public prescription drug
plan coverage for antiretrovirals and the potential cost to people living
with HIV in Canada: a descriptive study. CMAJ. 2018;6(4): E551–E560.
https://doi.org/10.9778/cmajo.20180058.

120 Rachlis B, Light L, Gardner S, et al. The impact of drug coverage on viral
suppression among people living with HIV in Ontario, Canada. Can J
Public Health. 2018;109:800–9. https://doi.org/10.17269/s41997
-018-0104-z; McAllister J, Beardsworth G, Lavie E, et al. Financial stress is
associated with reduced treatment adherence in HIV-infected adults in a
resource-rich setting. HIV Med. 2013;14(2):120–4. https://doi
.org/10.1111/j.1468-1293.2012.01034.x.

121 See Canada's source for HIV and hepatitis C information (CATIE). Access
to HIV and hepatitis C drugs: federal, provincial and territorial drug
access programs [Internet]. Toronto: CATIE; n.d. [cited 2022 July 21].
Available from: https://www.catie.ca/treatment-care-hepatitis-c
-treatment-care-and-support/access-to-hiv-and-hepatitis-c-drugs-federal.

122 Health Canada. About pharmacare [Internet]. Ottawa: Health Canada;
2024. Available from: https://www.canada.ca/en/health-canada
/services/health-care-systems/national-pharmacare/about.html?utm
_campaign=hc-sc-vurl-24-25&utm_medium=vanity-url&utm_source
=canada-ca_pharmacare.

123 Yoong D, Bayoumi AM, Robinson L, et al. Public prescription drug
plan coverage for antiretrovirals and the potential cost to people living
with HIV in Canada: a descriptive study. CMAJ. 2018;6(4): E551–E560.
https://doi.org/10.9778/cmajo.20180058.

124 Canada's source for HIV and hepatitis C information (CATIE). Your guide to HIV treatment: paying for treatment [Internet]. Toronto: CATIE; n.d. [cited 2022 July 21]. Available from: https://www.catie.ca/your -guide-to-hiv-treatment/paying-for-treatment.

125 Yoong D, Naccarato M, Gough K, et al. Use of compassionate supply of antiretroviral drugs to avoid treatment interruptions or delayed treatment initiation among HIV-positive patients living in Ontario: a retrospective review. Healthc Policy. 2015;10(3):64–77. http://www.ncbi .nlm.nih.gov/pmc/articles/pmc4748343/.

126 Canada's source for HIV and hepatitis C information (CATIE). Where to? [Internet]. Toronto: CATIE; 2022 [cited 2022 July 21]. Available from: https://whereto.catie.ca/.

127 For a more detailed overview of immigration and refugee law in Canada, please see chapter 7 of this volume.

128 *Immigration and Refugee Protection Act*, SC 2001, c 27, s 38(1)(a).

129 *Immigration and Refugee Protection Act*, SC 2001, c 27, s 38(1)(b).

130 *Immigration and Refugee Protection Act*, SC 2001, c 27, s 38(1)(c).

131 Immigration, Refugees and Citizenship Canada (IRCC). Danger to public health or public safety [Internet]. Ottawa: IRCC; 2013. Available from: https://www.canada.ca/en/immigration-refugees-citizenship /corporate/publications-manuals/operational-bulletins-manuals /standard-requirements/medical-requirements/refusals-inadmissibility /danger-public-health-public-safety.html.

132 *Immigration and Refugee Protection Regulations*, SOR/2002-227, s 1(1).

133 *Immigration and Refugee Protection Regulations*, SOR/2002-227, s 1(1).

134 *Immigration and Refugee Protection Regulations*, SOR/2002-227, s 1(1).

135 *Immigration and Refugee Protection Regulations*, SOR/2002-227, s 1(1).

136 Immigration, Refugees and Citizenship Canada (IRCC). Temporary public policy regarding excessive demand on health and social service. Ottawa: IRCC; 2018. Available from: https://www.canada.ca/en /immigration-refugees-citizenship/corporate/mandate/policies -operational-instructions-agreements/excessive-demand-june-2018.html.

137 Immigration, Refugees and Citizenship Canada (IRCC). Program delivery update [Internet]. Ottawa: IRCC; 2022. Available from: https:// www.canada.ca/en/immigration-refugees-citizenship/services /immigrate-canada/inadmissibility/reasons/medical-inadmissibility.html.

138 Immigration, Refugees and Citizenship Canada (IRCC). Excessive demand on health services and on social services [Internet]. Ottawa: IRCC; 2022. Available from: https://www.canada.ca/en/immigration -refugees-citizenship/corporate/publications-manuals/operational -bulletins-manuals/standard-requirements/medical-requirements /refusals-inadmissibility/excessive-demand-on-health-social-services.html.

139 Immigration, Refugees and Citizenship Canada (IRCC). Mitigation plans for excessive demand [Internet]. Ottawa: IRCC; 2018. Available from: https://www.canada.ca/en/immigration-refugees-citizenship/services/immigrate-canada/inadmissibility/reasons/mitigation-plans.html.

140 *Immigration and Refugee Protection Act*, SC 2001, c 27, s 24(1). See also Immigration, Refugees and Citizenship Canada. Temporary Resident Permits (TRPs): considerations specific to inadmissibility on health grounds [Internet]. Ottawa: Immigration, Refugees and Citizenship Canada; 2015. Available from: https://www.canada.ca/en/immigration-refugees-citizenship/corporate/publications-manuals/operational-bulletins-manuals/temporary-residents/permits/considerations-specific-inadmissibility-on-health-grounds.html.

141 *Immigration and Refugee Protection Act*, SC 2001, c 27, s. 24(1). See also Immigration, Refugees and Citizenship Canada. Temporary Resident Permits (TRPs): considerations specific to inadmissibility on health grounds [Internet]. Ottawa: Immigration, Refugees and Citizenship Canada; 2015. Available from: https://www.canada.ca/en/immigration-refugees-citizenship/corporate/publications-manuals/operational-bulletins-manuals/temporary-residents/permits/considerations-specific-inadmissibility-on-health-grounds.html.

142 Please see chapter 7 for more information about challenging immigration decisions.

143 Please see chapter 7 for more information about challenging immigration decisions.

144 United Nations. Convention relating to the status of refugees (adopted 1951 July 28, entered into force 1954 Apr 22). Treaty Series, vol. 189, p. 137 [cited 2023 Jan 31]. Available from: https://www.refworld.org/docid/3be01b964.html; *Immigration and Refugee Protection Act*, SC 2001, c 27, s 39(2).

145 Immigration, Refugees and Citizenship Canada. Canadian Panel Member guide to immigration medical examinations [Internet]. Ottawa: Immigration, Refugees and Citizenship Canada; 2024. Available from: https://www.canada.ca/en/immigration-refugees-citizenship/corporate/publications-manuals/panel-members-guide.html.

146 Panel physicians are instructed that they must request HIV screening for children aged younger than 15 years in certain circumstances, including children born to a mother living with HIV; children showing failure to thrive; children with suspected active tuberculous, hepatitis B, or hepatitis C; and when there is a history of another sexually transmitted infection. A full list can be found in Immigration, Refugees and Citizenship Canada. Canadian Panel Member guide to immigration medical examinations [Internet]. Ottawa: Immigration, Refugees and

Citizenship Canada; 2024. Available from: https://www.canada.ca/en
/immigration-refugees-citizenship/corporate/publications-manuals
/panel-members-guide.html.

147 Immigration, Refugees and Citizenship Canada. Canadian Panel
Member guide to immigration medical examinations [Internet]. Ottawa:
Immigration, Refugees and Citizenship Canada; 2024. Available from:
https://www.canada.ca/en/immigration-refugees-citizenship
/corporate/publications-manuals/panel-members-guide.html. In Quebec,
physicians do not normally report the name of the person testing positive
for HIV (see regulation under the *Public Health Act*, CQLR c S-2.2, r 2.1, ss
11–13). It is currently unknown whether panel physicians conducting IMEs
in Quebec report the person's name to public health authorities.

148 Immigration, Refugees and Citizenship Canada. Canadian Panel
Member guide to immigration medical examinations [Internet]. Ottawa:
Immigration, Refugees and Citizenship Canada; 2024. Available from:
https://www.canada.ca/en/immigration-refugees-citizenship
/corporate/publications-manuals/panel-members-guide.html.

149 Immigration, Refugees and Citizenship Canada. Canadian Panel
Member guide to immigration medical examinations [Internet]. Ottawa:
Immigration, Refugees and Citizenship Canada; 2024. Available from:
https://www.canada.ca/en/immigration-refugees-citizenship
/corporate/publications-manuals/panel-members-guide.html.

150 Immigration, Refugees and Citizenship Canada. Program delivery
update: Termination of the automatic partner notification policy
for applicants who test positive for HIV in the sponsored family or
dependent refugee classes [Internet]. Ottawa: Immigration, Refugees and
Citizenship Canada; 2023. Available from: https://www.canada.ca
/en/immigration-refugees-citizenship/corporate/publications
-manuals/operational-bulletins-manuals/updates/2023-hiv-partner
-notification.html.

151 *Social assistance* is defined in section 2 of the *Immigration and Refugee
Protection Regulations* as "any benefit in the form of money, goods or
services provided to or on behalf of a person by a province under a
program of social assistance, including a program of social assistance
designated by a province to provide for basic requirements including
food, shelter, clothing, fuel, utilities, household supplies, personal
requirements and health care not provided by public health care,
including dental care and eye care." Social assistance does not include
Employment Insurance, provincial student loans, subsidized housing, tax
credits, childcare subsidies, and temporary programs put in place during
the COVID-19 pandemic, such as the Canadian Emergency Response
Benefit. See also Immigration, Refugees and Citizenship Canada.

Applications under family classes: assessing the sponsor [Internet]. Ottawa: Immigration, Refugees and Citizenship Canada; 2022. Available from: https://www.canada.ca/en/immigration-refugees-citizenship /corporate/publications-manuals/operational-bulletins-manuals /permanent-residence/non-economic-classes/family-class-assessing -sponsor.html.

152 *Immigration and Refugee Protection Regulations*, SOR/2002-227, s 1(3).

153 *Immigration and Refugee Protection Regulations*, SOR/2002-227, s 2.

154 *Immigration and Refugee Protection Act*, SC 2001, c 27, s 96.

155 *Immigration and Refugee Protection Act*, SC 2001, c 27, s 97.

156 *Convention* refugees and persons in need of protection must demonstrate that there is nowhere in their country where they can live without facing persecution or a risk to their life, a risk of torture, or a risk of cruel or unusual treatment or punishment. An IFA must be reasonable, meaning that a claimant cannot be expected to risk their life or safety by traveling to and living in a proposed IFA.

157 *Covarrubias et al v Canada (Minister of Citizenship and Immigration) et al*, (2006) 354 NR 367 (FCA).

158 Please see chapter 7 for a discussion of applications for permanent residence from within Canada on humanitarian and compassionate grounds.

159 Positive Destinations. Information and advocacy on travelling and relocating with HIV [Internet]. 2024. Available from: https://www .positivedestinations.info/.

160 Exceptions exist for residents returning to Canada with a personal quantity of prescription medications prescribed and filled in Canada for their use or for a person or animal for whom they are responsible, Canadian residents returning to Canada with prescription medications who are continuing medical treatment that was initiated abroad for themselves or a person or animal under their care with whom they are travelling, and Canadian residents and temporary residents who are part of a foreign-sponsored clinical trial. For more details, see Health Canada. Bringing health products into Canada for personal use (GUI-0116) [Internet]. Ottawa: Health Canada; 2021. Available from: https://www .canada.ca/en/health-canada/services/drugs-health-products /compliance-enforcement/importation-exportation/personal-use-health -products-guidance/document.html.

161 Health Canada. Bringing health products into Canada for personal use (GUI-0116) [Internet]. Ottawa: Health Canada; 2021. Available from: https://www.canada.ca/en/health-canada/services/drugs-health -products/compliance-enforcement/importation-exportation/personal -use-health-products-guidance/document.html.

162 Health Canada. Bringing health products into Canada for personal use (GUI-0116) [Internet]. Ottawa: Health Canada; 2021. Available from: https://www.canada.ca/en/health-canada/services/drugs-health -products/compliance-enforcement/importation-exportation/personal -use-health-products-guidance/document.html.

163 Health Canada. Bringing health products into Canada for personal use (GUI-0116) [Internet]. Ottawa: Health Canada; 2021. Available from: https://www.canada.ca/en/health-canada/services/drugs-health -products/compliance-enforcement/importation-exportation/personal -use-health-products-guidance/document.html.

164 Health Canada. Bringing health products into Canada for personal use (GUI-0116) [Internet]. Ottawa: Health Canada; 2021. Available from: https://www.canada.ca/en/health-canada/services/drugs-health -products/compliance-enforcement/importation-exportation/personal -use-health-products-guidance/document.html.

11 Health Justice in Paediatric Practice: Children's Rights and Social Justice for Patients and Their Families

SARAH GANDER, LEE ANN CHAPMAN,
AND MELANIE LAKING

Numerous studies have shown that child health and development are affected by more than just biological factors. The social determinants of health (SDOHs) are integral to the development, health, and wellness of all Canadians, especially children. These conditions of daily life are in some cases equal to biological factors in explaining health disparities; the World Health Organization estimates that 30–55 per cent of health disparities are dictated by social factors.[1]

Children and youth represent a population particularly at risk because of social factors, given the profound consequences of adverse childhood experiences (ACEs), which are defined as traumatic childhood events, such as abuse, negligence, or household dysfunction, that can affect a child's current and future adult health, as well as the importance of healthy attachment, nurturing, literacy, nutrition, and health surveillance in the early years.[2] All of these factors come together to form the future person and affect their ability to thrive in society and reach their full potential. Data from across Canada show that almost all caregivers (96.8 per cent) reported at least one social need when they were screened for factors that would affect child health.[3,4] Furthermore, ACEs and unmet social needs, which are risk factors for toxic stress and poor health outcomes, disproportionately affect children from racialized communitiees.[5] Although early identification and management can mitigate harmful effects, health providers often feel helpless and frustrated when faced with the intertwined health and social challenges their young patients experience.[6]

To address these health-harming risk factors that often have a legal solution, health care providers and legal communities began to formally collaborate. The earliest partnerships, first in the United States and then in Canada, began in paediatrics and, in particular, in children's hospitals.[7]

However, although several children's hospitals have access to legal help on site, it is helpful for health care providers to first spot the social issues that may have a legal solution and then to know that there are resources and even free legal services available to patients and their families should an intervention be required. See Appendix 1 for a summary of legal aid and pro bono services found across Canada.

Using relevant case examples, this chapter highlights some of the factors that affect a child's health, followed by those that affect a family's ability to care for a child. Within this framework, we address interventions that health providers can use to support improving health outcomes. This may help to reduce disparities and thereby move towards more equitable access to health and health care for children and youth.

In the first section, we provide through case examples an overview of the rights of all children to equitable health, which include equity in health care decision-making, safety and protection, education, and the youth criminal justice (YCJ) system. We then focus on the particular experiences of discrimination, racism, and historical trauma as SDOHs for Indigenous and 2SLGBTQ+ children and youth.[8,9] The second section explores social factors related to the family's ability to care for the child, such as immigration status, employment, tax-related benefits, income supports, and housing safety and stability. The chapter concludes with sample letters that health care providers may use as templates for education, immigration, and employment matters to help access resources or rights for their minor patients and their caregivers.

Children's Rights as Social Determinants of Health

Children's Rights to Decision-Making and Privacy about Their Health

Mia is an 11-year-old girl. Her parents are in a high-conflict separation. They have made an application to family court, both claiming sole custody (decision-making responsibility). Mia requires a tonsillectomy and adenoidectomy for obstructive sleep apnoea. One parent wants her to have surgery that is essential to treat her health condition; the other refuses to consent to the surgery.

Consent

In Canada the legal age of majority is almost universally irrelevant in determining when a young person may consent to medical treatment.

> The concept of capacity flows from the ability to consent rather than chronological age. Although some jurisdictions in Canada may have a presumed age of consent to treatment, this does not preclude a person younger than that age from consenting when they are judged capable (with the exception of Quebec, where the age of consent is 14 years). The Supreme Court of Canada has affirmed that the ability to make health care decisions must be based on the capacity of the person, rather than the person's age, as a recognition of constitutional rights and the best interests of the child, a legal principle with respect to services to children in both domestic and international law (explained further in the text).

The right to have one's autonomy respected[10] is not only a basic principle of health equity, but according to paediatric patients it is also one of the most common criticisms related to accessing health care. Feedback from paediatric patients has critiqued the failure of health care providers to assess and respect their capacity to make health care decisions and the tendency to make assumptions based on age. This is commonly heard across many jurisdictions. In an Australian study surveying young patients aged 8–17 years, fewer than half answered "yes, definitely" to the question "Were you involved, as much as you wanted to be [should be], in decisions about your care and treatment?"[11]

However, certain legal documents, such as an advance directive of care or the appointment of a substitute decision maker under a power of attorney for personal care, may have defined age stipulations. For more detailed information, including a chart of the age in each province or territory at which a child can provide an advance health care directive, please consult the Canadian Paediatric Society's position statement, "Medical Decision-Making in Paediatrics: Infancy to Adolescence."[12]

Furthermore, it is important to remember that the right to make personal health decisions overrides family court orders granting custody (also called decision-making) to a parent. If the child has capacity, the decision-making right of the parent does not apply to personal health decisions. That is because the right of the capable person (regardless of age) is constitutionally protected under section 7 of the *Charter of Rights and Freedoms*,[13] which guarantees protection of personal autonomy and bodily integrity, as well as section 15, which grants equality rights.

When the health care provider has assessed that their minor patient is capable of providing valid consent, then the minor will have control over the disclosure of their information. Any release of personal health information of a so-called mature minor will need to be consented to by the mature minor, even if the request is made by a parent (unless disclosure is otherwise permitted by law, for example, when there is a possibility of imminent harm to themselves or others or when the provider is required to report to a child welfare authority).

(Note that legislation does not yet recognize the right of even capable or mature minors to access medical assistance in dying [MAID] in Canada, even in cases of intolerable suffering that cannot be alleviated as result of an incurable life-limiting disease or injury. At the time of writing, a patient must be aged 18 years to be eligible for MAID.)

In the case of paediatric patients, it is particularly important to note that the right of the capable person to make decisions about health care also extends to the right to privacy protection of personal health information. Exceptions to the right to privacy are the same as for adults, with an additional exception for the duty to report to a child welfare agency when a child is in need of protection.

If a health care provider finds the patient is not capable of making decisions regarding their health care, the patient will in most cases have a right to legally challenge that finding. Once incapacity is established, the decision will then fall to the substitute decision maker as determined by a hierarchy under provincial law.[14] In cases in which there is no court-appointed decision-maker or power of attorney, the decision-maker, most often a parent, will be the legal guardian for all other decisions. With respect to separated families, if the child is not capable of making their own health care decisions, then the provider should ask for a copy of the most recent court-endorsed order or separation agreement, outlining who has the right to make health care decisions (called custody or decision making).

Many families, in particular parents, are not aware of the laws with respect to consent and privacy. Informing patients and families at the outset in an objective manner is generally conducive to less stress, hurt feelings, and possible future disputes. When health care providers insist that the child's consent is required, parents can feel defensive. Primary health care providers should ensure that information is displayed and provided to families at the outset of the services.

Best Interests of the Child

Like all other substitute decision-makers, parents must act in the best interests of the child, as defined by various provincial statutes, the content of which is generally not reflective of family religious or cultural values or other personal preferences but rather seeks the best health outcomes and reduction of harm for the patient. Note that in January 2020, *An Act respecting First Nations, Inuit and Métis Children, Youth and Families* came into force.[a] It recognized that Indigenous Peoples have sole jurisdiction over child welfare matters. It is too early to say what impact it will have on health care; however, it is expected that in all contexts, the interpretation of the best interests of Indigenous children will include best health outcomes and harm reduction and will also be inclusive of traditional customs and values. In circumstances in which the substitute decision-maker is not acting in the best interests of the patient, the provider must contact the local child welfare agency (for Indigenous patients, jurisdiction lies with Indigenous child welfare agencies), if the patient is of an age in their jurisdiction, or the Consent and Capacity Board.

[a] *An Act respecting First Nations, Inuit and Métis children, youth and families*, SC 2019, c24.

With respect to the case example of Mia at the beginning of this section, we propose the following as best practice:

- First, determine whether Mia has capacity: Does she understand what treatment is proposed, the consequences of refusing treatment, and the likely outcome of consenting to treatment, and is she able to make the decision freely? To determine this, she should be seen without the parents present.

If she has capacity, Mia makes the health care decision even if there is a family court order giving one or both parents the right to custody (decision making).

If Mia does not have capacity,

- then determine whether there is a court order for custody (decision-making). Even though they are still in court, there may be an interim order. Most interim orders do not have expiry dates.
- If there is no court order and parents are equal decision-makers, ask them to go to court as soon as possible for an interim order, if time allows.
- If there is no order and Mia's parents refuse to go to court, ask child welfare services to become involved.

- If child welfare services will not intervene, contact the provincial health care Consent and Capacity Board, the provincial or territorial Office of the Public Guardian and Trustee, or both.
- You may also contact the child and youth advocate for guidance, if there is one in your province.

Children's Rights to Safety and Protection

Casey is eight years old. He has repeatedly presented to your clinic and the emergency department for asthma exacerbations related to household cigarette smoke, mould, and other environmental triggers. His caregivers have struggled to fill prescribed medications (e.g., expensive metred dose inhalers) and to follow up with other medical recommendations (e.g., an aero chamber) or lifesaving interventions (e.g., ensuring there is a commercial injectable epinephrine device available in the case of immunoglobulin e–mediated allergies).

In clinical practice, health care providers may see children and youth who they believe to be in an environment that is unsafe or not sufficiently nourishing to support cognitive, emotional, and physical development.

Every child has a right to be cared for in a safe environment and to receive necessary medical care. The United Nations *Convention on the Rights of the Child*[15] (UNCRC), as well as various child protection laws across the provinces and territories, sets out the rights of the child to be protected and the obligations of others, including government agencies, to assist children in need of protection. Interventions to protect children do not require evidence of harm. One could argue the child could have a bad asthma flare regardless of the level of care or conditions at home, but that does not vindicate the potentially harmful exacerbating factors.

Children are in need of protection when there is a risk that the child is likely to be sexually molested or exploited, experience physical harm, or experience emotional harm. Neglect (including medical neglect), abuse, violence, parental substance use disorder, and homelessness are all issues that engage the health professional's duty to report when a child is at risk to police or local child welfare agencies under various provincial and territorial statutes.

It is worth noting that the statutory duty to report, as defined by provincial child welfare legislation, does not necessarily result in the most extreme interventions, such as the apprehension of a child, but rather flags that the child and by extension the family needs further resources. Child welfare agencies should be sources of support for families to ensure children do not end up in care for lack of resources or information. The standards for the duty to report, as well as ages for interventions by child welfare authorities, vary according to province or territory and can be found in the Public Health Agency of Canada's *Provincial and Territorial Child Protection Legislation and Policy, 2018*.[16]

If a child welfare agency is getting involved with your patient's family, it is good practice to let the parent or guardian know they should seek legal advice. In Ontario, Legal Aid Ontario will provide a limited certificate for parents when a child protection matter is in the works.

In the case of Casey, we do not recommend reporting this family without trying to support them first. We propose the following as best practices:

- Provide the family with a medical letter describing the child's medical condition and the requirements to accommodate their needs. This can help the family to ask their landlord to remediate any mould or to transfer or move up the waiting list for subsidized housing.
- Connect Casey's family to a community legal resource. This could help them stabilize their income and ensure they have appropriate medication coverage.

Amina, a 15-year-old girl, presents to your office with fever, vaginal discharge, and pain on urination. She arrives with an older person described as a friend or distant relative. She makes little to no eye contact with you, and when you suggest that you need to speak to her alone, the accompanying person and the patient decline, stating that you can talk openly in front of the other person. When you insist the other person leave, and you ask the patient about any sexual activity that is inappropriate or puts her at risk, she denies it. Furthermore, she does not easily answer questions about school and how and where she can pick up a prescription. She consents to a urine test, and the result is positive for chlamydia.

There are cases in which the health care provider may have a sense that their patient is a possible victim of child trafficking or their patient may tell them so. Many people believe that victims of trafficking are newcomers to Canada. It shocks many people to learn that in Canada the most common victims of child trafficking are Canadian-born and that 25 per cent of trafficking victims in Canada reported to the police are younger than age 18 years, and 96 per cent are female.[17]

Possible indications of trafficking may include

- contradictory personal information about address, school, family, and source of funds;
- evidence or suspicion of multiple sex partners;

- the appearance of an older friend or unspecified family member; and
- refusing to make eye contact.

A common presentation by children and youth may be some type of elimination dysfunction, for example, constipation, diarrhoea, dysuria, or discomfort in the genital region. It can be straightforwardly and simply addressed if there are no suspicions about the origin of the presentation. It is particularly important to take any signs or symptoms of sexually transmitted infections (STIs) very seriously, especially in young children and youth unable to consent by age or by capacity.

In Amina's case, you wonder whether she may possibly be a victim of sexual exploitation (trafficking). How do you proceed beyond medical treatment?

- Make it clear that not just this patient, but all patients, must be examined without the friend or relative, to thereby not raise the suspicions of the accompanying person.
- There are cases in which you may be told by the patient that they are a victim; if the patient is underage, you have a duty to report to child welfare authorities. You can also call the police, and you should if you believe imminent harm is possible, from either the accompanying trafficker or the young person fleeing them. Even if you may only have a suspicion, you should also report.
- You can also provide your young patient with information about the Canadian Human Trafficking Hotline,[18] which can be reached toll-free at 1-833-900-1010. Even if they say they will not contact it, they may change their minds at some future time.

It is also possible that a health care provider may have concerns that their patient may be forced into a marriage in Canada or will possibly be sent to another country for that purpose. Forcing someone into marriage without their consent is a criminal offence. Furthermore, nobody younger than age 16 is allowed to get married in Canada. It is also a crime to take anyone who is younger than 16 out of Canada for the purpose of a marriage in another country, even if the person wants to get married. In cases of both suspected child trafficking and forced marriage, the local child welfare agency, police, or both should be contacted. Resources for the health care provider and patient may be found on the Government of Canada's website.[19]

Children's Rights in Education

*Tarron is a 10-year-old boy in grade 4. He has a presumed learning disabil-
ity, attention deficit hyperactivity disorder, generalized anxiety disorder, and
Tourette syndrome. He has been bullied by some fellow classmates, who tease
him because of his tics. The school has provided some extra time for him to fin-
ish work, but no other academic supports, and has said they cannot do anything
about the bullying because they have not seen it.*

Primary health care providers are frequently asked to help when their
minor patients have difficulties in school connected to their health
issues. These can present as social issues, such as bullying; behavioural
issues, resulting in school discipline actions such as suspensions or
expulsions; and, most often, shortfalls in schools' accommodation of
students with special needs, which may be intertwined with all of these.

All children in Canada have equal rights to education under the
UNCRC; the *UN Convention on Persons with Disabilities, 2006;*[20] the
equality provisions of the *Charter of Rights and Freedoms*; and provincial
and territorial human rights codes, and as confirmed by the Supreme
Court of Canada.[21]

Equality is to be understood as substantive (equitable treatment), not
formal (same treatment); the core of substantive equality is the duty to
accommodate. This concept is examined in more detail in chapter 2,
but for the purposes of this discussion, the task of accommodation is
to remove barriers that may impede students with special needs from
fully participating in all aspects of education. The legal duty to accommodate is not a matter of convenience, but up to the point of undue
hardship. This applies to all aspects of learning – not just cognitive and
affective learning functions, but also social inclusion. As well as equal
access, all decisions by schools and school boards must be made in the
best interests of the child.[22]

The right of children with special needs to access accommodations
can be done through an assessment process to identify and then place
children. Most provinces have a committee charged with placing and
identifying the special need, often through a placement review committee. This process is triggered when a parent requests an identification in
writing to the principal, but it can also be the result of evidence of a disability and the need to accommodate from other sources. Evidence can
be provided by an external health care provider; the legal right derives
from the identification of the special need, not a particular process that
may take months or longer to access. Therefore, a letter from the health
care provider outlining the diagnosis and the types of accommodations

that can aid the child in achieving equal access to learning is valuable evidence in support of accommodations. If a school continues to deny accommodations, parents should be referred to the provincial or territorial human rights commission.

Special needs education is carried out in a variety of placements, including the regular classroom with supports, with withdrawal to a resource room as needed; in special classes; and, depending on the disability, in special schools (e.g., for those who are deaf or visually impaired).

Parents and students may request letters of support from health care providers to use as evidence in meetings, with respect to identification of the disability, the most appropriate placement, and special services that may be required to ensure equitable access. Decisions on special education can be appealed, either through an internal process within the school board or to the appropriate provincial human rights tribunal.

Once a special need has been identified, schools are then required to produce an Individual Education Plan that contains the goals set for the student that year; a list of the support services required to achieve those goals; and a list of the adaptations to educational materials, instructional strategies, or assessment methods.

Children also have the right to be free from bullying in school. Across the country, schools have a duty to address bullying both systemically and on a case-by-case basis. When schools ignore or are not effective in addressing bullying, primary care providers may be asked to provide evidentiary support to address harm or potential harm to students stemming from bullying. The student should be consulted in advance of providing evidence, to ensure their voice is heard regarding not only the effects of bullying, but what end results they wish to achieve. Beyond the obvious wish for the bullying to stop, this may include a wish that either the bully or the victim transfer schools, particularly if the bullying has been sustained and from multiple offenders. A letter from the health care provider outlining what harm the child is experiencing from bullying and the necessity for the issue to be addressed is helpful in alerting the school to their obligation to protect the child to prevent harm.

Anti-bullying resources across Canada, including helplines, can be found online:

- Ontario Secondary School Teachers' Federation, Canadian Bullying Resources Online: https://www.osstf.on.ca/en-CA/publications /research-studies/bullying/canadian-bullying-resources-online.aspx;

- Kids Help Phone Mental Health Resources: https://kidshelpphone
  .ca/; and
- Bullying Canada: https://www.bullyingcanada.ca/get-help.

The primary health care provider who wants to help with advocacy should be aware that education, like many other institutions, has a clear chain-of-command structure; it is best to find out with whom to speak before spending the time. Generally, it is best to start with the principal; if that is not helpful, then speak with the appropriate superintendent.

In the case example of Tarron at the beginning of the section, our best-practice suggestions include the following:

- Ask parents whether they have advocated on their own or whether they have received help.
- Children have a right to education and care if living with a disability. Ask whether the school has recommended or completed a psycho-educational assessment to confirm the learning disability or created a personal learning plan to guide Tarron's curriculum needs.
- Tarron requires extra supports, and the health care provider can inform the school of the kinds of supports needed if they are conversant in what may be required. Examples of supports might include different seating arrangements, additional time for testing, or computer accommodations for children who have problems with writing. Tarron may also require occupational therapy or counselling, which should also be accessible to meet his medical needs. A sample letter is provided at the end of this chapter.
- If identification of the disability has not yet taken place, the health care provider can support the parents' request for a psycho-educational assessment as soon as possible.
- Children have a legal right to be protected from bullying; this includes bullying outside of school that may be school related (students attending the same school, on school trips, etc.). The school may need to hear that message in clear terms. The school must address the bullying by meeting with the students and parents as well as implementing progressive discipline. Tarron has a disability; not only is he protected under education law, but he can also bring a human rights complaint if the school fails to take action.
- It is important not only to listen to the parents, but to speak to Tarron about possible outcomes he would like. Students' wishes should be respected, and you can write a letter of support based on health needs and the appropriate accommodation for the disability. Provide Tarron with the bullying hotline information listed earlier.

- Ask Tarron whether he thinks it would help if the other students were educated about Tourette syndrome. If so, you can suggest the family contact the Tourette Society of Canada to see whether someone could come speak at the school or provide educational pamphlets.

Children's Rights under the Youth Criminal Justice System

Tye is a young man with impulse control issues related to foetal alcohol spectrum disorder (FASD). In Tye's case, he has partial FASD. Tye became frustrated and upset when students were playing softball at recess. He believed they were not taking turns, and he became upset and yelled. He then pushed the student ahead of him in line, who as a result fell and cut his head on a rock. The other student's parents called the police, and Tye was charged with assault.

Sometimes young people (or their guardians) disclose that they have been, or expect to be, charged by the police and may ask their health care provider for help. If the young person has a disability that the health care provider believes may be associated with their actions, such as an impulse control disorder, a letter describing the condition and manifestations may be helpful to present to the patient or their lawyer with their consent, to help the courts determine an appropriate course of action. Similarly, it may be very helpful in cases in which the young person may not be capable of understanding their actions or when the provider is aware of past circumstances resulting in posttraumatic stress disorder that need to be taken into account.

All youth aged 12–17 fall under the *Youth Criminal Justice Act*.[23] Although the act recognizes that young persons must be held accountable for criminal acts, it acknowledges that young people lack the maturity of adults, and therefore they are not treated in the same way as adults. It is in society's interest to ensure that as many young offenders as possible are rehabilitated and become productive members of society.

First, it is important for the primary health care provider to understand that all information with respect to any youth's involvement with YCJ, whether as a witness or an offender, is subject to strict laws of confidentiality. This includes a ban on the sharing of any identifying information that a youth is involved with the YCJ system with the general public, unless under permissible exceptions.[24] Similarly, access to youth records (as opposed to adult criminal records) is subject to strict privacy guidelines to ensure young people have the best chance of successful rehabilitation.

If the family is concerned about not having a lawyer because they cannot afford to pay for one and do not qualify for legal aid, the court can order legal aid to provide a certificate for a lawyer because of the youth's vulnerability and the family's inability to direct family resources (note that the majority of YCJ lawyers take legal aid).

Most often youth are diverted from the system into programs that support rehabilitation health (these are known as extrajudicial measures or sanctions). As stated earlier, health care providers can be helpful in providing relevant health information to the youth's lawyer, and they may also be able to suggest the most appropriate diversion programs and help access those services.

Information on YCJ for young people can be found through the website of Ontario's specialty legal aid clinic, Justice for Children and Youth, https://jfcy.org/en/.

In Tye's case, our best-practice suggestions include the following:

- Provide a letter explaining that, as Tye's primary health care provider for several years, you know that he has been diagnosed with partial FASD. Explain how this can affect impulse control and social judgment and how stress can exacerbate his behaviours.
- Ask that this be taken into account and suggest that an appropriate diversion program with respect to Tye's condition and resulting behaviour would provide support to him with respect to behaviour modification and social skills training.

Indigenous Children's Rights to Equitable Health Care

William is an 11-year-old Anishinaabe child who lives with his parents and siblings in Toronto. William is registered under the Indian Act. *Three months ago, William and his family were involved in a motor vehicle accident while on the way to school. William's mother was seriously injured and is still recovering. The rest of the family was physically unscathed. During a visit with his family physician, William's parents share that he is falling behind his peers at school. He has started to complain of belly aches on weekday mornings, and getting him up and ready for school is a growing struggle. William shares that he is having a hard time falling asleep and is having nightmares about the accident. His teacher recently called home to discuss William's reluctance to participate in group activities. His parents have noticed changes in William's mood and are concerned about his increased anxiety. The family does not have the means to pay for private mental health counselling. They reached out to the federal Non-Insured Health Benefits (NIHB) program and learned that there are no NIHB-registered child therapists taking new patients in their area.*

Indigenous people experience substantial health disparities in Canada; this has been particularly acute in the paediatric population. Indigenous children and youth do not have the same access to health care as other Canadians.[25(p. 13)] This health gap is a direct result of the ongoing process of settler colonialism. "The historical settler colonial era deeply entrenched a racial hierarchy through a plethora of policies, systems, and structures based on racial hierarchies that have no evidentiary basis."[26(p. 2)] Anti-Indigenous racism, the *Indian Act*,[27] government policies aimed at assimilating Indigenous people (contrary to treaties that recognized the unique nation-to-nation relationship of Indigenous peoples and the Crown), and the so-called discovery doctrine have created structural inequalities that continue to negatively affect the health and wellness of Indigenous peoples in Canada.

Jordan's Principle

Jordan's Principle was named in response to the death of five-year-old Jordan River Anderson, a child from Norway Cree Nation who had a diagnosis of Carey-Fineman-Ziter syndrome. Jordan died in 2005 after spending all five years of his life in hospital as a result of federal and provincial authorities disputing who had responsibility for funding resources at home. Jordan's Principle is now law; it holds that First Nations children should not be denied access to public services while governments fight over who should pay for them. To ensure substantive equality, this can also include services that are not ordinarily available to other children.

The ongoing legacy of colonialism continues to negatively affect key SDOHs for Indigenous people, such as poor housing, lack of clean water, and food insecurity. The disproportionately low funding, particularly for Indigenous children, in health care, child welfare, and other services was the subject of years-long litigation at the Canadian Human Rights Tribunal (CHRT), led by Professor Cindy Blackstock, the First Nations Caring Society, and the Assembly of First Nations. On 26 January 2016, the CHRT ruled that the federal government's long-standing underfunding of child and family services on First Nations reserves, and its failure to ensure First Nations children can access government services on the same terms as other children, discriminates against First Nations children on the grounds of race and national and ethnic origin.[28] The federal government subsequently challenged CHRT's jurisdiction to deal with this matter, and not until late 2021 did the federal government finally agree to negotiate a settlement. This principle of equitable treatment in funding for Indigenous children is known as Jordan's Principle.

Access to funding through Jordan's Principle can include health-care-related needs but also other social and educational supports, such as laptops, tablets, or other e-learning tools if they meet an identified health, education, or social need. Jordan's Principle applies to First Nations children as well as some Métis children on reserve. To make a request for resources under Jordan's Principle, contact the Jordan's Principle Call Centre at 1-855-JP-CHILD (1-855-572-4453; open 24 hours/day, 7 days/week) or refer to the Government of Canada's Indigenous Services Jordan's Principle website (https://www.sac-isc.gc.ca/eng/1568 396296543/1582657596387). The Inuit Child First Initiative applies to Inuit children. To access benefits, call the national call centre at 1-855-572-4453 (also available 24 hours/day, 7 days/week).

With respect to health care insurance, to access the federal NIHB program an individual must be a resident of Canada and a registered First Nations person under the *Indian Act*, an Inuk recognized by one of the Inuit Land Claim organizations, or an infant younger than age 18 months whose parent is an eligible client. NIHB coverage includes many prescription medications; mental health counselling; some prescribed devices, such as glucometers and orthotics; and some over-the-counter products, such as vitamins. Not all prescribed medications are covered. If a prescribed medication is not covered, prescribers can apply for an exception. To initiate this process, prescribers should call the NIHB Drug Exception Centre at 1-800-580-0950.

Navigating NIHB coverage can be complex for both service users and care providers. Those experiencing challenges accessing NIHB-covered products and services, including both the appeals processes and coverage denials, can reach out to an NIHB navigator for support. In most jurisdictions NIHB navigators are located in various organizations, such as the Chiefs of Ontario. All Indigenous Peoples also have a right to access provincial and territorial health care.

INDIGENOUS CULTURAL SAFETY IN HEALTH CARE PROVISION

To provide equitable health care services to Indigenous people, which is the responsibility of all health care providers, more is needed than access to appropriate resources. Creating culturally safe health care spaces and interactions is also required. The process of creating culturally safe spaces for Indigenous people includes a recalibration of existing power dynamics between Indigenous people and health care providers. As such, culturally safe practices "require critical thinking and self-reflection about power, privilege and racism in educational and clinical settings."[29(p. 9)]

Note that Canada recognizes that First Nations, Inuit, and Métis have an inherent right of self-government protected by section 35 of the *Constitution Act, 1982* as well as the United Nations *Declaration on the Rights of Indigenous Peoples*,[30] which Canada endorsed without reservation in 2016, paving the way for 2021 implementation of the declaration into Canadian law. Providing culturally safe care includes recognizing the self-determination of Indigenous people in their own health and wellness, respecting Indigenous health and wellness practices, being aware of the impacts of settler colonialism on the health of Indigenous people, and providing care that is free of anti-Indigenous racism and bias. It is important to note that it is the service user who determines whether an interaction with a health care provider or service was culturally safe.

Our recommendations for supporting the development of a culturally safe environment for Indigenous patients include the following:

- Increase your own awareness and understanding of providing culturally safe care by participating in Indigenous-focused cultural safety training and workshops and through learning opportunities provided by professional regulatory bodies. See San'yas Indigenous Cultural Safety Training (https://sanyas.ca). Also see *Indigenous Health: the Royal College of Physicians and Surgeons of Canada*[31] for learning resources on supporting Indigenous health.
- Maintain a stance of cultural curiosity and humility when working with Indigenous people. Respect Indigenous perspectives on what it means to be healthy and the role of ceremony, traditional medicines, community, and culture in wellness.
- Advocate for the implementation of policies that create timely access to smudging and other Indigenous healing practices in clinical settings, so that Indigenous patients and families can use both biomedical and traditional healing practices when accessing care.
- Implement clear, easy-to-access processes for reporting culturally unsafe care. This will help to identify areas of practice that need improvement and can create opportunities for staff and health care settings to repair damaged relationships with Indigenous patients, families, and staff.

Our suggestions to approach the case example of William are as follows:

- To assist in securing funding for mental health counselling, ask the family whether they are aware of Jordan's Principle. Describe it if needed.
  - Share the Jordan's Principle Call Centre number (currently 1-855-572-4453) so that the family can initiate their application.
- Assist the family by writing a letter that clearly describes the unmet health need. At a minimum, William's unmet need is access to psychotherapy. Other needs might include a psycho-educational assessment, tutoring services, and a computer and headphones to access virtual psychotherapy. You can view instructions on how to write an appropriate documentation letter at https://www.sac-isc .gc.ca/eng/1620743040769/1620743088435
- Share that NIHB covers virtual mental health counselling. Explore whether this is a viable option for William and determine whether there are barriers to access. Include any barriers to access in the letter describing unmet need. Share information on how to connect with an NIHB navigator to get connected with a child therapist who offers virtual sessions.
- Share information on Indigenous-focused agencies and services in the area that can provide support. This requires developing and maintaining an awareness of local Indigenous agencies and the programs and services they offer. Many Indigenous organizations offer direct services such as counselling, youth programming, cultural programming, and education supports.
- Share information on community based mental health services offered by local hospitals and health care centers and offer to make a direct referral.
- Encourage the family to reach out to their reserve community to inquire whether any additional supports are available.

2SLGBTQ+ Children's Rights to Equitable Health Care

Your patient Christopher (name and male gender assigned at birth) is transitioning and asks to be addressed as Christina with she/her pronouns. Repeatedly when she attends bloodwork appointments at the hospital, the registering clerk loudly says "Christopher" when her turn is called. This requires more than one call out before Christina realizes they are calling her; she then looks at the ground as she shrugs and heads in for the appointment. To make matters worse, your front administrative staff have said more than once, "I can't bill under that name because it's not the legal name," and your colleague has often been heard saying, "I don't get this pronoun thing, it doesn't even make grammatical sense." The microaggressions pile on; last month the publisher of the school yearbook did not note her name change, and her picture was labelled Christopher.

Young people who identify as sexual minority youth have higher rates of depression, anxiety, and suicide than the general population because of the negative impacts of discrimination, harassment, and other forms of victimization.[32] In an online survey conducted in Canada, transgender youth had a higher reported risk of psychological distress, self-harm, major depressive episodes, suicidal ideation, and suicide attempts. Risk ratios ranged from 3.8 to 16.1.[33]

As a health care provider, you are perfectly positioned to be a powerful ally for your 2SLGBTQ+ patients. You can start by creating a safe environment. When your patients visit your office, something as simple as a pride flag sticker or rainbow is an instant signal of recognition. Having trained frontline staff who ask rather than assume pronouns and who ensure a safe and private space for health-related questions is imperative.

Because of past negative experiences with the health care system, 2SLGBTQ+ people may delay or avoid seeking health and mental health supports, or they may choose to withhold personal information from health care providers. In a Canadian study, participants reported considerable unmet needs or delays in primary, general, and gender-affirming care, with significant regional variation. Despite efforts towards equity in access to care for trans and non-binary people in Canada, including the introduction of province-wide continuing medical education and care navigation initiatives and increased coverage for gender-affirming surgical care under provincial and territorial health insurance plans, inequities persist.[34] Only 52.3 per cent of transgender youth had a primary care provider with whom they were comfortable discussing trans health issues, and 44.4 per cent reported an unmet health care need.[35] 2SLGBTQ+ youth are also more likely to face parental rejection or other trauma and are therefore more likely to be homeless or underhoused.[36]

An adolescent coming to a primary care office provides a unique opportunity to acquire not only treatment but information and affirmation (because they rarely want to come to the doctor). Regardless of the reason for the visit, youth may appreciate an opportunity to speak to you alone. It is good practice for paediatricians to prioritize some alone time to allow for private discussion with youth starting around age 11 or 12. This is often the developmental stage of seeking out and confirming gender identity or sexual orientation. In addition, puberty has likely begun. This is an ideal time to talk about safe practices and also allow youth to ask questions that they may be too apprehensive or embarrassed to ask other people in their lives. For youth transitioning from their assigned gender at birth, early puberty is when a consultation for hormone therapy could be considered.

Gender-affirming health care must be individualized according to a patient's needs. The first step towards inclusiveness in the health care provider's practice is letting the young person know up front that the practice is inclusive and welcoming. Something as small as having a poster supporting 2SLGBTQ+ health services can send a message to patients that they are in a safe, supportive environment.[37]

However, this visual acceptance should extend to all areas of the practice, including office administrators and all staff. Not assuming all patients are heterosexual and binary is a positive step towards helping all patients feel safe in accessing health care. Patients should not feel ostracized or stigmatized when identifying their gender; pronouns need not be assumed; and forms should reflect the young person's identity, even if health practice necessitates also identifying gender assigned at birth.

Patient confidentiality, which is always a legal right in patient care, must extend to ensuring against even unintentional slips, which can be extremely crucial to a young person who is not ready to identify to the broader community, or even to family members. Primary health care providers have an important role to play in supporting trans and gender-diverse children and youth throughout their gender journey. In addition to discussions about medical and surgical options, this may include conversations about non-medical and non-surgical aspects of gender affirmation (e.g., safe chest binding, voice therapy).

Various organizations representing sexual minority patients have provided tool kits and guidelines for primary care providers to help provide a safe environment that may prove helpful.[38] Asking patients, in particular young people, to disclose their sexual orientation can be sensitive even when the purpose is to ensure equal access to health care.

2SLGBTQ+ patients may have unmet social and legal needs that may include changing their name and changing gender markers in schools, as well as on legal documents such as health cards. Depending on provincial or territorial laws, changing their gender marker on their own or with the consent of their legal guardian may be an option that the young person can pursue, depending on their age. In some cases, it may require confirmation by a health care provider. Most federal documents, including passports, now allow for gender marker changes (as well as name changes), with three options, M, F, and X.[39]

Most provinces have enacted laws ensuring gender-affirming policies in publicly funded schools. This allows students to self-identify, change names, and initiate a group or other school activity that focuses on diversity in attraction, gender identity, or gender expression consistent with the promotion of a positive school climate that is inclusive and accepting of all students. However, in some cases the student may have to provide supporting documentation of their identity, which health care providers may provide. This could include a letter with a simple statement about the name change, but the requirements may differ from province to province.

It is helpful for young sexual minority patients to have access to resources to support health and safety through counselling and information services outside your office. Young patients may be directed to various agencies across the country that support young people; for example,

- the Lesbian, Gay, Bi & Trans Youthline (https://www.youthline.ca/) offers free peer support for youth aged 26 and younger (1-800-268-9688) and
- children and youth ages five to 20 can speak with trained counsellors at Kids Health Phone (1-800-668-6868; https://kidshelpphone.ca/).

As a health care provider, it is important that you take the time to understand your own bias and be mindful of not only your language but that of staff and colleagues in order to provide a safe space for all patients. Although it is human nature to make mistakes, a simple apology can often go a long way. Once you know better, you can try to do better every day. It is also important to be knowledgeable about local resources that youth may be interested in or require. Specifically, educate yourself about local community groups and other allied professionals who provide safe spaces for 2SLGBTQ+ youth. Last, understand not only local hormone and surgical options, but also limitations to access in the community. That way all options are presented to the youth, who may want more information than you can provide. It is critical to not put your own judgments on youth with the idea that they are too young, have not stopped growing yet, or it may just be a phase. Adolescence is one of the most stressful times for gender-fluid or transgender children as their body changes to reflect their biological and hormonal milieu.

The Family's Ability to Care for the Child

Note that in each category in this section, the focus on the issues relates to the child, caregivers of the child, or both. For more detailed information, see chapter 7 on immigration and health and chapters 5 and 6 on employment and social assistance and health.

Immigration Status

> *Natalia is a refugee claimant from Nation X who wants to have her daughter seen by a paediatrician. Your administrative assistant explains that this is not a primary care office, and paediatricians are often seen only on a referral basis. Natalia does not have a family doctor because they just arrived three weeks ago, and they cannot receive interim federal health coverage until they are determined eligible to make their refugee claim, which could take many weeks. Natalia's experience in Nation X was that specialty services especially for children were readily accessible, and she starts to cry because she does not have the money or energy to go all the way to the downtown emergency department to wait for a referral for her daughter's chronic medical issues.*

Often the parent's or child's immigration status affects the family's ability to access resources to support the child's health and adds to psychosocial stress that can also affect health. It is therefore important that primary health care providers understand that the immigration status of the patient and their family can affect their entitlement to benefits and resources. This section focuses on some unique aspects of immigration status with respect to paediatrics. This is especially true in areas in which paediatricians act as consultants and do not provide primary care, which is very common in Canada. It is important to understand the expectations of families given their prior experience and their home country's medical system.

As a caveat when speaking to families, in our experience people who refer to themselves as refugees are often refugee claimants – those who have applied for refugee status, but whose status has not yet been determined. Refugee claimants' health care is paid for through the Interim Federal Health Program rather than provincial plans, and providers should be aware that access to some health care covered by provincial plans may require pre-approval. Many services provided under supplemental coverage also require pre-approval. Please see chapter 7 for a more comprehensive treatment of immigration issues, including status categories, which are often related to access to benefits.

CLAIMS FOR STATUS FROM WITHIN CANADA, BASED ON THE BEST INTERESTS OF THE CHILD

Although risk to life due to lack of health care in the home country is not a ground for refugee status, it is a ground for making a humanitarian and compassionate (H&C) claim for permanent residence. A decision on an H&C application must include an assessment of the best interests of any child directly affected. In this context, *any child directly affected* could include children outside Canada.

Primary health care providers may be asked to provide supporting documentation when they have knowledge that a child cannot receive treatment in the home country or that the child cannot travel for the foreseeable future because of health issues. The health care provider may also be asked to provide evidence supporting a special need of the child that may not directly include medical care but is related to the child's health needs. Such things might include, for example, accommodation in education or specialized housing. Those interests need to be well identified and defined. Such information may include

- a diagnosis and treatment plan for any medical condition, and – if you have knowledge – whether that care could be provided in the country of origin;
- proof of a medical condition (e.g., person is living with HIV), and – if you have knowledge – that they would suffer discrimination in the country of origin as a result; and
- mental health assessment of past trauma or future trauma, should the child be returned to the country of origin.

REMOVAL ORDERS AND STAYS OF DEPORTATION

Caregivers may be asked to provide a letter in support of an order staying removal from Canada in cases in which children are receiving urgent ongoing care or the child should not travel for health reasons. The letter can be brief. It requires only the name of the child, the diagnosis or treatment that requires the child to remain in Canada for treatment, and identification of the treatment or, if no further treatment, why the child cannot travel outside of Canada. Where possible, an estimate of the length of time required for the child to remain in Canada should be included.

As discussed in chapter 7, immigration status and access to health care can be complicated. Best practice is to work with a legal professional to ensure that your letter provides the clinical opinion needed for the lawyer to make the case.

Our suggested best practices for Natalia are as follows:

- In response to the increasing number of people new to Canada, many areas are responding to their health care needs by creating clinics and designated health care access for newcomers and their families. Screening medical intakes and responses for newcomers with distinct needs fails to meet those needs or direct patients to the right service. In addition, lengthy wait times and differing expectations about the Canadian system are barriers to meeting health care needs. Referral to a newcomer-type clinic would be very appropriate and also ensure that the family is registered to be in line to receive a primary care provider should one exist.
- Having information in your office describing pathways to receive care and the different avenues (acute care services, walk-in clinics, virtual or e-consult-type services) may provide some accessible short-term solutions.
- From a humanitarian standpoint, you may choose to assess and treat the patient and save the information for future billing. You might ask Medavie Blue Cross, a private insurance company that is currently the administrator for the Interim Federal Health Program for refugee claimants and refugees for a deadline extension because of refugee eligibility wait times and the need for care.[40] This is a situation in need of powerful advocacy from health care providers to ensure resources are available to meet the needs of those we welcome to Canada.

Employment Issues

Divya is a single parent with a seriously ill child undergoing treatment. They will need to take several weeks (if not longer) off work to stay with the child in hospital and then several weeks afterwards to provide follow-up care at home. They are very concerned about losing their job or being demoted because of this. They are also concerned about the financial implications.

Parents and legal guardians whose children become ill, especially those with a serious chronic illness or who are critically ill or injured, may find that employment becomes precarious. This is especially the case for those who are new to the job or do not have secure employment. Often employers warn parents of job loss if they continue to take time off work to attend multiple appointments or take leaves of absence for extended periods to care for a sick child.

All Canadian workers are covered by employment standards acts or codes in their province or territory, or by the *Canada Labour Code*[41], if they are a federally regulated employee. These codes include provisions for medical certificates that physicians and nurse practitioners can provide to ensure job protection for workers because of illness. This differs from Employment Insurance (EI) medical certificates because provincial and territorial certificates provide only job protection, not payment.

If a parent or guardian continues to be off work beyond the amount of time protected by the *Employment Standards Act*, they may still be protected under the *Canadian Human Rights Act* on the basis of family status (parent or guardian of a sick child).[42] Parents can contact an employment lawyer or their human rights commission if they are fired or if the employer fails to accommodate their request for different shifts. Primary health care providers may be asked for supporting documentation. All parents who belong to a union should be directed first to their union representative for any questions related to work law. In Ontario, families can contact the free Pro Bono Ontario hotline (toll-free, 1-855-255-7256; https://www.probonoontario .org/hotline/) for questions related to employment rights (as well as other issues, such as housing and debt), as well as their local community legal aid clinic (see Appendix 1 for more information).

EMPLOYMENT INSURANCE

Physicians and nurse practitioners may be asked to sign medical certificates for patients to access EI. It is worth reminding parents that EI is a federal insurance scheme to provide income replacement under certain conditions, but it does not protect jobs. As discussed earlier, job protection flows from various provincial and territorial employment standards acts, employment contracts, and human rights codes.

There are three types of EI benefits: regular EI, sickness EI, and special benefits EI. Sickness EI and regular EI are specific to the employee, not to the employee as a caregiver. At the time of writing, special benefits EI requires the applicant to have 600 hours of insurable earnings. Several EI benefits are directed to caregivers such as parents and legal guardians. These benefits include the following:

- Maternity benefits are payable to the person who has given birth; they cannot be shared. These benefits commence as early as 12 weeks before the due date or the actual date on which the person gives birth. Under most circumstances, a person cannot receive these benefits for more than 17 weeks after their due date or the date they gave birth, whichever is later. However, parents should be directed to Service Canada for any possible exceptions for extending the period with respect to a critically ill child, in particular a child in hospital.

- Parental benefits are available to parents of a newborn or adopted child. The two kinds of benefit periods are (a) standard, taken within 52 weeks of birth, and (b) extended, taken within 78 weeks. There are some exceptions that allow for extension of the period, for example, when a newborn is hospitalized. Parents should be directed to Service Canada if asking for an extension. Parental benefits are shared.
- Family critical caregiver benefits are available to the caregiver of someone whose life is at risk and needs care and support. Up to 35 weeks can be paid within a 52-week period.[43]
- Compassionate care benefits are available to the caregiver of someone at the end of life, with a significant risk of death within 6 months.[44]

Please also see chapter 5 on work and health for further information about these benefits.

Primary health care providers may be asked to complete a medical certificate for any of these special benefits; the medical certificates are self-explanatory. There are specific and complex rules on taking special benefits. If all requirements are followed, parents or caregivers may be able to take up to 102 weeks in total (as long as these benefits are not combined with any regular EI). Parents with questions about accessing EI should be directed to call Service Canada to ensure they qualify and to understand the interaction between benefits. Your local legal aid clinic (if you have one) should be able to provide some legal advice as well.

With respect to Divya and their concerns about job protections as well as the financial implications of taking time off work, our best-practice suggestions are as follows:

- If the child's health is critical (i.e., their life is at risk), the physician or nurse practitioner can sign the medical form for the family caregiver benefit (FCB). The FCB provides for up to 35 weeks of remuneration, including both while the child is in hospital and critical and during the follow-up supporting care at home as a result of the critical injury or illness.
- Many provinces and territories have statutory job protection corresponding to FCB leave. If so, the medical practitioner may be asked to sign that medical certificate as well, because employers can request the employment standards certificate.

- If the province or territory does not provide job protection, the parent may have to file a human rights complaint if the employer threatens action, and the health care provider may be asked for further information to support a claim.

Tax-Related Benefits

CANADA CHILD TAX BENEFIT

All children whose parents qualify (have the necessary immigration status, file income tax, are within financial eligibility) are eligible for the Canada Child Benefit as well as various provincial or territorial benefits.[45] See chapter 6 on health and access to benefits for further detail.

DISABILITY TAX CREDIT AND THE CANADA DISABILITY BENEFIT

Those persons whose children have a severe and prolonged impairment in one category, significant limitations in two or more categories, or receive therapy to support a vital function may also qualify for disability benefits, for example the Canada Disability Benefit, which is automatic on being granted the Disability Tax Credit (DTC). The vital functions affected are walking, hearing, vision, speaking, dressing, feeding, bladder bowel functions, mental functions, and life-sustaining therapies. The DTC can be provided to only one parent.

Eligible primary health care providers may be asked to help apply for the DTC. It is not for every child with a chronic disability; it has particular qualifications and is rarely provided to children aged younger than one year because all babies require help with at least one of the preceding daily functions.

A child is eligible for the DTC when a medical practitioner certifies, on Form T2201, the Disability Tax Credit Certificate, that the child has a severe and prolonged impairment in physical or mental functions and is impaired at least 90 per cent of the time, and the Canada Revenue Agency (CRA) approves the form. The Canadian Paediatric Society and the CRA have guides on appropriately filling out the application form for the DTC.[46]

Parents should be cautioned not to pay agencies charging a percentage of the benefits (including retroactive benefits) for filling out the DTC. There are community agencies and CRA free tax clinics that can help without charge. To access benefits, parents must file their income tax.

Health care providers can refer their patients to free tax clinics in their area to help them.

As well as the DTC and attenuated provincial disability benefits, some provinces provide financial assistance to parents to help with extraordinary cost related to their child's severe disability, such as Assistance for Children with a Severe Disability (ACSD) in Ontario, which is a direct funding program for low- and moderate-income families.[47] Note that ACSD is not considered social assistance for immigration sponsorship purposes; for more information, see chapter 7 on immigration law and health.

HENSON TRUST

There is a particular trust in Canadian law that can be set up to benefit people with a chronic disability. Specifically, it protects the assets (usually an inheritance) of the person and allows the person the right to collect government benefits and entitlements because it is an absolute discretionary trust, meaning that the trustee has absolute discretion in dispensing money from the trust. Because the assets do not vest with the beneficiary, they cannot be used to deny means-tested government benefits, including various disability support programs. It also has income tax relief implications.

A Henson trust can be established as either a living trust or a testamentary trust. Refer your patient to legal advice if they are considering this option.

Conclusion

Primary care practitioners are often in the best place to observe the impact SDOHs have on their patients and therefore often take on the role of advocates in pursuit of their patients' health. They are in a unique relationship based on trust and privacy, and they have the professional expertise to listen and translate patients' stories into a diagnosis of illness. What often emerges is a complex story, which may explain, for example, a patient's non-compliance with medical treatment. However, often the factors that emerge are reasons that go beyond choice and are based on multiple social factors impeding access and compliance. Once heard and understood, the health care provider may feel overwhelmed by their patient's complex needs while wishing to reduce health disparities. The intention of this chapter is to provide insights into paediatric patients' rights and to support patient-centred care in the pursuit of optimizing health.

Resources

Sample Letters

Ensure you obtain consent from a capable patient before releasing information.

Letter to Principal: Accommodation of Child's Special Needs
To ___________ Date

I am the physician/nurse practitioner for ______________ D.O.B., ___ a student in grade ___.

This letter is to confirm that________________ has received the diagnosis of _______________________. Accordingly, ___________will require certain accommodations to assist with their studies, in order to provide them with the best opportunity to access equitable education. [If time limited, include the expected duration of needs.]
The following accommodations for_______________ will best help _______

[When not clear from diagnosis, include the reasons for recommending each accommodation.]
Equipment: _________________
Additional time for assignments, classwork, tests __________________
A quiet environment to write exams and tests___________________
Assistant for learning, personal care, etc. _________________
Thank you for your attention to this matter. Should you have any questions, please do not hesitate to contact me.

Sincerely,

Letter to Principal: Child Being Bullied
To _______________ Date: __

I am the physician/nurse practitioner for ______________ D.O.B., ___ a student in grade __

___________ [or parents] *has reported to me that they have been bullied by various* students/named student(s) [at school, in the classroom, at recess, on the bus, etc.]. *I understand that the parents have reported this to the teacher, and the bullying is ongoing despite any interventions that may or may not have taken place.*
The bullying has had a detrimental impact on the health of ______, who is experiencing increased anxiety, as well as other symptoms related to the ongoing

incidents. I am requesting that you conduct a prompt investigation and address the issue before ______'s health continues to deteriorate.

(As you are aware, ____ is a special needs student; therefore you have the added duty to protect ____ from bullying based on these special needs under the Human Rights Code *as well as the* Education Act.*)*

Sincerely,

Immigration Letter Accompanying a Humanitarian and Compassionate Application in the Child's Best Interest with Respect to a Child's Need to Remain in Canada for Health Care

To Immigration Refugee & Citizenship Canada Date:

Re: Humanitarian & Compassionate Application for _______________

I am writing in support of the Application for H&C based on the best interests of the child.

_______ has been diagnosed with _________. [Describe condition, severity, duration, etc.]

Accordingly, _______ will require [procedures, medications, social supports, etc.]. *It has come to my attention that ________'s home country ___________ cannot provide the necessary* [health care, social supports, etc.] *necessary to treat ____'s condition, and therefore we strongly urge that ____be allowed to remain in Canada for treatment.*

Please contact me if you have any further questions.

Sincerely,

Letter for Employer: Caregivers Require Accommodation at Work Due to Child's Illness or Disability

To Whom It May Concern

Request for Workplace Accommodations for ___________________ Date __

_________ is the parent [guardian] of a child who is [ill, injured, has a disability, etc.]. *Accordingly, due to their health, the child must remain at home and cannot attend* [school, daycare, multiple appointments] *at this time until at least* [duration]. *A parent must remain with them to provide care. Therefore, the parent is* [unable to attend work, must change shifts, needs to leave work early, etc.].

Thank you for your consideration. Please contact me if you have further questions.

Sincerely,

Screening Tools

One of the most effective ways to assess the impact of the everyday living conditions of patients is to use a few key questions as the first step in positive interventions. Multiple screening and poverty tools have been developed across the country to aid providers, as well as provide the links to key government and community resources to support positive interventions, some specific to paediatric practice.[48] Screening does not have to be overly demanding on time or overly intrusive, and it can inform a case finding approach that is discussed in chapter 1. Typical questions from child poverty tools follow.

> Families tell us that caring for a very ill child can mean extra financial stress. We want to help understand and see whether we can make suggestions or referrals to access help for you. Please feel free to answer any or none of the following questions:
>
> 1. Do you have trouble feeding your family?
> 2. Do you have trouble paying for medications?
> 3. Do you receive the child tax benefit?
> 4. Do you have a safe place to live?
> 5. Is your child experiencing any difficulties in school?
> 6. Do you have any other challenges you wish to disclose?

NOTES

1 World Health Organization. Social determinants of health [Internet]. Geneva: World Health Organization; n.d. [cited 2023 May 2]. Available from: https://www.who.int/health-topics/social-determinants-of-health#tab=tab_1.

2 For further discussion, see the Canadian Paediatric Society Position Statement on ACEs: Williams RC. Position statement from ACEs to early relational health: implications for clinical practice. Paediatr Child Health. 2023;28(6):377–84. https//doi.org/10.1093/pch/pxad025.

3 Gottlien L, Hessler D, Long D, et al. A randomized trial on screening for social determinants of health: the iScreen Study. Pediatrics. 2014;134(6): ee1611–e1618. https://doi.org/10.1542/peds.2014-1439.

4 Jackson SF, Miller W, Chapman LA, et al. Hospital-legal partnership at Toronto Hospital for Sick Children: the first Canadian experience. Healthc Q. 2012;15(4):55–61.

5 Selvaraj K, Ruiz MJ, Aschkenasy J, et al. Screening for toxic stress risk factors at well-child visits: The Addressing Social Key Questions for Health Study. J Pediatr. 2019 Feb;205:244–249.e4. https://doi.org10.1016/j.jpeds.2018.09.004.

6 European Public Health Alliance. Social determinants of health – what can doctors do? [Internet]. London: British Medical Association; 2011 [cited 2023 May 3]. Available from: https://epha.org/social-determinants-of-health-what-can-doctors-do/.

7 The first medical–legal partnership at Boston Children's Hospital was established in 1993 by Dr. Barry Zuckerman. Canada's first Medical Legal Partnership in 2009, at the Hospital for Sick Children, in partnership with Pro Bono Ontario.

8 These two groups receive special focus because their rights and resources are differentiated from those of other groups (e.g., racialized peoples, newcomers) who are also, as stated earlier, differentially affected by SDOHs.

9 Government of Canada. Social determinants of health and health inequalities [Internet]. Ottawa: Government of Canada; 2022 [cited 2023 May 2]. Available from: https://www.canada.ca/en/public-health/services/health-promotion/population-health/what-determines-health.html.

10 In *A.C. v Manitoba (Director of Child and Family Services)*, 2009 SCC 30, the Supreme Court of Canada found that the legal obligation to act in the best interests of the child required recognizing the autonomy of the capable child (regardless of age) to make their own health care decisions. Various provincial legislations recognize this right. With respect to health care, under the UN *Convention on the Rights of the Child*, children have the right both to the best health care possible and to have their right to decision-making on all matters concerning themselves be given due weight according to capacity (United Nations. Convention on the Rights of the Child [adopted 20 November 20], Treaty Series, vol. 1577, p. 3 [cited 2023 May 2]. Available from: https://www.refworld.org/docid/3ae6b38f0.html).

11 Bureau of Health Information. Admitted Children and Young Patients Survey results [Internet]. St. Leonards (NSW): The Bureau; 2014 [cited 2019 Dec 24]. Available from: http://www.bhi.nsw.gov.au/BHI_reports/patient_survey_results/admitted_children_and_young_patients_survey_results_2014. Similar questions were asked in an unpublished survey of grade 11 and 12 high school students from across Toronto attending a workshop on consent and capacity with similar results.

12 Coughlin KW. Medical decision-making in paediatrics: infancy to adolescence. Paediatr Child Health [Internet]. 2018 May;23(2):138–46 [cited 2023 Apr 11]. Available from: https://cps.ca/en/documents/position/medical-decision-making-in-paediatrics-infancy-to-adolescence.

13 *Canadian Charter of Rights and Freedoms*, s 7, Part 1 of the *Constitution Act*, 1982, being Schedule B to the Canada Act 1982 (UK), 1982, c 11.

14 In Ontario, this is governed by the *Health Care Consent Act*, 1996, SO 1996, c 2, Sched A. Available from: https://www.ontario.ca/laws/statute/96h02.

15 United Nations. Convention on the Rights of the Child (adopted 1989 November 20), Treaty Series, vol. 1577, p. 3 [cited 2023 May 2]. Available from: https://www.refworld.org/docid/3ae6b38f0.html.

16 Public Health Agency of Canada (PHAC). Provincial and territorial child protection legislation and policy [Internet]. Ottawa: PHAC; 2018 [cited 2023 Apr 11]. Available from: https://cps.ca/en/documents/position/medical-decision-making-in-paediatrics-infancy-to-adolescence.

17 Ally Global Foundation. Human trafficking happens in Canada too [Internet]. Vancouver (BC): The Foundation; n.d. [cited 2023 May 2] Available from: https://ally.org/canada?gclid=EAIaIQobChMI5I3xmo uB_QIVpsiUCR3mdQcLEAAYASAAEgLckvD_BwE.

18 Canadian Human Trafficking Hotline. About us [Internet]. The Hotline; n.d. [2023 Apr 11]. Available from: www.canadianhumantraffickinghotline.ca.

19 Government of Canada. Forced marriage [Internet]. Ottawa: Government of Canada; 2023 [cited 2023 May 2]. Available from: https://travel.gc.ca /assistance/emergency-info/forced-marriage.

20 United Nations. Convention on the rights of persons with disabilities (2007 Jan 24). Treaty Series, vol. 2513, 3 [cited 2023 May 2]. Available from: https://www.refworld.org/docid/45f973632.html.

21 See, for example, *Eaton v Brant County Board of Education*, [1997] 1 SCR 241.

22 *Eaton v Brant County Board of Education*, [1997] 1 SCR 241.

23 *Youth Criminal Justice Act*, SC 2002, c 1.

24 Department of Justice Canada. Publication bans [Internet]. Ottawa: The Department; n.d. [cited 2023 May 2]. Available from: https://www.justice .gc.ca/eng/cj-jp/victims-victimes/factsheets-fiches/publication.html.

25 Halseth R, Murdock L. Supporting Indigenous self-determination in health: lessons learned from a review of best practices in health governance in Canada and internationally. Prince George (BC): National Collaborating Centre for Collaborative Health; 2020.

26 Smylie J, Harris R, Paine SJ, et al. Beyond shame, sorrow, and apologies – action to address Indigenous health inequities. BMJ. 2022;378:o1688.

27 *Indian Act*, RSC, 1985, c I-5.

28 *First Nations Child and Family Caring Society of Canada and the Assembly of First Nations v Attorney General of Canada*, 2016 CHRT 2.

29 Royal College of Physicians and Surgeons of Canada. Indigenous health values and principles statement: the Indigenous Health Writing Group of the Royal College. 2nd ed. Ottawa: The College; 2019.

30 United Nations. Declaration on the rights of Indigenous Peoples (adopted 2 October 2007) [cited 2023 2 May]. Available from: https://www.refworld .org/docid/471355a82.html.

31 Royal College of Physicians and Surgeons of Canada. Indigenous health [Internet]. Ottawa: Royal College of Physicians and Surgeons of Canada; n.d. [cited 2023 May 2]. Available from: https://www.royalcollege.ca/en /about/strategic-themes/indigenous-health.

32 Burton CM, Marshal MP, Chisolm DJ, et al. Sexual minority-related victimization as a mediator of mental health disparities in sexual minority

youth: a longitudinal analysis. J Youth Adolesc. 2013 Mar;42(3):394–402. https://doi.org/10.1007/s10964-012-9901-5.

33 Veale JF, Watson RJ, Peter T, et al. Mental health disparities among Canadian transgender youth. J Adolesc Health. 2017 Jan;60(1):44–49. https://doi.org/10.1016/j.jadohealth.2016.09.014.

34 Scheim AI, Coleman T, Lachowsky N, et al. Health care access among transgender and nonbinary people in Canada, 2019: a cross-sectional survey. CMAJ Open. 2021 Dec 21;9(4):E1213–E1222. https://doi.org/10.9778/cmajo.20210061.

35 Scheim AI, Coleman T, Lachowsky N, et al. Health care access among transgender and nonbinary people in Canada, 2019: a cross-sectional survey. CMAJ Open. 2021 Dec 21;9(4):E1213–E1222. https://doi.org/10.9778/cmajo.20210061.

36 Whitbeck LB, Chen X, Hoyt DR, et al. Mental disorder, subsistence strategies, and victimization among gay, lesbian, and bisexual homeless and runaway adolescents. J Sex Res. 2004 Nov;41(4):329–42. https://doi.org/10.1080/00224490409552240.

37 Collier R. Promoting pride in practice. CMAJ. 2012 Oct 16;184(15):E789–E790. https://doi.org/10.1503/cmaj.109-4296.

38 See, for example, Bourns A. Sherbourne's guidelines for gender-affirming primary care. 4th ed. Toronto: Rainbow Health Ontario; 2019. Available from: https://www.rainbowhealthontario.ca/product/4th-edition -sherbournes-guidelines-for-gender-affirming-primary-care-with-trans-and -non-binary-patients/; Bourns A. Guidelines for gender-affirming primary care with trans and non-binary patients [Internet]. Toronto: Rainbow Health Ontario; 2019. Available from: http://www.transforumquinte.ca /downloads/Guidelines-and-Protocols-for-Comprehensive-Primary-Care -for-Trans-Clients-2019.pdf; Trans Care BC. Health professionals [Internet]. Vancouver (BC): Trans Care BC; n.d. Available from: http://www.phsa .ca/transcarebc/Documents/HealthProf/Primary-Care-Toolkit.pdf; and Clarkstone C. Working with lesbian, gay and bisexual youth: information for primary care [Internet]. eMentalHealth.ca Available from: https:// primarycare.ementalhealth.ca/index.php?m=fpArticle&ID=52746.

39 Government of Canada Help Centre. How do I change the sex or gender identifier on my application or document? [Internet]. Ottawa: Government of Canada; 2023 [modified 2024 June 10; cited 2023 May 2]. Available from: https://www.cic.gc.ca/english/helpcentre/answer.asp?qnum=1253&top=32.

40 For further information on the Interim Federal Health Program, visit https://www.canada.ca/en/immigration-refugees-citizenship/services /refugees/help-within-canada/health-care/interim-federal-health -program/coverage-summary.html or contact Medavie IFHP toll-free at 1-888-614-1880.

41 *Canada Labour Code*, RSC, 1985, c. L-2.

42 *Employment Standards Act,* 2000, SO 2000, c 41; *Canadian Human Rights Act,* RSC, 1985, c H-6.

43 Government of Canada. Medical certificate for family caregiver benefits. Ottawa: Government of Canada; 2017 [cited 2023 May 7]. Available from: https://catalogue.servicecanada.gc.ca/content/EForms/en/Detail .html?Form=INS5242B.

44 Government of Canada. Medical certificate for family caregiver benefits. Ottawa: Government of Canada; 2017 [cited 2023 May 7]. Available from: https://catalogue.servicecanada.gc.ca/content/EForms/en/Detail .html?Form=INS5242B.

45 Government of Canada. Apply for the Canada Child Benefit [Internet]. Ottawa: Government of Canada 2023 [cited 2023 May 7]. Available from: https://www.canada.ca/en/revenue-agency/services/child-family -benefits/canada-child-benefit-overview/canada-child-benefit-apply .html.

46 Canadian Paediatric Society. Tips for paediatricians completing the Disability Tax Credit (DTC) form [Internet]. Ottawa: The Society; n.d. [cited 2023 May 7]. Available from: https://canfasd.ca/wp-content /uploads/2016/11/DTC_Tips_for_Paediatricians_June_22_2016.pdf; Canada Revenue Agency. Disability tax credit [Internet]. Toronto: The Agency; n.d. [cited 2023 May 7]. Available from: https://www.canada .ca/en/revenue-agency/services/tax/individuals/segments/tax-credits -deductions-persons-disabilities/disability-tax-credit.html.

47 ACSD Ontario. Assistance for Children with Severe Disabilities Program [Internet]. Toronto: ACSD Ontario; n.d. [cited 2023 May 2]. Available from: https://www.ontario.ca/page/assistance-children -severe-disabilities-program; FCSD Alberta. Family Support for Children with Disabilities (FCSD) [Internet]. Edmonton: FCSD Alberta; n.d. [cited 2023 May 2]. Available from: https://www.alberta.ca/fscd .aspx; Department of Community Services. Direct family support for children [Internet]. Halifax: Government of Nova Scotia; 2013 [cited 2023 May 2]. Available from: https://novascotia.ca/coms/disabilities /DirectFamilySupportForChildren.html; Government of Yukon. Find supports for your child with a disability [Internet]. Whitehorse: Government of Yukon; n.d. [cited 2023 May 2]. Available from: https:// yukon.ca/en/health-and-wellness/babies-and-childrens-health/find -supports-your-child-disability.

48 Centre for Effective Practice (CEP). Poverty: a clinical tool for primary care providers [Internet]. Toronto: CEP; 2016 [cited 2024 Jan 28]. Available from: https://cep.health/clinical-products/poverty-a-clinical-tool-for-primary -care-providers/#pc_page_44.

12 Estate, Financial, and Personal Care Planning for Marginalized and Isolated Populations

NAHEED DOSANI, EDGAR-ANDRE MONTIGNY,
AND MERCEDES PEREZ

This book focuses on issues relevant to low-income persons, marginalized individuals, persons who are isolated and lack social networks or social supports, and persons who experience homelessness or housing insecurity. Therefore, the comments that follow in this chapter apply to persons with limited income and assets who are not likely to possess more complicated forms of property, such as investments, business properties, stocks, bonds, a Registered Retirement Savings Plan (RRSP), or other financial instruments that are more common among the holdings of persons with higher income and easy access to social and other supports.

For individuals who own property and have a sufficient income, a stable home, and family or friends they can rely on for support, end-of-life planning can often be less complex. In these cases, decisions often focus on who will make decisions about property or medical and personal care should a person become unable to do so for themselves and who will inherit their property when they die. Individuals with supportive family and friends usually have no problem identifying people they can rely on for support and therefore name as attorneys for personal care or property or as executor of their will.

In most of these cases, estate planning is about making decisions, recording those decisions through legal documents, and keeping the documents safe and accessible until they are needed. Generally, when the people named as attorneys or executors are also individuals from a stable background with resources and support systems, they can be relied on to step up and perform the functions they were named to perform when required.

Individuals with stable homes and resources are usually able to store important documents over time to ensure they are kept safe until needed. They can put in place plans to ensure that their attorneys or executor can access these documents when required. They can usually trust that their executor will have access to the resources necessary to cover the costs of administering their estate, including the cost of hiring a lawyer to assist with the process. Therefore, having created a will, most people with resources and supports can be satisfied that their wishes will be honoured and carried out upon their death.

People without stable housing, reliable family ties, or social networks often have no one they can turn to perform the functions of attorney or executor. Furthermore, homeless or marginalized individuals rarely have access to legal advice or services to help them with such issues. Even if a person creates the necessary documents to express their end-of-life needs, people without stable housing face huge challenges keeping these documents safe and ensuring that others will know where to find them in an emergency. If the documents cannot be found when needed, all the effort that went into preparing them may be wasted.

Even when an individual is able to start planning for incapacity or end-of-life situations, the questions they need to consider and the options they have to explore are usually quite different from the issues faced by persons in more financially secure and supported circumstances.

For instance, the usual assumption that everyone should have a will may not apply to many marginalized low-income persons. There are costs associated with using a will to transfer property, and, when a person's assets are limited, the costs of pursuing the necessary court processes may eat up a large share of the estate or surpass its value. Transferring property through means other than a will, such as the use of joint property options, can pose some risk but may nevertheless offer a more effective means of ensuring that the property of a marginalized and isolated person goes where the individual wants it to go.[1]

The lack of options for low-income persons may partially explain why they are less likely to have undertaken any end-of-life planning. Many low-income persons might not turn their minds to estate matters or to future situations in which they might lose capacity unless someone such as a health care provider (HCP) tells them it might be necessary.

For this reason, HCPs (especially those in primary care) can play a key role in helping low-income patients understand the importance of end-of-life planning as well as directing them to service providers who are best placed to assist with their unique needs.

When a HCP identifies that a patient may be near the end of life or is at risk of losing personal care or financial capacity and may soon require others to make decisions for them, it is important to determine whether the patient has made any plans to deal with such situations. It is useful to know whether the patient has family members (or caregivers) who can assist them, whether the patient has named attorneys for personal care or property, or whether they have a will. It is important to raise the question of what can be done to financially protect their spouse or children. At this point, it may become apparent that the patient has no end-of-life plans in place, nor any plans to deal with potential future or imminent incapacity. In these situations, unless a HCP steps in to impress upon the patient how important it is to take action and offers some guidance as to where to find help, the patient may be unable to take the necessary steps.

People with little money often feel it is pointless to worry about their estate. People with children may not realize the challenges in getting the money in their bank account to their children if they die. Other individuals who are estranged from their closest family members may not realize that they can give their property and even the power to make decisions for them to a friend, rather than relying on family members they do not trust.

For low-income and marginalized patients, a more in-depth probe into the person's living circumstances and social situation may be required to identify their needs. This will allow a health care worker to determine how best to assist.

Although it is not a HCP's role to create legal documents for a patient, in many cases a HCP may be the only source a low-income person has to learn about what they need or what they can do to control what happens to them and their property when they die or who will make decisions for them if they become unable to make decisions for themselves. A HCP may also be a patient's only available resource for links to appropriate services in the community. In this sense, HCPs become a vital conduit between vulnerable patients and the legal services they require.

Unfortunately, locating affordable and accessible legal services is often very challenging. The sad truth is that until a more robust system of social and legal supports is available to assist with incapacity and end-of-life planning, marginalized populations will face major hurdles at every stage of the process. Where some level of ongoing support is available, there are steps that support workers, HCPs, and community groups can take to ensure people in unstable marginalized circumstances

- can make plans for future illness, incapacity, and end-of-life care;
- can make plans for the disposition of their property after they die;

- are offered the dignity of deciding what happens to their body; and
- are offered the comfort of knowing their wishes will be carried out if they become incapable or upon their death.

When told that they should start thinking about their long-term care needs and end-of-life planning because they may be facing a treatment or condition that could result in their death or incapacity, most people are concerned about three issues:

1. Who will make decisions about their medical care if they are unable to do so themselves?
2. Who will pay their bills and what will happen to their property if they die?
3. What will happen to their body after they die?

Issues related to who will make decisions or pay bills for a patient if they become incapable of doing so for themselves fall under substitute decision-making, which involves processes outlined in legislation such as Ontario's *Health Care Consent, 1996*[2] and *Substitute Decisions Act, 1992*,[3] as discussed later.

This chapter closes with a review of the issues related to estates and the transfer of property after a person's death.

Each section contains substantive information respecting the applicable laws, followed by analyses of scenarios replicating issues that may arise in regular practice.

Powers of Attorney, Guardianship, and Substitute Decision-Making

Planning for Financial and Health Care Decision-Making in the Event of Incapacity

INTRODUCTION

Although many people understand the basic concept that a will determines what is done with property after death, many do not realize that if they lose capacity to make decisions while they are still alive, because of illness or accident, a substitute decision-maker (SDM) may have to step in and manage their property or consent to treatment or personal care on their behalf. A person can require a SDM temporarily, while they recover from an illness or medical treatment, or more long term, when their condition is such that they are not likely to regain capacity.

Whether a SDM is required depends on a person's capacity to make the decision at issue.

WHAT IS CAPACITY?

Capacity relates to decision-making ability. The law recognizes that capacity as a concept is issue specific. This means that a person's capacity relates to the decision that needs to be made, for example, capacity to make financial decisions, capacity to make treatment decisions, and capacity to make decisions about where a person lives and what supports (medical or otherwise) might be needed to keep the person safe and healthy.

Capacity is generally defined as the ability to understand information relevant to the decision being made and the ability to appreciate the reasonably foreseeable consequences of the decision.[4] Capacity as understood in law is a concept that recognizes that some persons may be capable of making certain types of decisions (e.g., managing their property) but incapable of making other types of decisions (e.g., about whether to take antipsychotic medication or not) at any given time.[5]

Capacity is also understood to be time specific.[6] This means that a person may be incapable today but regain capacity at a later date (e.g., a person who is in a coma because of a car accident but later regains consciousness). The opposite is also captured in the definition of *capacity* – a person may be capable today but lose capacity down the road because of illness or accident.

Typically, *capacity* refers to the ability to make a type of decision, not the wisdom of the decision being made. In other words, a capable person can make decisions that others might deem foolish. Capacity is concerned with ability, not a person's best interests.[7]

PRESUMPTION OF CAPACITY

A person is generally presumed to be capable, and mental disorder does not automatically equate with incapacity.[8] A person does not lose capacity or the right to make decisions just because a relative or other individual thinks they are incapable. There must be a good reason to challenge this presumption.

Only certain people can declare another person incapable of making a particular type of decision. For instance, HCPs can make determinations of treatment capacity. Most jurisdictions also have specially trained individuals, such as Ontario's designated capacity assessors,[9] who can assess the capacity of individuals and make findings of incapacity. Such a finding of incapacity often means that a SDM must make certain decisions on behalf of the incapable person. Most jurisdictions also offer a means to challenge these findings.[10]

CONSENT

Consent is the key reason capacity matters. Whether the issue is medical treatment or a major financial decision, a person must consent or agree to whatever action is taken. Given the potential consequences of consenting to or refusing medical treatment or the impact of giving away large sums of money, it is important to ensure that a person is capable of giving consent. If a person lacks capacity, their consent is not valid.

SUBSTITUTE DECISION-MAKERS

If a person loses capacity to make financial or personal care decisions, a SDM will need to step in to make decisions on their behalf. This person may be an attorney for property or an attorney for personal care, named in power-of-attorney documents, or it may be a person who is designated as a SDM in legislation. The key difference between the different types of SDM is that attorneys for property and attorneys for personal care are selected and appointed by an individual while they are still capable. This allows the individual to exert some control over who will make decisions for them if they become incapable in the future. An individual grantor can provide instructions to their attorney to guide them when making future decisions.[11]

SDMs are also bound to follow any known prior capable wishes of the individual. However, it can be far more difficult to confirm these wishes when the SDM was not chosen by the individual.[12]

ATTORNEYS FOR PROPERTY AND PERSONAL CARE

A capable individual can grant a power of attorney for property (POAP) or a power of attorney for personal care (POAPC) to a friend or relative, meaning that the named individual will have the authority to make financial or medical care decisions for that person, should the grantor become incapable of doing so themselves. The precise rules as to what is required for a valid grant of a power of attorney vary from province to province. Certain provinces may have different signing requirements for power-of-attorney documents, and the documents and roles may have different names. We have included a brief description of the names of power-of-attorney documents in several provinces in Table 12.1 to illustrate some of the differences. Each province may also have different

Table 12.1. Some Unique Aspects of Powers of Attorney across Canada

Province	Key points
Alberta	In Alberta, for financial and legal matters, you make an enduring power of attorney and nominate an attorney. For personal and medical care, you make a personal directive and nominate an agent.[a]
British Columbia	In British Columbia, for financial and legal matters, you make an enduring power of attorney and nominate an attorney. For personal and medical care, you make a representation agreement and nominate a representative.[b]
Manitoba	In Manitoba, for financial and legal matters, you make an enduring power of attorney and nominate an attorney. For personal and medical care, you make a health care directive.[c]
New Brunswick	In New Brunswick, for financial and legal matters, you make an enduring power of attorney and nominate an attorney. For personal and medical care, you make a power of attorney for personal care and nominate an attorney for personal care. You can choose to create an advance health care directive to accompany your power of attorney for personal care, which is simply a list of additional instructions that is incorporated into the power-of-attorney document.[d]
Nova Scotia	In Nova Scotia, for financial and legal matters, you make an enduring power of attorney and nominate an attorney. For personal and medical care, you make a personal directive and nominate an agent.[e]
Ontario	In Ontario, for financial and legal matters, you make a power of attorney for property and nominate an attorney for property. For personal and medical care, you make a power of attorney for personal care and nominate an attorney for personal care.[f]
Quebec	In Quebec, a power of attorney only applies to property, allowing your attorney to act on your behalf while you are still capable (e.g., if you are going on vacation and need someone to manage your financial affairs during your absence). A power of attorney for personal care is called a protection mandate, which comes into effect if you become mentally incapable.[g]
Saskatchewan	In Saskatchewan, for financial and legal matters, you make an enduring power of attorney and nominate an attorney. For personal and medical care, you make a health care directive.[h]

[a] Government of Alberta. Enduring powers of attorney [Internet]. Edmonton: Government of Alberta; 2023. Available from: https://www.alberta.ca/enduring-power-of-attorney.aspx.

[b] Government of British Columbia. What every older Canadian should know about powers of attorney for financial matters and joint bank accounts [Internet]. Vancouver: Government of British Columbia; n.d. Available from: https://www2.gov.bc.ca/assets/gov/people/seniors/financial-legal-matters/pdf/powersofattorney_bc_web_final.pdf#; Government of British Columbia. Incapacity planning [Internet]. Victoria: Government of British Columbia; 2023: Available from: https://www2.gov.bc.ca/gov/content/health/managing-your-health/incapacity-planning.

c Public Guardian and Trustee of Manitoba. Enduring power of attorney: a guidebook for donors and attorneys [Internet]. Winnipeg: Public Guardian and Trustee of Manitoba; 2014. Available from: https:/www.gov.mb.ca/publictrustee/pdf/power_of_attorney _guidebook.pdf.

d Financial and Consumer Services Commission. Understanding powers of attorney [Internet]. Fredricton: Government of New Brunswick; 2024. Available from: https:// www.fcnb.ca/sites/default/files/2024-12/understanding-the-power-of-attorney.pdf.

e Legal Info Nova Scotia. Power of attorney [Internet]. Tantallon: Legal Info Nova Scotia; 2017. Available from: https://www.legalinfo.org/wills-and-estates-law/power-of-attorney.

f Ministry of Attorney General. Powers of attorney [Internet]. Toronto: Queen's Printer; 2021. Available from: https:www.publications.gov.on.ca.

g Government of Quebec. Power of attorney contract [Internet]. Montreal: Government of Quebec; 2023. Available from: http://www.quebec.ca/finance-income-and-other-taxes /power-attorney-legal-protection/power-attorney/power-attorney-contract.

h Government of Saskatchewan. Powers of attorney for adults [Internet]. Regina: Government of Saskatchewan; 2023. Available from: https://www.saskatchewan .ca/residents/justice-crime-and-the-law/power-of-attorney-guardianship-and-trusts /powers-of-attorney-for-adults.

nomination, signing, and witnessing requirements. Therefore, a power-of-attorney document that is valid in one province is not always valid in other provinces, unless the province's legislation recognizes valid powers of attorney from other provinces.

VALIDATING POWER OF ATTORNEY FOR PROPERTY AT BANKS

Banks can create problems when it comes to activating a POAP. It is always a good idea for the grantor of a POAP to inform their bank of their decision and to provide a copy of the document to the bank soon after executing it. This way the bank can review the document and inform the grantor if there are any potential problems, thus allowing the grantor to correct the problem. Otherwise, the problem may not be identified until the grantor is incapable and unable to correct the problem.

RESOURCES

Ontario has numerous resources available that offer information and guidance on preparing wills and powers of attorney, for example,

- Steps to Justice (wills and powers of attorney): https://stepstojustice .ca/legal-topic/wills-and-powers-of-attorney/;
- Community Legal Education Ontario: https://www.cleo.on.ca/en /publications/power;

- Advocacy Centre for the Elderly (power of attorney for personal care): https://www.acelaw.ca/legal-topic/powers-of-attorney/; and
- Government of Ontario (making a power of attorney): https://www.ontario.ca/page/make-power-attorney.

Ontario has many services to assist people in the preparation of wills, such as some community legal aid clinics, Pro Bono Students Canada's Wills Project, Queen's University's Elder Law Clinic, The 519 (Toronto), and Justice Net.

Personal Care Decisions When No POAPC Is Granted

Many people do not name anyone as their attorney for personal care. In such cases, if the person is found to be incapable of consenting to medical treatment, most jurisdictions allow a doctor to turn to family members to seek consent. For example, in Ontario the *Health Care Consent Act, 1996* provides a hierarchy of relatives a doctor can turn to for consent.[13] First in line are spouses, followed by parents and children aged older than 16 years.

As long as a person trusts their spouse, children, or parents to consent to treatment on their behalf, there may be no need to create a POAPC. However, if a person does not want their family making such decisions for them, or if they prefer a family member who is lower down in the statutory hierarchy, they will need to formally grant a power of attorney to another person.

Property Decisions When No POAP Is Granted

If a person does not name anyone as their attorney for property, and they become incapable of managing their property, the public guardian and trustee (PGT) can step in to become statutory guardian for property.[14]

It is also possible for a relative to apply to take over a statutory guardianship from the PGT. In most jurisdictions, a relative can also apply to the court to be appointed guardian for property (see the "Court-Appointed Guardians" section).

PUBLIC GUARDIAN AND TRUSTEE

The PGT and court-appointed guardian perform the same function as attorneys, but they are selected and appointed by statute or court order, usually when the individual in question no longer has capacity.[15] In most cases, the PGT can step in to play the role of statutory guardian of property.[16] This means that the PGT controls the person's property and is responsible for paying the individual's rent and other bills to the extent possible given their resources. There is an Office of the Public Guardian in every province that carries out a similar role, although practice and procedure vary from province to province.[17]

The precise details of who can act as a SDM and under what circumstances can vary from province to province. British Columbia and Alberta, for example, offer a wider range of options in terms of supported or co-decision-making alternatives, and other provinces focus on substitute decision-making.[18]

COURT-APPOINTED GUARDIANS

In some instances, a person, usually a close relative, may have gone to court to be appointed as guardian of the person or guardian for property. In such cases, the court-appointed guardian would have the authority to make decisions in any areas covered by the court order.[19] Given the considerable cost associated with obtaining a court-ordered guardianship, they are not common among low-income populations.

Powers of Attorney and Substitute Decision-Making Case Scenarios

KAMALJIT: WHO CAN MAKE FINANCIAL DECISIONS FOR AN INCAPABLE PATIENT?

Issues to Canvass
- Role of the PGT
- Role of an attorney for property
- What is a valid power-of-attorney document?

Background: Your patient Kamaljit is very upset. He claims that he cannot get enough to eat because the PGT refuses to give him enough money. He insists that he has a lot more money than the PGT admits.

You are aware that Kamaljit is subject to a PGT guardianship. You know that Kamaljit has a gambling addiction and has an extensive history of using whatever money is provided to him to purchase lottery tickets. You are not surprised that he is not buying enough food. You are also doubtful that the PGT is hiding anything. Kamaljit, as far as you are aware, receives Ontario Disability Support Program (ODSP) benefits.

Kamaljit produces a paper. It states in large printed letters "I, Kamaljit Chada, appoint my friend Juhel Smith as my attorney for property." He has signed the paper.

When asked, Kamaljit explains that Juhel is someone he met while buying lottery tickets. He is sure Juhel will give him all the money the

PGT has been hiding from him. Kamaljit wants you to call the PGT to tell them to give his money to Juhel.

Question: Can Kamaljit grant a power of attorney to Juhel while he is subject to PGT property guardianship?
   Answer: No.
   Discussion: The PGT can only act as statutory guardian of property if Kamaljit was found incapable of managing his property in the past. A person can be incapable of managing their property but still be capable of appointing someone to manage their property for them. However, once the PGT becomes statutory guardian, they are not likely to renounce this role without some proof that their client is indeed capable of granting a POAP.

In this case there is reason to be concerned that Kamaljit does not really understand what an attorney for property is supposed to do. He appears to be selecting Juhel solely because Juhel will do what he wants. Kamaljit does not seem to appreciate the risk involved in giving Juhel control over his income.

The PGT would also require some assurance that the proposed attorney is able to act in the best interests of the incapable person. In this case it is doubtful the PGT would feel that Juhel would be a suitable SDM for Kamaljit.

Question: Is the document Kamaljit gave you a valid power of attorney?
   Answer: No.
   Discussion: There is no specific form or format for a valid power of attorney. However, in most provinces, a power of attorney must be signed before two witnesses. In this case, a handwritten note with no witness signatures is not a valid grant of decision-making power.

Question: Could Juhel become a guardian or SDM for Kamaljit?
   Answer: It is possible, but not likely.
   Discussion: Juhel could apply to become Kamaljit's statutory guardian of property in place of the PGT. He would have to prepare a detailed management plan outlining his specific plans for managing Kamljit's property. Although it is possible for family members to take over the role of guardian from the PGT, it is not likely that Juhel, as a non-relative, would be allowed to take over the guardianship, especially in circumstances in which Kamaljit seems to want Juhel to take over simply to access money to spend on lottery tickets.

Juhel could also apply to the Superior Court of Justice to be appointed guardian of property for Kamaljit. This process would require considerable legal fees. Juhel would also have to satisfy the court that he is a suitable guardian for Kamaljit, and, as part of his application, he would also have to provide a detailed property management plan. It does not appear likely that he would be able to do this.

ALI: WHEN IS A POWER OF ATTORNEY NEEDED, AND WHAT IS REQUIRED TO GRANT A POWER OF ATTORNEY?

Issues to Canvass
- Language, communication issues, and their impact on capacity and the ability to understand and appreciate
- Proper accommodation and limits of accommodation
- Obtaining proper instructions – power of attorney and consent to treatment.

Background: Ali is a refugee. He is 66 years old and has been in Canada for five years.

Ali does not understand English very well. He can understand only very basic phrases. His mother tongue is not a common language, and there are no professionals and very few individuals in the area who speak his language. All attempts to locate an interpreter have failed.

Ali lives with his nephew, Vardar, who can speak Ali's language, but only to a limited extent. Ali's sister, Vardar's mother, spoke Ali's language, but she died last year. Ali has no financial resources and relies on his nephew for support. He has not accessed any public social services. He has no income and no bank account.

Ali also has almost no contact with other people beyond his visits with his doctor. His doctor struggles to communicate with Ali and is increasingly worried that Ali's health issues will require some complex treatments. He is not sure how to explain the issues to Ali. He feels Vardar should make treatment decisions for Ali.

Ali's doctor admits that without a better means of communicating with Ali, it is not possible to determine with any certainty whether Ali is capable of making his own treatment decisions – specifically, whether he cannot understand information because of a language barrier or whether he lacks the mental or cognitive ability to understand regardless of the language used.

A hospital social worker suggested to Vardar that Ali should grant powers of attorney for both personal care and property to Vardar to allow him to communicate with doctors and other third parties on Ali's behalf. She wrote a note in English addressed "to whom it may concern," stating that Ali wanted to grant a power of attorney to Vardar.

Vardar brought Ali to a legal clinic and asked them to produce power-of-attorney documents for Ali.

It was clear to the clinic lawyer that Ali has only a limited understanding of what a power-of-attorney document authorizes. In English, Ali can express that he "wants POA" (holding and gesturing with the note from the social worker). He can also say, "Vardar – do all."

It is not clear whether Ali is asking for what he wants or whether he is simply doing what he has been told to do. The clinic lawyer fears that it is not possible to determine what Ali does or does not understand. For that reason, the clinic lawyer is not able to create a power-of-attorney document for Ali.

Question: What will happen to Ali if he cannot grant a POAPC? Will his medical treatment be affected?

Answer: It is not legally necessary for Ali to grant a power of attorney for treatment decisions to be made on his behalf should he be found treatment incapable.

The need for substitute consent in the event that Ali is found to be treatment incapable can be addressed by virtue of the statutory hierarchy of SDMs in Ontario's *Health Care Consent Act, 1996*. The hierarchy prioritizes guardians of the person and attorneys for personal care, but if neither of these exist, the hierarchy prioritizes family members. If a person is content to allow one of these relatives to consent to treatment on their behalf, then no further steps are necessary.

In this case, Ali's doctor can seek consent from Vardar pursuant to Ontario's *Health Care Consent Act, 1996*. In the absence of other relatives, Vardar would be the highest-ranked SDM in the statutory hierarchy.

If Ali does not want Vardar to make treatment decisions for him if he becomes incapable, then Ali would have to grant a power of attorney to someone else.

Furthermore, if Ali were able to grant a power of attorney to Vardar, this would provide Vardar with a broader scope of authority. Ontario's *Health Care Consent Act, 1996* grants SDMs the authority to make decisions in delineated areas only, specifically respecting treatment, personal assistance service, and admission to long-term care. In contrast, a POAPC provides authority to consent in all areas of personal care, including shelter, nutrition, and safety.

It does not appear that Vardar needs the authority of a POAPC to make treatment decisions for Ali if Ali is incapable of making his own treatment decisions.

Question: If Ali is unable to grant a POAP to his nephew, what happens?

Answer: Because Ali has no financial resources and Vardar supports him, it is not necessary for Vardar to make any decisions for the management of Ali's property. If Vardar were not supporting his uncle, Ali would be in far more vulnerable and isolated position financially.

Question: Is this a situation in which the PGT could help?

Answer: The PGT could step in to manage Ali's property if Ali were found incapable of doing so himself, but there is currently no need because Vardar is supporting Ali financially.

Question: If Ali cannot grant powers of attorney, could Vardar apply to become his uncle's court-appointed guardian?

Answer: Vardar could apply to become Ali's guardian for property and guardian of the person. However, this is a very costly process and would require Ali to undergo capacity assessments. Currently, Ali's medical care and property issues can be dealt with through other means, and it is not clear that he is incapable of making his own treatment or financial decisions.

Question: Who would pay the costs of a guardianship application?

Answer: Vardar would have to pay the full cost of guardianship applications, which would likely cost upwards of $10,000 in court and legal fees, so there is good reason to pursue other solutions.

MARGE: PREVENTING RELATIVES FROM MAKING TREATMENT DECISIONS

Issues to Canvass
- Capacity and mental health
- Diagnosis and capacity
- Choosing one's own decision-maker
- Obligations of attorney
- Prior capable wishes

Background: Marge, aged 56, has a variety of chronic health issues, including a mental health condition. Marge manages fairly well, but there have been times when she required hospitalization in a mental health facility for short periods.

Marge is intelligent and thoughtful. She is knowledgeable about treatments and has clear opinions on which medications she is willing to consent to and which she would never allow.

Some of the treatments and medications that Marge refuses to accept are among the treatments most often recommended by doctors for persons with her conditions. As her primary health care worker, you have recommended these treatments, and you have not had reason to question the presumption of her capacity.

Marge lives with her sister, Hilda, her only living relative. Although Hilda is generally supportive, she has made it clear that she disagrees with Marge's refusal to consent to certain medications, and if she had her way, Marge would be forced to take the medications her doctors recommend.

Marge wants to ensure that her sister does not become her SDM for treatment decisions in the event that Marge is found to be treatment incapable. She wants to ensure that her doctors will not give her medications she does not want in the event of her own treatment incapacity. Instead of her sister, she wants her friend Astral to be her SDM for treatment decisions. What can Marge do?

Question: Can Marge's doctor take instruction from a friend rather than a sister of a patient?
Answer: Maybe.

It is possible for a physician to seek consent for a treatment from an incapable patient's friend, but only if the friend has been appointed Marge's attorney for personal care pursuant to a valid POAPC. If Marge does not create a POAPC granting decision-making authority to a person of her choice, her doctor will be obliged to turn to a relative in the hierarchy of SDMs listed in legislation such as Ontario's *Health Care Consent Act, 1996*.[20] In Ontario, in the absence of a spouse, children aged older than 16, or parents, Marge's sister Hilda would be the highest-ranked relative in the statutory hierarchy. Again, it is important to note that this would only occur if Marge were deemed a treatment-incapable patient by a HCP.

Question: Is Hilda allowed to impose her wishes on Marge?
Answer: No.

Once a person has the authority to consent to treatment and make other medical decisions on behalf of another person, there is always a risk that they will make decisions based on their own views and wishes rather than those the incapable person would have made were they able. There are some protections against this.

As explained earlier, capable individuals may express wishes respecting personal care issues, such as treatment that will govern substitute decision-making in the event of future incapacity. "Prior capable wishes" may be expressed in a POAPC as an advance care directive, in any written form or orally.[21] All SDMs must make treatment decisions in keeping with any known prior capable wishes (e.g., a living will), even those that have been expressed orally.[22]

Given that Marge made her wishes about certain medications clear to her doctor and her sister, both would be bound to follow Marge's prior capable wishes, regardless of whether her sister agreed with them.

In Ontario, there is also a process before the Consent and Capacity Board that allows someone to challenge a SDM's authority to make decisions. In this case, Astral could apply to replace Marge as SDM on the basis that Hilda is ignoring Marge's prior capable wishes and consenting to treatments that Marge would never accept. This can, however, be a complex process (these applications are known as Form C applications to the Consent and Capacity Board).[23]

The best way for Marge to ensure that Hilda has no ability to influence or impact the medications she receives is to name Astral as her SDM of choice in a POAPC. As long as Marge remains capable with regard to medical and treatment decisions, she can detail her wishes about medications in her POAPC.

Even if her wishes were not recorded in a formal document, Marge could write out her instructions, but she would have to make sure to give copies to all relevant individuals (family, physician, friends, etc.). If Marge were to become unable to make medical decisions for herself, whether she created a POAPC document or not, whether her friend Astral or her sister became her SDM, both would be bound by her prior capable wishes.

Question: Does Marge's mental health condition mean she is not capable of granting a power of attorney?

Answer: No.

Capacity to grant a power of attorney is not determined by a person's diagnosis. Although in some cases a mental health condition can render a person incapable of making certain decisions for a certain period of time, one cannot assume incapacity simply because a person has a mental health diagnosis. Even if a condition periodically renders a person incapable for varying lengths of time, it does not mean that the person was incapable at the time they granted a power of attorney.

Capacity is both task and time specific. As long as the person was capable to perform the specific function at the time it was done, the fact that the person may have been incapable days before or became incapable shortly after executing a document will not affect the validity of the document. It is possible for a person to be incapable of managing their property but still capable to grant a POAP to allow someone else to manage their property for them.[24] The same is true for a POAPC.[25] For persons with fluctuating capacity, or for whom capacity is otherwise a concern, it would be prudent to have the POAPC created and executed with the assistance of a lawyer.

In Ontario, capacity to give a POAPC is present if the grantor (a) has the ability to understand that the proposed attorney has a genuine concern for the grantor's welfare and (b) appreciates that the grantor may need the attorney to make personal care decisions for them.[26] A POAPC can be revoked by the grantor at any time as long as the grantor is capable of giving the power of attorney.[27] Both the granting and the revocation of a POAPC must be in writing but need not be in any particular or prescribed form.[28] Forms are available online.[29] However, the POAPC will only be valid if (a) the grantor has capacity to give a POAPC, (b) a specific person or persons have been named as the attorney or attorneys, (c) it is signed and dated by the grantor, and (d) it has been witnessed by two persons.[30]

URSULA: IMPACT OF INCAPACITY

Issues to Canvass
- Impact of failure to plan for incapacity on family
- Impact of intestacy

Background: Ursula is 58 years old. She lives with her husband, Norbert. She and Norbert have no children. Both her parents and Norbert's parents are deceased. They both have siblings who live in Europe. Ursula has one adult daughter, Nadia (aged 34), from her first marriage to Nicolas. Nadia lives in Ontario. Three months ago, Norbert had a major stroke. He was left in a coma. He has been placed in a long-term care facility.

Norbert was very traditional. He controlled the finances. All property is in his name alone, and Ursula was dependent on him. She has not worked or had an income of her own since she married Norbert 25 years ago. She has no knowledge of what property Norbert has. He paid the bills each month and gave her a cash allowance to buy groceries.

Ursula has just been sent a notice that the rent has not been paid for three months. The landlord is threatening her with eviction. Ursula has no money at all. She has no way to access the funds in Norbert's bank account. Norbert's pension is being deposited into a bank account she cannot access. The bank refuses to release any funds to Ursula unless she can provide documentation, such as a POAP, showing that she has the authority to control Norbert's accounts.

Question: What will happen to Ursula?

Answer: In this situation, Norbert's primary health care worker, the bank, or Ursula herself should contact the PGT. The PGT can investigate and determine that a guardianship is required to manage Norbert's property for the good of his dependent spouse. The PGT will be able to deal with the landlord and resolve the unpaid rent issue. The PGT can also provide a weekly allowance to Ursula from Norbert's income to cover her daily living expenses.

Question: Could this have been avoided?

Answer: Yes.

Had Norbert granted a POAP to his wife, she would have been able to access and manage his property during his illness and incapacity. Had Norbert named Ursula as joint holder on his bank account, nothing further would have been required. Ursula would have been able to support herself and Norbert during his illness.

Wills and Estate Issues

What Is a Will, and Do I Need One?

In a narrow sense, wills and estate issues refer to plans and options related to transferring one's property after death, but they can implicate a wide range of questions, including who decides where property goes in the case of intestacy, what financial rights accrue to a spouse or common-law partner after one's death, and who decides what happens to the body of the deceased. These issues are canvassed here.

A will or, more formally, a last will and testament, is essentially a person's instructions to others as to what they want done with their property after they die. The concept of property includes the body of the deceased person. Many people assume that as long as they create a will leaving their property to their spouse or children, their family will have no problem accessing their funds. Unfortunately, this is not the case.

For the purposes of this discussion, there are two basic types of will:

1. *Formal will*: This type of will is usually typed and signed by the testator as well as two witnesses and is usually prepared by a lawyer or other legal professional. However, a will does not need to be typed. It will be valid even if handwritten as long as it is signed

and witnessed by two people. For those individuals who can afford to consult a lawyer, this is a sound way to record and enforce the person's wishes concerning the distribution of their property after death.

Many will templates are available for free online, encouraging people to create their own will without involving a lawyer. The problem with using these will templates, however, is that it is easy to make a mistake, such as having a beneficiary witness the document. Without anyone reviewing the document once it is prepared, the errors may not be detected until it is too late to correct them. Whether the errors will have a major impact on the estate depends, of course, on the type of error.

2. *Holographic will*: This type of will is entirely handwritten by the testator, dated, and signed at the bottom. There is no need for witnesses. Such wills are accepted in most Canadian jurisdictions but not all. British Columbia and Prince Edward Island do not accept wills that are handwritten and unwitnessed.[31]

There are some rules that must be followed.[32] Failure to properly prepare a holographic will can mean that it will be found to be invalid. However, the range of errors is more limited than with a homemade formal will.

A holographic will
- should state that the document is intended to be the last will and testament of the writer;
- should clearly identify the writer by name;
- should be dated;
- can have no typed parts; and
- should have every word in the handwriting of the testator; in addition,
- anything written below the signature will not be valid.

Holographic wills are often used in emergency situations in which a person may not live long enough or remain capable (or of sound mind) long enough to prepare a formal will. If the situation is urgent, a person can write out their holographic will on the spot. Holographic wills are not limited to emergency situations and can also be prepared as a replacement for, or instead of, a formal will.

A holographic will is usually short and intended to state the essential details. The more detail a person wants to include, the less appropriate a holographic will may be. A holographic will is most effective when the instructions as to the distribution of the person's property are clear and simple, for example, "I wish my property to be distributed to my wife" or "to my friend." If the instructions are more complex, it is best to prepare a formal will. It is useful to name an executor in the holographic will, but not essential.

If a holographic will is used, it is a good idea for the testator to provide a sample of their handwriting and signature to someone they trust. To probate a holographic will, it is necessary for someone to swear an affidavit stating that they recognize the person's signature and can confirm that the handwriting of the will is that of the deceased testator.

Whether the will is formal or holographic, it is still usually necessary for a named executor or anyone stepping in to act as executor (in the absence of one being named) to apply to the court to obtain a certificate of appointment of estate trustee to actually administer the estate. For another person to take control of or dictate what happens to a deceased person's estate, they will have to demonstrate that the deceased gave them that authority. This authority is usually granted in a will. A person named as executor of the will and trustee of the estate is assumed to have the authority to claim and distribute estate assets. However, a will alone is usually not sufficient to allow an executor to gain control of estate property. For more details on executors and estate trustees, see the "Executors and Estate Trustees" section.

In the Canadian legal system, a will, whether formal or holographic, cannot usually be used to transfer or distribute property until it has been probated. This means that the person intending to act as the executor or estate trustee (or manager) of the deceased's property (or estate) is obliged to file an application with the court to obtain a certificate; in Ontario, this is called a certificate of appointment as estate trustee (with or without a will).[33] Each province has its own estate or probate process, requirements, and fees.[34] However, the general process requires that the original will, along with documents such as proof of death and some form of application, be filed with the court or a court office. The court will review the application material and grant authority to the executor, allowing them to claim the assets of the estate and distribute them. The time required for this process also varies greatly not only from province to province but also from one region of a province to another. In most cases, until this certificate is granted, most property of the deceased cannot be accessed, real estate cannot be sold, and bank account funds cannot be distributed to beneficiaries. Obtaining a certificate costs money. In some cases in which the funds in a bank account are minimal, the cost of obtaining a certificate could amount to 50 per cent or more of the funds, imposing a major penalty on the family. In addition, in larger centres with busier courts, it can take several months to obtain a certificate. In the meantime, the family has to find a way to manage without the funds.

There was a time when most banks would, upon the production of a formal will naming an estate trustee or executor, release to the executor small sums (usually under $20,000) in a deceased's bank account without demanding a certificate. This could, in many cases, allow a low-income family to quickly access the funds they needed to survive. Increasingly, however, banks are demanding a certificate in all cases, even when the sums in an account are small and it is clear that the family has an urgent need to access them.

There are some concessions to small estates. In Ontario, for example, estates valued at less than $50,000 pay no estate administration tax. There is a special small estate certificate for estates valued at less than $150,000 that offers a more streamlined application process. Nevertheless, there are still costs associated with seeking probate, even for a small estate.[35]

Although it is not necessary that a lawyer complete the application forms, many people will hire lawyers to assist with this process because it is very time-consuming and can be challenging. If a person's assets in the bank or elsewhere amount to less than approximately $3,000, the process related to using a will to transfer those funds to a family member, friend, or charity could prove unduly complicated, and the costs involved could equal or surpass the funds being obtained. Also, an executor is entitled to a fee for the work involved in administering an estate. This can amount to between 3 per cent and 5 per cent of the total value of the estate. Although it is important to have an executor to manage the estate, an executor's fees could further reduce the portion of the estate actually available to distribute to beneficiaries.

WHEN NO EXECUTOR OR TRUSTEE IS NAMED

When no executor or estate trustee is either named in a will or appointed by the court, it will be very difficult to take any action with the property of the deceased.

A spouse may be able to claim funds from a bank account or take charge of the deceased's body, but a person, even a spouse, who has not been named executor in a will or appointed estate trustee by the court will usually not be able to take any action with the property or body of the deceased.

People often expect that if they have named a person as their attorney for property under a POAP, that person will be able to deal with their apartment and personal possessions after they die. This is not the case. An attorney for property only has the authority to deal with the property of the person who granted them the power while that person is alive. Once the grantor dies, the authority of the attorney ends. Therefore, an attorney for property would not have any authority to empty bank accounts, seize assets, or even enter the apartment of a deceased grantor or dispose of that person's possessions after the person's death.

In certain instances, the PGT may step in to probate an estate when no one else is available to act as executor. In some limited cases, the PGT may also take responsibility for disposing of a body, if the person was a client of the PGT and no family members come forward to claim it.

If a person dies without a will or there is no person who can be appointed pursuant to section 29 of Ontario's *Estates Act*,[36] then the court may, pursuant to the *Crown Administration of Estates Act*,[37] appoint the PGT to act as estate trustee.

PERSONAL POSSESSIONS

If the bulk of an individual's estate consists of personal possessions, they can instruct anyone they trust to carry out their wishes concerning those personal possessions. No special certificate or other authority is required to allow a person to disperse the property of a friend or relative.

The problem is that a person's decision to privately give informal permission to a friend or even a family member to take their possessions or empty their apartment may not be respected by others. There is no way for these people to defend or enforce their authority. An individual can provide the person with a written document to show to others, such as a landlord, to prove that they were asked to step in. A person can also provide a letter to their landlord indicating that they have asked someone to deal with their property if they die. Most landlords are anxious to have the apartment of a deceased person emptied and ready to re-rent, so they may not place too many hurdles in the way of anyone trying to help.

Unfortunately, the cost and time involved in using a will to transfer property means that wills are often not an effective tool for many low-income persons to use to protect their family's financial needs and interests after their death.

DEBTS

It is also useful to note that if a person's debts exceed the sums they leave behind at death, a will may serve no purpose other than setting up the estate and any person named as executor as targets for debt collectors.

ESTATES OF INDIGENOUS PERSONS

When an individual is Indigenous, and usually a resident of a reserve, the rules and processes for making a will, what constitutes a valid will, and who administers the estate are all controlled by the *Indian Act* rather than provincial legislation, such as the *Succession Law Reform Act* in Ontario. Estates of Indigenous persons on reserve are handled by the Federal Department of Crown-Indigenous Relations and Northern Affairs Canada. Reserve lands are also transferred according to different rules than non-reserve land. The Government of Canada offers estate services for First Nations.[38]

Alternatives to Wills

JOINT OWNERSHIP OF REAL ESTATE OR BANK ACCOUNTS

If a key bank account is solely in the name of someone who dies, the bank will usually freeze the account, meaning the funds in the account cannot be accessed or dispersed without bank approval.[39] If a number of people are dependent on the income of one family member, the best way to protect the financial well-being of the family in the event of the account holder's death or incapacity is to have another person as joint holder of the account.

Similarly, if real estate is in the sole name of the deceased, transferring the property may involve paying estate administration tax and other fees. If the property is held jointly, the survivor retains the property, and no estate or other fees must be paid.

With a joint account, upon the death of one owner, the funds become the property of the survivor or survivors. This means the funds in a jointly held account can still be accessed if one of the holders dies or becomes incapable.[40]

Although there are always risks involved in giving another person access to one's bank account, in most family situations the risks of having the family's entire income tied up in an account they cannot access are far greater.

NAMED BENEFICIARIES

Although it may not be an option for all, a life insurance policy or pension plan that pays a death benefit can be a useful tool to help family members and others access cash to cover the costs of burial and other expenses related to a death.

When a person is permitted to name a beneficiary on a financial product, such as a pension, RRSP, or life insurance policy, the named beneficiary will typically receive the funds in question within a few weeks of the institution or agency being notified of the death of the policy holder. This is often a far quicker process than the probate process. Furthermore, because the funds do not form part of the estate, there is no need to pay estate administration taxes.

Some individuals name their estate as their beneficiary. This is not a good idea. Naming the estate as a beneficiary of a life insurance policy will serve little purpose, because funds that go into the estate will be trapped in the estate until the certificate has been granted. Also, there may be estate administration tax payable on the funds if they go into the estate.

When a Will May Be Useful

Despite the problems of probate, a will may be necessary or useful under certain circumstances, namely,

- a common-law spouse is involved or
- a person wants to name non-relatives as beneficiaries.

INTESTACY: SHOULD IT BE AVOIDED?

Although a certificate of estate trustee is generally required to allow the sale of real estate in the name of a deceased person or to access funds in a solely held bank account, a will is not necessary to obtain a certificate. The process of obtaining a certificate when there is no will is not that different from the process used when there is a will.

For persons who are married or who have adult children and who wish these family members to benefit from their estate, it may not be necessary to create a will. If no will is created, there is an intestacy (property of the deceased with nowhere to go). In such situations, the distribution of the estate is dictated in Ontario by the *Succession Law Reform Act*.[41] A legal surviving spouse would be entitled to the entire estate (assuming the estate is worth less than $300,000). If there is no surviving spouse but adult children, the children would share in the estate equally.

One problem, however, is that similar to instances in which there is a will, someone has to apply to the court to obtain a certificate for an estate without a will. The costs and time involved are also similar.

The rules relating to intestacy can be complex, and they vary from province to province, especially with respect to the entitlements of common-law spouses.[42]

COMMON-LAW SPOUSES: HOW TO PROTECT THEM

In some provinces, such as Alberta, British Columbia, and Saskatchewan, a common-law spouse or domestic partner can inherit under an intestacy. In other provinces, notably Ontario, a common-law spouse cannot rely on the rules of intestacy to ensure that their partner benefits from their estate. To ensure a common-law spouse can access any part of an estate, their partner has to create a will naming them as their heir or, when possible, as joint owner of property.

FRIENDS RATHER THAN FAMILY

As with a common-law spouse, non-relatives cannot inherit under an intestacy. For persons who have no immediate family or who are estranged from their family and do not wish them to obtain any benefit from their estate, it is necessary to create a will. In an intestacy even distant relatives may inherit the patient's property rather than a close friend or common-law spouse.

CHARITABLE DONATIONS

If a person wishes to leave their estate to a charity rather than their family members, they need to create a will to state this; a charity cannot inherit in an intestacy.

Wills and Estates Scenarios

JAMIE

Issues to Canvass
- Joint accounts
- Named beneficiaries
- Powers of attorney
- Is a will necessary?

Background: Jamie, aged 53, is married with two teenage sons. He was injured at work several years ago and has been living on disability and pension benefits. Jamie has recently been diagnosed with an aggressive terminal condition. As part of a palliative approach to care, you tell him he should start to consider what he needs to do to ensure his family can manage financially in the event of his death.

Jamie reports that his wife, Susan, manages much of the household expenses and pays most of the bills. They share a joint chequing account and a joint savings account. Jamie has no other property beyond his personal possessions.

Jamie has named his wife as the beneficiary of a small work-related pension he is entitled to, and he has also named her the beneficiary of a life insurance policy. Jamie is very concerned that he has no will.

Question: Is it urgent that Jamie make a will?
   Answer: No.

Although a will may be helpful, in this case should Jamie die without a will, his wife and children will be protected and able to access the funds they require to support themselves.

Discussion: On a practical level, Jamie has ensured that his wife Susan will have access to funds to pay the bills when he dies.

- As joint holder of their bank account, Susan would automatically become the owner of the joint property upon Jamie's death. At the very least, this will give her access to funds in the immediate aftermath of Jamie's death, allowing her time to reorganize the family's finances.
- Jamie has also ensured that some money will come to Susan soon after his death via his life insurance policy and pension funds. This will allow Susan to pay bills related to Jamie's death and burial without undue hardship.

Both of these options get funds into Susan's hands far more quickly than if she obtains a certificate through the probate process (either with or without a will).

Question: What happens if Jamie dies without a will?

   Answer: Whether Jamie creates a will leaving his estate to his wife or he dies intestate (without a will), Susan would still inherit Jamie's estate, because in the case of an intestacy in Ontario, Susan, as surviving spouse, would be entitled to the first $300,000 of his estate. The problem is that, with or without a will, the process to obtain a certificate can be slow and costly; at times it can take several months to get any money into the hands of a surviving spouse or children.

Question: Can Jamie create a holographic will?

   Answer: Yes (but not in every province).

If Jamie's instructions for his estate are simply that he wishes his wife Susan to receive his entire estate, he can create a handwritten (or holographic) will as long as he is careful to ensure that his holographic will is entirely in his own handwriting and is signed and dated. A more formal will signed before witnesses may not be required. Holographic wills are accepted in most provinces, but not British Columbia or Prince Edward Island.

Question: Would Jamie's estate still require probate?

Answer: Yes.

Whether a will is formal or holographic, it is still necessary to pursue the probate process to obtain legal authority to claim estate assets. The process is not usually much different whether the will is formal or holographic.

When limited assets are involved and the desire is to ensure that a spouse or children inherit the estate, creating a will does not necessarily create any advantages as far as the time or effort required to administer the estate.

A will that names an executor can make it clear who should make decisions about the body. However, in the absence of a will stating otherwise, most will accept instruction from a surviving spouse concerning issues such as cremation or burial.

Question: What if Jamie becomes incapable of making decisions before he dies?

Answer: In this situation, Jamie has already ensured that Susan can access their bank accounts and keep the family going during any incapacity on his part. Because Susan is already joint owner of the bank accounts, the bank should not require Susan to produce any power-of-attorney document to allow her to access her own accounts.

Should Jamie become incapable of making treatment decisions, Ontario's *Health Care Consent Act, 1996* allows a HCP to turn to his spouse to obtain consent. A POAPC is not required in such cases.

JAI

Issues to Canvass
- Intestacy
- Non-relatives as beneficiaries
- Probate issues and costs
- Bank issues
- Risks and benefits of joint assets
- Holographic wills

Background: Your patient Jai, aged 72, is not eating. You discover that she is grieving. Her friend of some 50 years, Alice, has died.

You remember Jai mentioning Alice during her last visit when she was asking how to help Alice access some home care services. You sense that Alice and Jai were a couple, but Jai does not seem comfortable acknowledging that. It is clear, however, that Jai depended upon Alice a great deal.

Jai mentions that her savings are gone. She helped pay for some of the services Alice required while she was terminally ill. She trusted she would be reimbursed because Alice had always told her that any money she left behind would be hers. Jai also notes that since Alice's death she can no longer rely on Alice helping her out with grocery money. Jai seems to be struggling to feed herself.

Jai reports that she went to the bank, the same bank that she and Alice went to together for years, to tell them that Alice had died. She knew that Alice had about $40,000 in her account with the bank. Jai then asked when she could get access to the money in Alice's account because she had no other way to pay for a small memorial service for Alice. She adds she was too embarrassed to tell the bank she needed the money to buy food. The bank told Jai that they could not give her the money without seeing Alice's will or some other evidence that Jai was entitled to the funds.

Jai is sure Alice never made a will. Alice always said she had one bank account, and the people at the bank were well aware of her wish that Jai get it all after she died.

Jai wants you to intervene and tell the bank to give her the money Alice wanted her to have. She cannot understand why the people at the bank who knew both of them well are now treating her like she is some stranger trying to steal money.

Question: Is there a way for Jai to get access to the funds in Alice's bank account?

Answer: No, the bank will not release funds to Jai.

Discussion: In situations in which no will has been created, there is an intestacy. In most provinces, there is legislation that details who benefits from an estate in the case of intestacies.

Most intestacy processes privilege immediate family. Surviving legal (or formally married) spouses and children of the deceased share the estate. Only if no immediate family exists will parents, siblings, or cousins share the estate. Under an intestacy, unrelated friends and, in many jurisdictions, even common-law spouses, have no right to a share of the estate.

To ensure that unrelated persons can benefit from an estate, a person must create a will of some form. In a will, a person may leave their property to a friend, a charity, or even a stranger. For persons with no family or those who are estranged from their relatives, a will may be the only way to ensure that their estate benefits someone of their choice.

Question: What if Jai were to obtain a certificate of appointment as estate trustee without a will from the court. Would the bank release the funds to her?

Answer: Yes.

If Jai produced a certificate granted by the court, the bank would release the funds in Alice's account. However, the funds would be placed in an estate account that Jai could administer as estate trustee. The problem is that even as estate trustee, Jai could not give the funds to herself as Alice may have wished. Jai would instead be bound to distribute the estate according to the intestacy rules, which means she would have to locate any relatives of Alice and distribute the funds to them. If, after sufficient effort has been made to locate relatives, it becomes clear that it is not possible, Jai may then be able to apply to the court for permission to release the funds to herself. The challenge is that the entire process of obtaining the certificate, following the process to identify relatives, and finally obtaining permission from the court to do what Alice always wanted done could take months, if not years, and the cost of these processes could amount to a large portion of the value of the estate funds (or even exceed them).

In the meantime, none of this would be of any assistance to Jai in meeting her immediate need for funds to purchase food.

Question: Would it matter if Alice was receiving some form of provincial social assistance, such as ODSP benefits and Jai was her ODSP trustee, also called a representative?

Answer: No.

If Alice was a recipient of provincial social assistance, such as Ontario's ODSP benefits, a plan specific to persons with disabilities, that provincial program may assist with the cost of Alice's burial, but it is not likely that much more could be done to help Jai beyond referring her to relevant social services.

Some programs, such as ODSP, will appoint a relative or other person as an ODSP trustee or representative, particularly when the recipient may have a cognitive or mental health disability, which essentially allows the person to act in a role similar to that of an attorney for property, receiving the person's benefits and ensuring the funds are used for the benefit of the ODSP recipient. The appointment is generally only recognized by ODSP and only in relation to the receipt of ODSP benefits. Therefore, it is doubtful that either the bank or the court would accept Jai's status as ODSP representative as sufficient to allow her to inherit from Alice. Even if, as ODSP representative, Jai had access to Alice's bank account while Alice was alive, this access would end with Alice's death.

Question: Would it matter if, during her last illness, Alice's personal support worker was willing to swear an affidavit that Alice told her she wanted Jai to get her money?

Answer: No.

The affidavit on its own would not be sufficient. It may be sufficient to guide an executor if there was a will; however, even if someone were to apply to be appointed as estate trustee, as long as there is no will, that executor would still be obliged to distribute the estate according to the provisions of Ontario's *Succession Law Reform Act*. It is doubtful the sworn affadavit would override the provisions of the act. Although this situation could be resolved with a court order, the cost of obtaining such an order would likely exceed the value of the estate.

Question: Would it matter if Alice left a handwritten note stating, "I want my friend Jai to have all my money and other stuff when I die" (signed "A")?

Answer: Yes.

It is possible that such a document would be accepted as a holographic will. Jai could seek appointment as estate trustee with a will, allowing her to obtain the funds from the bank and distribute the funds to herself. The will would have to be verified, which would involve finding someone other than Jai to attest to the authenticity of Alice's handwriting and signature, as well as attesting that "A" was one of the ways that Alice signed her name. In this situation, an affidavit from Alice's personal support worker might be useful in confirming that the handwritten will reflects Alice's wishes.

Question: If Jai does not get the funds in Alice's bank account, what happens to that money?

Answer: Given that it is unlikely that anyone else would apply to administer Alice's estate, the funds may sit in the account for some time. They will eventually be transferred to a federal system that manages unclaimed funds from bank accounts.[43]

The funds will, unfortunately, be of no use to Jai.

Question: What could Alice have done to ensure her wishes concerning her bank account were realized?

Answer:

- *Joint bank accounts*: One way Alice could have ensured that Jai inherited her bank account funds would have been to make Jai a joint holder on the account. If Jai was providing care for Alice, this might have made it easier for Jai to make purchases for Alice while she was alive, and it would have meant that the bank funds would automatically have become Jai's property upon Alice's death with no need to obtain a certificate. Given the long-term relationship and clear level of trust between Jai and Alice, this option may have presented clear benefits to both with very limited risk to Alice.

  Alice's idea of creating a handwritten will was laudable. If she had sought help to ensure that her will met all of the guidelines without ambiguity, it would have been easier for Jai to use the will. However, it is likely that no bank would transfer funds to Jai based on the holographic will alone, even if it was perfectly executed. Jai would most likely still be forced to seek an appointment as estate trustee to get the funds out of the bank.

- *Named beneficiaries*: If Alice had a life insurance policy, RRSP, or a pension, she might have been able to name Jai as her beneficiary. Most of these financial instruments allow you to name the person of your choice, not necessarily a family member, as a beneficiary. If this is done, the beneficiary should receive whatever funds are involved within a few weeks of the institution holding the funds being notified of the holder's death. There is no need to probate a will or fight with a bank to obtain access to the funds.

Question: What types of social services could have helped?

Answer: In this case, if Alice and Jai had had access to legal advice early on in Alice's illness, Alice may have been able to take some simple steps to ensure that her wishes concerning her bank account were honoured without forcing Jai to go to any great level of trouble to claim the funds upon her death. A short conversation of 15–20 minutes with a lawyer may have been sufficient to allow Alice to make her gift to Jai effective.

Given that Jai and Alice were long-time clients, it seems the bank could have done more to inquire about their clients' needs and level of estate planning. The bank could have asked about Alice's wishes for her estate and offered her some options to ensure her wishes were met rather than simply waiting until Alice died to tell Jai what should have been done.

A social worker may still be able to assist. Jai may be able to claim Alice's federal government death benefits, as her long-time common-law spouse. Common-law spouses are able to receive survivor benefits as well as death benefit.[44]

ALEXIS

Issues to Canvass
- Holographic wills
- Probating a holographic will
- Who can seek probate?
- Is probate is necessary, what is required, what is the cost, and who pays?
- Can property be transferred to a social service agency without probate?

Background: Your patient Alexis, aged 29, lives in a shelter. He receives ODSP benefits. You are treating him for a life-threatening hereditary condition.

Alexis recently inherited $25,000 from his mother who died from the same condition he has. He left the funds in his bank account but notes that ODSP has been insisting that he needs to do something with the money or his monthly benefits will be reduced. His ODSP worker suggested he give the money to his father to manage for him.

Alexis tells you he was very upset by this suggestion because his father, Dimitri, was abusive to both Alexis and his mother. Alexis knows his father lives in Ottawa with his second wife, but he has not had contact with him in many years.

When he mentioned this to a friend, the friend told him that if he died without a will, his father, as his only relative, would likely inherit everything he had just received from his mother. Alexis is certain his mother would never have wanted Dimitri to get her money.

Alexis shows you a piece of paper pulled from a notebook where he has written down the following:

> *I, Alexis Orlov, want this to be my will. I wish whatever money I have when I die to be given to ACME Social Services because they helped me. I do not want my father to inherit even one penny from me.*

He has dated it and signed the bottom of the sheet. After showing you the paper, Alexis stuffs it into his pocket.

Months later Alexis is brought to the hospital in distress. He dies soon after.

The document you saw last time he was in your office was found in his pocket, crumpled, torn, and smudged with what could be blood or food stains, but still readable.

Question: Will the beneficiary Alexis named in his handwritten will benefit from his estate?

Answer: Yes (probably).

Discussion: Alexis's handwritten document would most likely be found to be a valid holographic will in provinces where such wills are recognized. It should be possible to probate the will as long as there is evidence that Alexis was capable at the time that he wrote it. Since Alexis did not name an executor or trustee, it is unlikely that a bank or other institution holding any of his assets would release them without a certificate from the court.

Someone will have to step forward to apply to be appointed as executor of Alexis's estate. Once they obtain a certificate they could claim Alexis's assets, reimburse expenses paid to obtain the certificate, and then distribute the remaining funds to the ACME Social Service agency as Alexis wished.

The challenge will be to find a person willing to undertake the process to obtain a certificate. ACME Social Services would have an interest in locating a person to act as executor simply to receive the gift Alexis made to them.

If Alexis was subject to the guardianship of the PGT, the PGT could release funds on the basis of the holographic will alone, but this would be discretionary.

Question: If Alexis had not created a will, would ACME Social Services still receive his estate?

Answer: No.

Discussion: If Alexis had not created his holographic will, there would have been an intestacy. His estate would have been distributed according to the provincial intestacy laws, which usually dictate that immediate family, such as spouses, children, parents, or siblings, benefit from the estate. Non-relatives, friends, and charities usually have no rights under an intestacy. In this case, Dimitri might very well have inherited everything Alexis received from his mother.

For persons who wish to leave their property to people other than their immediate family members, such as friends or charities, a will is necessary.

Executors and Estate Trustees: Who Gets Things Done

Whether a person creates a formal will naming an executor or trustee,[45] leaves a holographic will or dies intestate, someone has to step in to administer the estate. An executor or trustee also has legal authority over the body of the deceased and therefore decides how the remains will be dealt with.

The position of executor or trustee is one of some importance. Many persons with little experience with court processes and legal matters may feel intimidated and may not want to take on this role.

Some individuals who wish to create a will are unable to do so simply because they cannot find anyone to name as executor or trustee. Some people may not want to burden their spouse or children with this process. Others simply have no suitable social contacts they trust or wish to impose upon in such a way.

If a person is already subject to the financial guardianship of the PGT, the PGT may assist with processing the estate, but in other cases in which there is no money to hire a lawyer to assist, the probate process may become a major barrier to ensuring that a person's property is actually disbursed appropriately and in a timely fashion.[46]

Marginalized and isolated people often do not have anyone they can ask to take on the role of estate trustee. Without such a person to rely on to carry out the wishes and instructions of the deceased person, it becomes very difficult to ensure those wishes will be respected.

As explained earlier, an estate trustee or executor is entitled to have their expenses reimbursed, and they can claim a small fee as payment for their efforts. Unfortunately, with a smaller estate, the executor's fees will be small, and there is no guarantee that there will be sufficient funds in the estate to cover all costs. In short, there are financial risks involved in being the executor of a small estate. This further reduces the number of people willing to take on this role.

If a person has no one to name as the attorney for property or personal care, there are alternatives. The PGT can step in to manage property, and legislation such as Ontario's *Health Care Consent Act, 1996* provides a list of potential SDMs for treatment decisions. In contrast, there is no alternative public process that offers executors or estate trustee services. Although in rare instances the PGT may step in to process an estate, this is not a service most can rely on.

Protecting Documents

Creating a will or power-of-attorney document is the first step. Unfortunately, this step alone will not accomplish much if the original signed documents cannot be found when they are needed.

Wills and power-of-attorney documents may not actually be required for many years. The challenge is to ensure that documents created today can be kept safe and made available to the persons who needs them five, 10, or 20 years in the future.

To activate a power of attorney or to obtain authority to deal with an estate, it is necessary to provide the original signed document, either a power-of-attorney document or a will, to a doctor, bank, or estate court. Even if a photocopy of the document is available, if the original signed document cannot be found, a bank, doctor, or estate court may not agree to take instruction from or recognize the authority of the attorney or executor named in the document.

For persons with more stable housing and social networks, documents can be placed in a safe place in the family home, and at least one other family member or friend can be made aware of that location and given whatever key or passcode may be required to access the documents. Documents can be stored in a safe deposit box at a bank, and in some cases a lawyer may keep the documents for their clients.

Short of some public service that allows people to store documents, most people with no stable housing will have a difficult time keeping documents safe and, furthermore, available to those named as attorney or executor or trustee.

One option may be to leave original documents with the person named as executor or attorney. If a person has been trusted enough to be named to one of these roles, they should also be trustworthy enough to store and protect valuable documents. Of course, for this option to work, the executor or attorney also has to have some degree of stable housing and long-term security.

The key risk with this option is that if the executor or attorney becomes too ill to function or dies, any documents they were keeping on behalf of another person may get lost. Even if the people dealing with the executor's or attorney's property find the documents, they may not know where to find the person who created them to give the documents back. The longer the documents are stored, the greater the chances that they will not be found when needed.

Disposal of the Body

Next to concerns about what happens to their property, the priority for most people faced with the prospect of death is what will be done with their body.

If a person has a will and has named an executor, the executor has the legal authority to decide what happens to the body of the deceased.[47] It is possible for a patient to provide oral or written instructions to their named executor or trustee as to their wishes. If no one steps forward as executor or trustee, it is less clear what happens to a body. If there are family members to claim the body, they are normally allowed to decide what is to be done.

Banks will at times agree to pay for funeral costs, burial costs, or both from the account of the deceased. This requires that the deceased had sufficient resources in the bank. In many cases, a lack of resources will prevent or limit an executor's or family member's ability to carry out all of the deceased's wishes concerning burial or funeral arrangements.

There are some programs to help cover the cost of burial for members of certain groups, such as veterans or Indigenous persons. For persons with some work history in Canada, the Canada Pension Plan provides a death benefit that is intended to help cover the cost of burial.[48] Someone would have to apply for this benefit on behalf of the deceased person. Public funding for burial is also available at the municipal or provincial level, although eligibility and the level of service provided vary from location to location. Most major centres also have social service agencies that can assist with burial processes for those who are indigent.

If a person dies in a shelter or while receiving social services, the social service agency involved may be able to arrange for the disposal of a person's body; some even strive to observe any special religious obligations or wishes of the deceased to the extent possible. However, in most cases all a social service agency can arrange is a basic burial in a plot paid for by the municipality or cremation. People who die while in receipt of provincial social assistance may also have access to public burial or cremation services.[49] Municipalities will also cover the costs of burial or cremation for persons whose bodies remain unclaimed.[50] Some cemeteries offer burial or cremation services for the indigent.[51]

There are other options as well:

- *Pre-paid funeral*: A person can pre-pay for a funeral. These plans are often expensive, and in some cases it may be difficult to ensure that the services paid for are actually provided.[52]
- *Donation of body to science*: While alive, a person can express their wish to donate their body to science.[53] For instance, in Ontario, the *Trillium Gift of Life Act*[54] outlines that a person can provide consent to donate their body by (a) filling out a consent form (Donation of Body to School of Anatomy) available from any school of anatomy; (b) in writing, as per section 4(1) of the act; or (c) orally, in the presence of at least two witnesses before death. If consent has not been given before death, next of kin may give consent after death, as per

section 5 of the act. A key issue is that a person must ensure that someone is aware of their desire to gift their body. The donation must be made soon after death for the body to be viable for research.

Executors and Estate Trustees Scenarios

GILBERT: ESTATES

Issues to Canvass
- Importance of updating documents
- Benefits and risks of naming an organization or person you do not know well as estate trustee
- Disposal of body: what is possible and how to implement wishes
- Obligations of estate trustees
- What happens in cases in which there is no estate trustee or anyone to claim a body or possessions?

Background: Gilbert was an elderly man who had immigrated to Canada in his youth. He was married but did not have children. His wife died a few years ago.

Gilbert always supported himself but entered retirement with a minimal income and no savings. He was able to obtain geared-to-income housing.

In 2008, when he turned 85, Gilbert signed forms to confirm that he wanted his body gifted to the University of Toronto for medical research. It was very important to him that he make some contribution to medicine and research; he felt his body was the only thing he had to offer.

In 2010, Gilbert created a will that also noted his wishes concerning the disposition of his body. He named his friend Jack as his executor. He did not name an alternate because he did not know anyone else that he trusted enough for this role. Gilbert also granted a POAP and a POAPC to Jack. Neither was ever activated because Gilbert remained alert and capable throughout his lifetime.

Jack suffered a stroke in 2019. He is alive but lives in a long-term-care facility. He is not capable of performing any functions, including acting as an estate trustee.

Gilbert intended to create new documents, but by 2019 he was largely housebound because of his age and infirmity. His social circle was small, and he could not identify anyone to take on the role for him. The COVID-19 pandemic left him further isolated.

Gilbert died in 2021, aged 97. He was destitute. His last rent cheque emptied his bank account.

Question: Who takes control of Gilbert's body?

Answer: In the absence of anyone stepping forward to claim a body, the coroner will take custody of it. With no family member stepping forward to make decisions and no executor who can take control, Gilbert will be buried by the municipality.

Question: Who ensures that Gilbert's body is donated to science as he wished?

Answer: Unfortunately, unless the university is notified quickly that there is a body to be donated, Gilbert's good intentions to donate his body to science may not be realized. Unless the transfer of the body happens within days of death, it may not be viable for scientific research.

Question: Who covers the cost of burial?

Answer: If the body was donated to science, the university will dispose of Gilbert's remains once their research is complete. Otherwise, the municipality will pay.

Question: What happens to Gilbert's possessions?

Answer: Without anyone to claim or dispose of Gilbert's possessions, the landlord will most likely have to empty the apartment and will either donate the contents to charity or simply have them thrown away.

Alternatives

Question: Would anything change if Gilbert left a note behind stating that he wanted his body donated to science and that any money he had left was to be given to the organization Senior Care that sent him a hot lunch once a week? The note was written on a typewriter since Gilbert's hands were too stiff to allow him to write with a pen. Gilbert signed the note.

Answer: No.

Discussion: A typed note does not meet the requirements for a holographic will. A more formal will has to be witnessed by two witnesses. Although it may be possible to have this note declared the equivalent of a holographic will by a court, the costs of doing so would most likely be prohibitive.

Question: Would anything change if Gilbert had named an alternate estate trustee in his will?

Answer: Yes.

Discussion: Had Gilbert named an alternative executor in his will, the alternate could come forward and act as executor and arrange for Gilbert's body to be donated expeditiously to the university.

Question: What if Gilbert had named a not-for-profit social service agency as an alternate trustee for his estate? When speaking to this agency, the executive director agreed that if Gilbert left his estate to them, they would act as estate trustee, empty his apartment, dispose of his belongings, and ensure his body went to the university.

Answer: Maybe.

Discussion: This might work, but not-for-profit social service agencies (e.g., the Salvation Army or United Way) can change their policies. Although one executive director may agree to act as estate trustee for people willing to donate their estate to the agency, a new executive director may refuse to honour such an agreement.

The sad truth is that unless the estate is large enough to provide some clear benefit to the organization, it is a rarely worth the cost to the organization to take on the role of estate trustee in return for a small inheritance or a room full of old furniture and clothes.

Possible solutions: Gilbert could have seen his wishes realized if he had had access to legal advice. A legal professional could have suggested ways for Gilbert to better protect himself.

However, the key problem for Gilbert was that he lacked anyone to turn to once his friend Jack became incapable of acting as his estate trustee because of his stroke. If there was an organization that could provide attorneys and executors to low-income people for free or for a low cost, numerous individuals would be better able to plan for incapacity or death.

People with no family or friends to rely on, to name as attorneys, trustees, or executors, cannot create plans for their future because all forms of planning involve naming an individual they trust and can rely on to carry out their wishes. Without someone to rely on, a person cannot create a will or grant powers of attorney.

The PGT can step in to manage a person's property if they become unable to do so and are unable to name anyone themselves to take on the job. The PGT, however, is less likely to step in to act as estate trustee for a small estate. Unless the estate is large enough to justify the costs of administration, the PGT is unlikely to act unless special circumstances compel it.

If a social service agency was able to supply persons able to act as executors or estate trustees as well as attorneys, far more people would be able to create a will knowing that someone would take responsibility for administering their estate and honouring their wishes.

Providing this service to people would resolve numerous problems faced by socially isolated and marginalized people when trying to plan for their end of life and have a say in what happens to their property and their body after death.[55]

MILDRED

Issues to Canvass
- Importance of protecting documents
- Impact of lost documents
- Importance of executor and trustee

Background: Mildred, aged 54, has died after a long illness. She told you months ago that she had taken care of everything; specifically, that she made a will and had pre-paid for a funeral. Mildred asked you to call her executor Rita to inform her of her death to ensure that Rita will approach the funeral home to carry out her plans. Mildred assured you that Rita knew what to do, and she had all the documents she needed to take care of everything for Mildred.

After several attempts to reach Rita, you become concerned that Rita is no longer available. You do not know where Mildred pre-paid for the funeral home services. There is some urgency to determine what is to be done with Mildred's body.

Question: Will Mildred be buried according to her wishes?
Answer: No.
Discussion: If no one claims Mildred's remains, nobody can locate any evidence that Mildred had a pre-paid funeral, and there is no evidence that Mildred left any instructions about her burial, she will be buried by the municipality in a public plot.

Question: What will happen to Mildred's property?
Answer: The PGT was Mildred's statutory guardian for property. The PGT had asked several times for a copy of Mildred's will and a copy of the pre-paid funeral plan. She refused to provide either. The PGT was also told that Rita had everything, but they were never able to locate Rita. There is a very small amount in Mildred's account with the PGT.

Because no relatives can be located, the funds may languish unclaimed for some time.

Question: What could have been done to help Mildred?

Answer: Had Mildred given copies of her will and the pre-paid funeral agreement to the PGT as requested, the PGT may have been able to enforce the agreement to ensure her funeral occurred as per her wishes. At the very least, the documents would have allowed the PGT to understand what Mildred's wishes were. Without the documents, no one had any clear idea of what Mildred had paid for and what she wanted.

NOTES

1 Government of British Columbia. What every older Canadian should know about powers of attorney (for financial matters and property) and joint bank accounts [Internet]. Victoria: Government of British Columbia; n.d. Available from: https://www2.gov.bc.ca/assets/gov/people/seniors/financial-legal-matters/pdf/powersofattorney_bc_web_final.pdf#.
2 *Health Care Consent*, 1996, SO 1996, c 2, sched A.
3 *Substitutes Decisions Act*, 1992, SO 1992, c 30.
4 See, for example, section 4(1) of the *Health Care Consent Act, 1996*, SO 1996, c 2, sched A, and sections 6 and 45 or the *Substitute Decisions Act, 1992*, SO 1992, c 30.
5 See, for example, section15(1) of the *Health Care Consent Act, 1996*, SO 1996, c 2, sched A.
6 See, for example, section 15(1) of the *Health Care Consent Act, 1996*, SO 1996, c 2, sched A.
7 *Starson v. Swayze*, 2003 SCC 32 (CanLII), at para. 76.
8 *Starson v. Swayze*, 2003 SCC 32 (CanLII), at para. 77; see also section 4(2) of the *Health Care Consent Act, 1996*, SO 1996, c 2, sched A.
9 Government of Ontario, Office of the Public Guardian and Trustee. The Capacity Assessment Office: questions and answers [Internet]. Toronto: Queen's Printer for Ontario; 2020. Available from: https://www.publications.gov.on.ca/store/20170501121/Free_Download_Files/300631.pdf. For another example, see Government of Alberta. About capacity assessments [Internet]. Edmonton: King's Printer for Alberta; 2023. Available from: https://www.alberta.ca/capacity-assessment.
10 See, for example, section 16 of the *Substitute Decisions Act, 1992*, SO 1992, c 30, and sections 20 and 32 *Health Care Consent Act, 1996*, SO 1996, c 2, sched A.

11 See Advance Care Planning Ontario. A clinician's guide to substitute decision making [Internet]. Toronto: Advance Care Planning Ontario; 2022. https://www.pcdm.ca/acp/clinicians-guide-for-substitute-decision -making.

12 *Substitute Decisions Act, 1992*, SO 1992, c 30, s 66(3).

13 See *Health Care Consent Act, 1996*, SO 1996, c 2, sched A, s 20.

14 See, for example, in Ontario, *Mental Health Act*, RSO 1990, c M.7, ss. 54–60 and *Substitute Decisions Act, 1992*, SO 1992, c 30, ss 15–21.

15 Ministry of Attorney General. Guardianship: learn about different types of guardianship available for mentally incapable adults [Internet]. Toronto: King's Printer; 2023. Available from: https://www.ontario.ca/page /guardianship.

16 Office of the Public Guardian and Trustee. The role of the public guardian and trustee [Internet]. Toronto: Queen's Printer; 2020. Available from: https://www.publications.gov.on.ca/store/20170501121/Free_Download _Files/300613.pdf.

17 See Chetner SL. Role of government substitute decision-makers: public guardians and public trustees [Internet]. Toronto: Office of the Public Guardian and Trustee; 2013; Available from: http://www.cba.org/CBA /cle/PDF/ELD13_slides_Chetner.pdf.

18 For example, see Government of Manitoba. Information for substitute decision makers: supported decision making vs. substitute decision making [Internet]. Winnipeg: King's Printer for Manitoba; n.d. Available from: https://www.gov.mb.ca/legal/copyright.html.

19 Office of the Public Guardian and Trustee. Guardianship: learn about different types of guardianship for mentally incapable adults [Internet]. Toronto: King's Printer for Ontario; 2023. Available from: https://www .ontario.ca/page/guardianship.

20 See *Health Care Consent Act, 1996*, SO 1996, c 2, sched A, s 20.

21 See, for example, *Health Care Consent Act, 1996*, SO 1996, c 2, sched A, s 5.

22 See, for example, *Health Care Consent Act, 1996*, SO 1996, c 2, sched A, s 5, and *Substitute Decisions Act, 1992*, SO 1992, c 30, s 66(3).

23 For example, see *Health Care Consent Act, 1996*, SO 1996, c 2, sched A, s 33(2), and Consent and Capacity Board. Applying to the board to be appointed a representative to make decisions with respect to treatment admission to a care facility and/or personal care service [Internet]. Toronto: King's Printer for Ontario; 2023. Available from: http://www .ccboard.on.ca/scripts/english/publications/formchtml.asp.

24 In Ontario, see *Substitute Decisions Act, 1992*, SO 1992, c 30, s 8.

25 In Ontario, see *Substitute Decisions Act, 1992*, SO 1992, c 30, s 47.

26 In Ontario, see *Substitute Decisions Act, 1992*, SO 1992, c 30, s 47.

27 *Substitute Decisions Act, 1992*, SO 1992, c 30, s 47(3).

28 *Substitute Decisions Act, 1992*, SO 1992, c 30, s 47(4).

29 Ministry of the Attorney General. Powers of attorney: continuing power of attorney for property and powers of attorney for personal care [Internet]. Toronto: Publications Ontario; 2021. Available from: https://www .publications.gov.on.ca/store/20170501121/Free_Download_Files/300975 .pdf.

30 *Substitute Decisions Act, 1992* SO 1992, c 30, ss 47, 48.

31 Rollenhagen L. Can you create a holographic will in British Columbia? [Internet]. Toronto: Clear Estate; 2021. Available from: https://www .clearestate.com/blog/can-you-create-a-holographic-will-in-british -columbia.

32 For example, see *The Wills Act*, CCSM, c W150, S 6, and Canada, Ontario, *Successional Law Reform Act*, RSO 1990, c S.26, s 6.

33 Ministry of Attorney General. Apply for probate of an estate [Internet]. Toronto: King's Printer; 2023. Available from: https://www.ontario.ca /page/apply-probate-estate.

34 For example, compare the Ontario system with that of British Columbia; see Government of British Columbia. Probating a will [Internet]. Victoria: Government of British Columbia; 2023. Available from: https://www2 .gov.bc.ca/gov/content/life-events/death/wills-estates/probating-a-will.

35 See Ministry of the Attorney General. Probate of a small estate [Internet]. Toronto: King's Printer for Ontario; 2023. Available from: https://www .ontario.ca/page/probate-small-estate.

36 *Estates Act*, RSO 1990, C E.21.

37 *Crown Administration of Estates Act*, RSO 1990, c C.47.

38 See Indigenous Services Canada. Estates services for First Nations [Internet]. Ottawa: Government of Canada; 2024. Available from: https://www.sac-isc .gc.ca/eng/1100100032357/1581866877231.

39 Daly B. What happens to bank accounts after death in Canada [Internet]. Toronto: Loans Canada, 2023 [updated 2024 Nov 11]. Available from: https://loanscanada.ca/debt/what-happens-to-my-bank-accounts-after -i-die/.

40 In cases in which one owner becomes incapable, there may be challenges, and the PGT may be involved, but these issues can usually be resolved.

41 *Succession Law Reform Act*, RSO, 1990 c S 26, Part II, Intestate Succession, ss 44–46. Also see Community Legal Education Ontario (CLEO). If your partner dies [Internet]. Toronto: CLEO; 2024. Available from: https:// www.cleo.on.ca/en/publications/property-division-common-law -couples/if-your-partner-dies.

42 For one example of the complexities of intestate succession, see Government of British Columbia. Part 3 – when a person dies without a will [Internet]. Victoria: Government of British Columbia; 2014. Available

from: https://www2.gov.bc.ca/assets/gov/law-crime-and-justice/about
-bc-justice-system/legislation-policy/wesa/part3.pdf.

43 See Financial Consumer Agency of Canada. Unclaimed bank balances
[Internet]. Ottawa: Government of Canada; 2023. Available from: https://
www.canada.ca/en/financial-consumer-agency/services/banking
/unclaimed-balances.html.

44 See Employment and Social Development Canada. Survivor's pension [Internet].
Ottawa: Government of Canada. Available from: https://www.canada.ca/en
/services/benefits/publicpensions/cpp/cpp-survivor-pension.html.

45 *Executor of my will and trustee of my estate* is the formal term.

46 Government of Ontario. Estates administration: the role of the public
guardian and trustee [Internet]. Toronto: Queen's Printer; 2020. Available
from: https://www.publications.gov.on.ca/store/20170501121/Free
_Download_Files/300621.pdf.

47 *Saleh v. Reichert*, 1993 CanLII 9394 (ON SC) at paras. 8 to 15.

48 Government of Canada. Death benefit [Internet]. Ottawa: Government of
Canada; 2023. Available from: https://cremationcare.ca/119/Government
-Benefits.html.

49 See Ministry of Community and Social Services. Ontario Disability
Support Program policy directives 7.2 death of a recipient [Internet].
Toronto: Queen's Printer; 2022. Available from: https://www.ontario.ca
/document/ontario-disability-support-program-policy-directives-income
-support/72-death-recipient.

50 City of Toronto. Funerals and burials [Internet]. Toronto: The City; 2023.
Available from: https://www.toronto.ca/community-people/employment
-social-support/support-for-people-in-financial-need/assistance-through
-ontario-works/policies-and-procedures/funerals-and-burials/.

51 Mount Pleasant Group. Financial assistance [Internet]. Toronto: The
Group, 2023. Available from: https://www.mountpleasantgroup.com
/en-CA/Resources/government-resources/financial-assistance.aspx.

52 Consumer Protection Ontario. Pre-plan and pre-pay final arrangements
[Internet]. Toronto: King's Printer Ontario; 2023. Available from: https://
www.ontario.ca/page/pre-plan-and-pre-pay-final-arrangements.

53 Minister of the Solicitor General. Whole body donation [Internet]. Toronto:
King's Printer for Ontario; 2023. Available from: https://www.ontario.ca
/page/whole-body-donation.

54 *Trillium Network Gift of Life Act*, RSO, 1990 c H-20.

55 See Young L, Russell A. Dying alone: hundreds of bodies are going
unclaimed in Ontario and Quebec [Internet]. Global News; 2017 Feb 22.
Available from: https://www.globalnews.ca/news/3262664/dying-alone
-more-peoples-remains-going-unclaimed-in-ontario-and-quebec.

Indigenous Legal Expert Reflection on Chapter 12

KATE FORGET

My name is Kate Forget, and I am a member of Matchewan First Nation and grew up in New Liskeard, Ontario. I am legal counsel at the Indigenous Justice Division (IJD) in the Ministry of the Attorney General. I joined IJD in 2016 to be on a team of counsel who represented Ontario before the National Inquiry into Missing and Murdered Indigenous Women and Girls.

During this time, I was seconded to the Office of the Independent Police Review Director's systemic review of the Thunder Bay Police Service. The systemic review examined existing policies, practices, and attitudes of the Thunder Bay Police Service as they related specifically to Indigenous missing persons and death investigations. The report *Broken Trust: Indigenous People and the Thunder Bay Police Service*[1] was released in December 2018.

I also act as inquest counsel on behalf of the Office of the Chief Coroner on inquests involving the deaths of both Indigenous and non-Indigenous people.

The opinions expressed here reflect my own personal experiences and observations.

At various points throughout my career and lifetime, I have unfortunately had to meet with Indigenous families who have lost a loved one. As can be expected, no one meeting looks the same, because each family and each individual grieves differently.

When it comes to end-of-life and death rights, some principles can be followed that will, it is hoped, offer comfort and support to Indigenous families, which we should all strive for in the work that we do.

First, it is important to understand the history and ongoing legacy of colonialism and how your profession in and of itself may have an impact on the initial interactions that you have with an Indigenous person. You may have the greatest bedside manner and an understanding of Canada's dark history and relationship to Indigenous Peoples, but you need to be mindful that this will not necessarily amount to a positive working relationship at the outset.

The profession that you are part of has a history of harming Indigenous people, whether it be through the forced sterilization of Indigenous women or nutritional experiments conducted on Indigenous children. Systemic racism continues to affect Indigenous people when it comes to accessing health care, and that is always the jumping off point.

As a result, you may be met with a lack of trust, disinterest, or fear when you meet with an Indigenous person. If you truly understand the history that you represent as a professional, you will form more positive relationships with Indigenous people and not respond out of surprise or frustration.

It is your duty to earn trust, and it is important to remember that you cannot walk into a room with an Indigenous person and assume that you should already have it. Being mindful of what you represent as a health care professional is critical in all that you do.

Although I myself am an Indigenous woman, I am also a government lawyer. And I know all too well the harms that government institutions have inflicted on Indigenous communities and people. I acknowledge this when I meet with Indigenous families and speak with them about what my intentions are and what their expectations of me may be. Acknowledging that the systems that I am part of – whether it be justice, education, child welfare, or health care – have not served Indigenous people well is an important first step in any discussion, and my hope is that it will assist in building trust.

Another practical approach is this: if you don't know, ask. It really is that simple. It is also important to not make assumptions about Indigenous people. Pan-Indigeneity does not exist. Indigenous Nations are all different. When it comes to death rites, which are separate and apart from legal rights, there is no one-size-fits-all approach. For example, some communities may follow traditional practices, and others may follow Christian practices. Certain ceremonies and protocols may be of utmost importance when a death occurs in an Indigenous community. You cannot assume that because an approach you previously took with an Indigenous person was a good one that it will work again in the future.

Asking someone what their wishes or preferences are goes a long way.

Acknowledging that you may not have all of the answers but that you will do your best to find them is also essential to working with Indigenous families in a respectful way.

It is important to be aware that some end-of-life processes, such as the division of property and wills and estates, may be different depending on whether the person lives on reserve or in an urban community. The *Indian Act* may apply,[2] depending on the individual's circumstances. Again, this goes back to not making assumptions and asking questions.

Being mindful of supports is also critical in using a trauma-informed approach when working with Indigenous families. The individual may benefit from having access to an Elder, a Knowledge Keeper, or a non-traditional support person when difficult discussions are taking place. Can this be offered or, at the very least, canvassed with the person?

In terms of making a difficult discussion a little bit easier, ask whether the individual requires translation services. Some Indigenous people who are language speakers (i.e., those who speak their Indigenous language) may prefer receiving information in their own first language. Different communities have different dialects, and making the appropriate arrangements to facilitate translation should be incorporated as a best practice.

Finally, think about how you would want to be approached and addressed when talking about end-of-life rites or rights, the death of a loved one, or both. How would you want your loved one to be referred to?

I have on more than one occasion witnessed health care professionals and lawyers using terms that are disrespectful when referring to individuals. Words such as the *decedent* or *addict* and phrases such as *the individual made poor lifestyle choices* should always be avoided. Ask the individual how they would like you to refer to them or their loved one. Language matters. And these small acts of consideration matter. We need to step back from the processes we are familiar with and take a more humane approach when serving individuals who are grieving or at their lowest moments.

Always remember that every single Indigenous person that you meet will have experienced the impacts of colonialism in one way or another. At present, Indigenous communities are in the process of recovering from unmarked graves children who never returned home from Indian residential schools across this country. We need to understand the harms that Indigenous Peoples have experienced and the trauma that continues to be inflicted on them by the institutions that we represent.

What does that mean to you? What are your responsibilities? And what will you do moving forward?

NOTES

1 Office of the Independent Police Review Director (OIPRD). Broken trust: Indigenous people and the Thunder Bay Police Service [Internet]. Toronto: OIPRD; 2018. Available from: https://leca.ca/wp-content/uploads/broken-trust-compressed-1.pdf.
2 *Indian Act*, RSC, 1985, c I-5.

13 Health Care Decision-Making Involving People with Intellectual and Developmental Disabilities in Primary Health Care: Solidarity to Promote Capabilities While Mitigating Vulnerabilities

WILLIAM F. SULLIVAN, MERCEDES PEREZ,
JOHN HENG, AND PAULA HUTCHINSON

The United Nations *Convention on the Rights of Persons with Disabilities* (UNCRPD) enshrines as guiding principles "respect for inherent dignity, individual autonomy including the freedom to make one's own choices, and independence of persons," "non-discrimination," and "full and effective participation and inclusion in society."[1] The UNCRPD also requires countries to recognize "that persons with disabilities enjoy legal capacity on an equal basis with others in all aspects of life."[2]

The UNCRPD was ratified by Canada in 2010. Even where provisions of international human rights laws have not been expressly incorporated into Canadian law, the presumption of conformity remains an established interpretive principle in delineating the breadth and scope of rights guaranteed in the Canadian *Charter of Rights and Freedoms*, including the rights to life, liberty, and security of the person in section 7 and the right to equality in section 15.[3] The Supreme Court of Canada has recognized that "our *Charter* is the primary vehicle through which international human rights achieve domestic effect" and that, in particular, sections 7 and 15 "embody the notion of respect of human dignity and integrity."[4]

The rights recognized in the UNCRPD and protected by sections 7 and 15 of the *Charter* underscore the need to recognize and support a presumption of capacity as well as a right to full participation in decision-making regarding all areas of life for people with disabilities. How this applies practically in health care and specifically in the health care of people with intellectual and developmental disabilities (IDD), however, is a question that calls for further reflection.

People with IDD have lifelong limitations in cognitive, adaptive, and social skills that result from differences in neuropsychological development that become manifest before adulthood.[5] These differences vary in type and severity among people with IDD. Known causes of IDD can be genetic (e.g., Down syndrome or fragile X spectrum disorder), environmental (e.g., foetal alcohol spectrum disorder), or prenatal and perinatal (e.g., some instances of cerebral palsy), or they could be linked to multiple causes (e.g., some instances of autism spectrum disorder). The cause of IDD is, however, unknown for roughly half of those who have been diagnosed with IDD, and people with IDD are not always diagnosed as such.[6] They can often go unrecognized in health and other systems. This can happen especially when a person's limitations in cognitive, adaptive, and social functions are mild or the person has concurrent mental health conditions. Mental illness is more common among people with IDD than among those without IDD.[7]

Like everyone in society, people with IDD have a range of capabilities and limitations in making various decisions regarding their health. These capabilities and limitations depend on the type of decision and on interacting individual, environmental, and social factors. In this chapter, we begin by introducing what we call a solidarity model of supportive relationships in health care to promote the health care decision-making capabilities of people with IDD while mitigating vulnerabilities. Using an illustrative case example of applying this solidarity model, we explore opportunities and challenges to implementing the right to, and presumption of, legal capacity of people with IDD in primary health care.

Our solidarity model builds on the deliberative model of Emanuel and Emanuel's four models of the physician–patient relationship.[8] This solidarity model can be regarded as a mean or midpoint between opposed tendencies of their informative and paternalistic models. Primary care providers operating in ways that have features of the informative model might tend to presume, without inquiring, that most people with IDD are always capable of identifying and communicating their health needs and making informed and voluntary health care decisions independently. Those who operate in ways that have features of the paternalistic model might presume that most people with IDD always lack the capability to make informed and voluntary health care decisions. Such primary care providers tend either to take over decision-making for people with IDD or engage substitute decision-makers to decide for such patients without adequately assessing these patients' needs for accommodations and supports. By contrast, we argue that those who operate according to the solidarity model will more likely directly engage with people with IDD by embracing a supported decision-making approach that focuses on the importance of patients' relationships to people who know and love them, to help inform and facilitate care that these patients need and want. Such an approach can promote the decision-making capabilities of people with IDD while mitigating vulnerabilities in many instances. However, a range of scenarios are possible in primary care. In some instances, advocacy and coaching by primary care providers might be necessary to build and develop such supportive relationships. In other cases, supported decision-making might not be feasible, for example when decision supporters are lacking for a person with IDD or there is great uncertainty as to whether such supporters are truly acting in solidarity with the person with IDD. In these instances, a substitute decision-making approach might be better suited.

Solidarity Model of Relationships in Health Care

Ezekiel J. Emanuel and Linda L. Emanuel argued that the physician–patient relationship, in the context of medicine in the United States, needed to be redefined to allow both the physician and the patient to take an active role in treatment decisions.[9] They proposed four models of the physician–patient relationship (paternalistic, informative, interpretive, and deliberative) and noted that a shift had occurred in the medical context of the United States from the paternalistic model towards the informative model. They concluded by recommending that a deliberative model is best for the physician–patient relationship. In the deliberative model, "the physician and patient jointly engage in deliberation about what kind of health-related values the patient could and ultimately should pursue."[10(p. 2222)]

The deliberative model rightly recognizes the importance of discussing patients' values or goals (not merely medical information) as the grounds of health care decisions. It also acknowledges that patients might sometimes need the help of physicians in reaching certain health care decisions. However, the deliberative model still presupposes a dyadic model of the physician–patient relationship, one that does not attend to and engage a wider circle of possible decision-making supporters of the patient. It also restricts discussions of values within this relationship to values that relate to biological or psychological health, without necessarily referring to a broader range of values or goals that might also be significant for patients in making decisions about their overall well-being. Overall well-being includes biological and psychological health but could encompass other values or goals such as environment, social relationships, and experiencing spiritual fulfilment through art, music, and nature.

For health care relationships that involve people with IDD, we recommend broadening the Emanuels' deliberative model to what we refer to as the *solidarity model*. This model recognizes, on one hand, the more complex contemporary Canadian primary health care context of multidisciplinary family health teams and multi-sectoral systems of services with which people with IDD engage. These typically include many different non-physician health care provider relationships with patients. On the other hand, the solidarity model also acknowledges the significance to people with IDD of their relationships with close and trusted family members, friends, and others who provide care and support in a professional or non-professional role. The solidarity model also envisions a shared purpose and commitment among this circle of supporters of a person with IDD to uphold the person's dignity and offer them as much support as needed to promote their health and overall well-being, including support for decision-making. Often such support is present to help inform and facilitate health care that people with IDD need and want.

How the Law Typically Conceptualizes Capacity to Give Informed Consent and Substitute Decision-Making

Ontario's *Health Care Consent Act, 1996 (HCCA)*[11] illustrates a typical legal understanding of a patient's capacity to give consent for health care. It codifies a presumption of capacity to make treatment decisions regardless of age or diagnosis.[12] All individuals, including people with IDD, are presumed capable of making their own treatment decisions. The presumption can only be displaced on the basis of a valid assessment conducted by a qualified assessor, typically the health care practitioner proposing a specific treatment.

Capacity to give consent for health care requires the ability to understand the information relevant to deciding about a specified treatment and the ability to appreciate the reasonably foreseeable consequences of accepting or refusing the proposed treatment.[13] Capacity is a legal construct, not a medical determination, and focuses on ability rather than the wisdom of any particular treatment decision.[14] The legal concept of capacity and the accompanying presumption of capacity seek to promote individual autonomy and self-determination. These are values that receive constitutional protection in Canada's *Charter of Rights and Freedoms*.[15] The law also codifies procedural and due process rights. Those found incapable of making treatment decisions can challenge that decision to the Consent and Capacity Board or the Superior Court of Justice, depending on the context of the finding of incapacity.[16]

A patient's capable consent to treatment must also be informed. For informed consent, the *HCCA* requires that, among other factors, consent must be given voluntarily and must not be obtained through misrepresentation or fraud.[17] Informed consent further requires that the person has received all relevant information respecting (a) the nature of the treatment; (b) the expected benefits, material risks, and side effects of the treatment; (c) alternative courses of action; and (d) the likely consequences of forgoing the treatment.[18]

The Ontario law applies a model of substitute decision-making in instances in which a person has been found to be incapable of giving informed consent to treatment. If a person is found incapable of making a treatment decision, consent must be obtained by the physician or other health care provider from a substitute decision-maker who is typically a close family member, a person previously appointed by the incapable person as their attorney for personal care, or a court-appointed guardian.[19]

For a more fulsome discussion of legal capacity and substitute decision-making in health care, please see chapter 12 on advance planning.

Supported Decision-Making

The solidarity model of health care relationships aims to promote patients' decision-making capabilities. Capabilities go beyond clinical and legal notions of an individual's capacity to make decisions independently, as determined by typical cognitive assessments and legal criteria. Such assessments of decision-making capacity focus on an individual's ability to perform certain cognitive tasks by themselves. Health care providers and ethicists are recognizing, however, that "healthcare decisions are always supported decisions."[20(p. 29)] The exercise of autonomy by any patient in reaching health care decisions is relational. That is, the process of reaching health care decisions is often interdependent and engages other people. It entails reciprocal interactions such as communicating, discussing, interpreting, and seeking or receiving guidance in various ways and to varying degrees, depending on the complexity of the decision and the gravity of its effects. The notion of capability encompasses these forms of support. A person's capability to reach a decision is a composite of individual efforts plus supports received from others. For people with IDD, such forms of support can be very important. They can increase opportunities to be involved in making decisions regarding their health and other areas of life from which they are too often excluded.[21]

Supported decision-making has been proposed as a legal alternative to substitute decision-making. An impetus for this shift in legal theory and law is article 12 of the UNCRPD, mentioned earlier, which obliges participating countries to recognize the right of persons with disabilities to equal standing with other persons before the law. This includes the right of all persons with disabilities to make decisions regarding health and other aspects of life, with the supports that they need, to be legally recognized and fully realized.

This approach is reflected, at least in part, even in Ontario's health care consent and substitute decision-making legal framework. Specifically, Ontario codifies a presumption of treatment capacity that applies to all individuals regardless of age or diagnosis.[22] Ontario law also requires that substitute decision-makers make treatment decisions in keeping with prior capable wishes or, if there are none, in keeping with the person's values and beliefs.[23] The law in Ontario also requires attorneys for personal care and guardians of the person to "encourage the person [for whom they are deciding] to participate, to the best of his or her abilities, in the guardian's decisions on his or her behalf."[24] However, mandatory legal requirements for substitute decision-makers to follow prior capable wishes, to encourage the participation of the person for whom they are deciding, and to weigh the person's values and beliefs in substitute decision-making only kick in after an incapacity finding is made. Also, although individuals in Ontario have significant legal avenues to appoint a substitute decision-maker of their choice,[25] the substitute decision-maker's role only takes effect after an incapacity finding is made.

Unlike Ontario, some jurisdictions have explicitly codified various frameworks of supported decision-making. For example, Alberta's *Adult Guardianship and Trusteeship Act* codifies a presumption of capacity and mandates that "where an adult requires assistance to make a decision or does not have the capacity to make a decision, the adult's autonomy must be preserved by ensuring that the least restrictive and least intrusive form of assisted or substitute decision-making that is likely to be effective is provided."[26] The Alberta act also provides that adults may appoint up to three people as supported decision-makers and that a decision that is "made with the assistance of a supporter or communicated by or with the assistance of a supporter is the decision of the supported adult for all purposes."[27] A supported decision may be refused if there is evidence of undue influence, fraud, or misrepresentation.[28]

The Yukon's *Adult Protection and Decision Making Act*[29] also incorporates a model of supported decision-making. For example, it stipulates that guardians of the person should not be appointed unless alternatives such as the provision of support and assistance have been tried, and it provides for supported decision-making agreements.[30] Associate decision-makers have codified responsibilities that include assisting the person to make and express a decision; advising the person by explaining relevant information and considerations; ascertaining the wishes and decisions of the adult and assisting them to communicate them; and endeavouring to ensure that the person's decision is implemented.[31] Decisions made or communicated with the assistance of the associate decision-maker must be recognized for all purposes as the decision of the person themself.[32]

Manitoba's *Vulnerable Persons Living with a Mental Disability Act*[33] applies only to persons with intellectual disabilities. It excludes persons diagnosed with a mental disorder. It recognizes "supported decision-making" (defined as a "process whereby a vulnerable person is enabled to make and communicate decisions with respect to personal care ... in which advice, support or assistance is provided ... by members of his or her support network"). A support network may include spouses, partners, family members, and others chosen by the vulnerable person.[34] The guiding purposes of this act recognize that a vulnerable person's support network "should be encouraged to assist the vulnerable person in making decisions so as to enhance his or her independence and self-determination" and that "substitute decision-making should be invoked only as a last resort."[35] A substitute decision-maker will only be appointed if it is determined that the vulnerable person is incapable of making personal care decisions either alone or with the involvement of a support network.[36]

Although Canada ratified the UNCRPD[37] in 2010, most provinces and territories in Canada, including Ontario, have yet to develop laws and regulations that explicitly recognize the right of people with disabilities to reach health care decisions through and with the assistance of support persons. Hence, family physicians and other health care providers often find themselves in a grey area of practice when seeking informed consent for health care interventions involving people with IDD through a supported decision-making framework.

It should be noted that accommodations are forms of support and are required under Ontario's *Human Rights Code*.[38] Although human rights legislation requires accommodation and supports to counteract discrimination on the basis of disability or other related grounds, this is not a fulsome recognition of supported decision-making because the approach of provinces and territories such as Ontario to health care consent is fundamentally grounded in functional assessments of capacity and a substitute decision-making model that comes into play upon a finding of incapacity.[39] As such, persons engaging in supported decision-making approaches are doing so informally and largely outside the existing framework established in legislation such as Ontario's *Health Care Consent Act, 1996* and the *Substitute Decisions Act.*

However, many aspects of supported decision-making are already implicit in the solidarity model of primary care, discussed earlier, that is widely accepted in health care practices for all patients. These practices centre on patients and their relationships with their caregivers. In such practices, family members of people with IDD and other caregivers are typically, and informally, given a role in helping with communicating, interpreting, and guiding people with IDD to reach health decisions, but not in taking over the decision-making.

Whether such informal supported decision-making arrangements should be formalized legally is a question that is disputed. For instance, Scholten et al. have argued that the risk of supported decision-making arrangements resulting in supporters exerting undue influences on a health care decision is higher than that of substitute decision-making arrangements.[40] In the latter, there are at least provisions for substitute decision-makers to be held legally accountable for the decisions that they make on behalf of the person concerned. Also, persons whose supports to reach health care decisions are informally recognized lose due process rights because they cannot legally challenge a finding of incapacity to make informed decisions independently when no formal assessment of this has been made.[41]

Peterson, Karlawish and Largent argue that, like substitute decision-making, it is important legally to regulate supported decision-making practices because "a formal agreement solemnizes the decision-making relationship, clarifies expectations, and allows third parties to independently check whether the beneficiary and supporter(s) are abiding by its conditions."[42(p. 12)] Kohn[43] and Blumenthal-Barby and Ubel[44] argue, however, that these expectations and safeguards can be achieved in most cases in health care without the need to formalize supported decision-making arrangements.

One key concern with both supported and substitute decision-making is that projection or undue influence by others can be difficult, if not impossible, to detect. Reasons for these challenges include that the health care decision-making process is often a very private exercise; it takes place within familial or close personal relationships marked by power and dependence. Separating out the interests and motives of supporters or substitute decision-makers from those of the person is limited because the person might not have a reliable means of communicating concerns to potentially impartial others.

Risks of rendering people with IDD vulnerable in supported and substitute decision-making arrangements should be mitigated. It is also important, however, to discuss what constitutes undue influence on the part of decision-makers. Understanding autonomy only in terms of independent decision-making can be a barrier to expressing solidarity with people who need assistance to reach health care decisions. In understanding when supported decision-making is appropriate, whether formalized or not, a solidarity model of the health care relationship avoids the extremes of paternalism (i.e., taking over the decision-making process entirely, without trying to engage the person with IDD or understand their goals, values, and preferences) and of presuming that any effort to interpret, guide, or coach the person with IDD on the part of decision-making supporters is necessarily biased or coercive (e.g., a projection and imposition of the supporter's own goals or values onto the person with IDD).

Decision-making is relational and interdependent. It is never value neutral, nor should this be expected. Douglas and Bigby acknowledge that supporters bring their own motivations, values, and beliefs when providing support,[45] but they propose that the risk that decision-making supporters are merely projecting and imposing their own motivations, values, and beliefs onto the person with IDD is minimized when their relationship to the person with IDD is close, when supporters are committed to upholding rights of the person with IDD, and when supporters engage in regular self-reflection and review. For the primary care provider, we also propose that assessing decision-making vulnerability using a tool, such as the one described later in this chapter, could include assessing, as far as possible, signs that decision-making supporters are unfamiliar with or inattentive to the goals or values of the patient.

A supported decision-making approach in primary health care, based on a solidarity model to promote the decision-making capabilities of people with IDD while mitigating vulnerabilities, is illustrated in the following story. The story draws from an actual clinical case, but the names and identifying features have been modified.

Pat's Story

Pat lives in a Canadian province in which supported decision-making is not legally formalized. Pat is a 38-year-old man with IDD (he has a mental age of five to seven years). Pat has a known history of gastroesophageal reflux disease, bronchial asthma, and a chronic cough. He lives in a group home, and his support workers assist him in all areas of his daily life. Pat has limited speech and uses a picture system to communicate. He also uses picture scripts to understand sequences, follow routines, consider options, and make decisions. Pat's parents are very involved in his life. They are his court-appointed guardians for health care decisions. They also believe that Pat has the right to make these decisions and seek support from other people whom he trusts.

Because of the spread of COVID-19 infection, Pat's group home has a policy that residents are not allowed to visit family or friends outside of their home if they are not vaccinated. Pat is not vaccinated. Pat's parents have asked his family physician to help them because Pat is fearful of medical procedures, including vaccination by means of injections. With the help of Pat's parents and a long-time support worker, together with input from the nurse on the health team who conducts the intake interview, his family physician establishes that Pat highly values his relationships and wants to be able to visit his parents and friends. By using pictures and simple language, his family physician describes the nature of the decision that Pat is being asked to make and the consequences of choosing or not choosing to be vaccinated. Pat at first states firmly that he does not want to be vaccinated. He pushes away the pictures that the family physician has been showing him. With some coaxing by his parents, Pat finally agrees to be vaccinated, but he still appears nervous and then asks his support worker to take him home. At this point, the family physician describes the various ways that Pat can be vaccinated, including receiving his vaccination at home. Pat nods, but the family physician is unsure whether Pat is just indicating that he wants to go home to end this stressful discussion or whether he is choosing to be given his vaccination in his home setting.

Pat's parents and support worker suggest that Pat needs more time to reflect on his options and reach a decision. His family physician suggests booking a second appointment, which will give Pat more time to consider his options and ensure that his decision is not being unduly influenced by wanting to please the people he cares about. In the meantime, Pat's support worker agrees to work with the nurse to develop a picture script to help Pat to review relevant information for his decision and to reflect on his options. The family physician also suggests some relaxation and distraction activities for Pat to try to reduce his fear of needles.

Commentary

Many people are involved in offering solidarity and support to Pat to make his decision regarding vaccination: the family physician and nurse on the health team, as well as Pat's parents and his support worker. All are committed to promoting Pat's decision-making capabilities. Given the uncertainty regarding whether Pat fully understands and appreciates the consequences of agreeing or refusing to be vaccinated, as well as questions regarding whether Pat's consent is voluntary, the physician could have deferred to the authority of Pat's parents as his legal attorneys for personal care to make this decision for Pat during the initial office visit. Likewise, Pat's parents could have insisted on their legal right to decide for their son to be vaccinated. They also need not have involved Pat's support worker. However, in this case, everyone works in solidarity with Pat to involve him in the decision and to offer him the supports that he needs to consider various options and to decide interdependently.

The main decision-making capability that Pat needs support for regarding this decision is choosing preferred proposed options for attaining what matters most to him in his situation. What matters most to Pat appears to be socializing with his family, friends, and others who love him and whose company he clearly enjoys. He can express this in simple language and by his behaviour. But he has difficulty weighing the transient dissatisfaction of being injected, which he fears, against the benefits of being vaccinated. The most important benefit of vaccination for him is being allowed to visit his family and friends again. The significance of what matters most to Pat could have been overlooked if the family physician had simply gone along with Pat's initial refusal to be vaccinated because of his fear of needles or had focused on discussing with Pat the decision to be vaccinated only in terms of the consequences of this decision for biological well-being. Here, Pat's social well-being appears to be what Pat relates to and should be the focus of communications with him regarding whether to be vaccinated.

At the same time, relaxation and distraction activities to help reduce Pat's fear of needles and the option of being vaccinated in a less stressful environment, such as at home in the company of his trusted support worker, are adjustments that can mitigate trauma to Pat of receiving an injection. As Cook and Hole note, trauma due to negative life experiences is a very common feature of the lives of people with IDD.[46] It is likely that Pat's fear of medical procedures, including being vaccinated by injection, is related to past negative medical experiences. Adjusting the ways in which vaccination is administered to Pat is not only an example of a trauma-informed approach to health care but also promotes his decision-making capabilities by expanding his range of options for deciding. Such adjustments make available to Pat alternatives that decrease the burden to him of being vaccinated, which he may be willing to accept, to attain the benefit of continuing to enjoy companionship, which he cherishes.

It is still necessary for the family physician and others on the health team to assess the appropriateness for Pat of using a supported decision-making approach. They should always check whether Pat would want the assistance of decision-making supporters for various aspects of the decision-making process, as far as this confirmation is possible. If Pat were entirely unable to confirm this, using his usual means of communication, then a supported decision-making approach is inappropriate. Solidarity, then, is best expressed by the family physician, health team, and Pat's substitute decision-makers working together to discern his goals or values to reach a decision on his behalf.

In this case, Pat does indicate that he requires assistance from his parents and support worker to reach a decision regarding being vaccinated. The additional supports that the health team, Pat's parents, and his support worker can offer (e.g., more time, coaching through picture scripts, and even coaxing by promising rewards, such as being able to visit family and friends) should not be regarded as ethically problematic in this context. These supports help Pat to choose a proposed medical intervention that will realize his goal of being allowed to visit his family and friends, which he hopes for and values the most. The approach taken by Pat's supporters should not be regarded as unduly influencing Pat's decision.

The family physician, however, should still use helpful tools, such as those described next, to document the decision-making process and to check for potential vulnerabilities regarding supported decision-making with Pat.

Conclusion of Pat's Story

At his second, in-home appointment with his nurse, Pat briefly showed the picture script that he created with his support worker, which outlined the steps that help Pat to connect a proposed medical option (being vaccinated) with his goal (being allowed to visit family and friends). Pat's parents and his support worker have gone over these steps with Pat to confirm Pat's decision to be vaccinated. Over the past two weeks, Pat and his support worker have read the picture script every day. They have also practised the steps and relaxation and distraction strategies to use during the vaccination. They talked about Pat's goal to visit his parents' house, why being vaccinated was important, and what he would be able to do once he is vaccinated.

When the nurse asks Pat if he is ready to be vaccinated, however, he again becomes agitated and says he wants to go his parents' house. This is a good reminder that the supported decision-making process may need to be iterative. Having practiced with Pat and knowing his limitations in comprehending and remembering sequences, Pat's support worker calmly intervenes by showing Pat the vaccination picture script and says, "Yes, we are going to Mom and Dad's house. First, calm body, then medicine, next visit Mom and Dad's house." Pat points to the calm body picture, begins his deep-breathing exercises, and uses his learned distraction strategies of looking away from the needle to watch his favourite spin toy while listening to calming music. The nurse begins to follow Pat's lead by also pointing to the pictures, using the words in the picture script and pausing to check Pat's understanding and desire to complete each step. They successfully complete all the steps together.

Although the approach taken in this story is an instance of informal supported decision-making, it nonetheless could meet legal standards for being accommodated to give informed and voluntary consent for health care decisions in Pat's province. Pat was eventually able to meet the threshold for legal capacity of understanding and appreciating the implications of his decision to be vaccinated in a manner that made sense to him, with the help of his supporters. He was also able to voluntarily undergo the procedure when accommodations, such as relaxation exercises, were offered.

Pat was fortunate to have a successful outcome because he had good supporters and available resources for accommodations. The protracted, iterative process of decision-making used, and the efforts by Pat's supporters to attend to his cues, follow his direction at each stage of the decision-making process, and accommodate his preferences as much as possible. It also mitigated the risks of projection and undue influence by his supporters on Pat's decision.

If circumstances had been different, this positive outcome may have been compromised by risk factors that affect decision-making, such the patient's limited ability to communicate and self-regulate, limited time available to the family health team, and supporters who are unfamiliar with or show signs of applying undue influence on the patient's decisions.

Additional barriers to applying a supported decision-making approach are raised when people with IDD have limited social supports due to life factors and certain social determinants of health (e.g., limited access to social services, poverty, lack of housing, social seclusion, and discrimination based on ableist or racist attitudes or structures and systems). Friedman, Rizzolo, and Spassiani found that persons with IDD experiencing these social determinants were less likely to receive support to make decisions about their health care.[47] A solidarity model includes advocacy by family physicians and the health team to address these barriers and to promote the dignity of the person with IDD, help the person to build social relationships, and have equitable access to supported decision-making processes. An example of an advocacy letter for Pat is offered in Appendix 3.

Tools for Primary Health Providers to Promote Decision-Making Capabilities

Pat's story is the story of one person with IDD in a specific context. It is important to recognize the range of life situations and related contextual risks, types of health decisions, and range of needs for decision-making supports of different people with IDD. People with IDD will require supported decision-making to varying degrees depending on the type of decision to be made. For some decisions, certain persons with IDD will be able, with minimal supports, to communicate, understand information, and appreciate possible benefits and burdens of various alternative interventions. They can also be guided by their goals or values to select a preferred medical intervention. This scenario is more likely if the decision involves a health issue and an intervention familiar to the person; when there is less uncertainty regarding the intervention's benefits, risks, or burdens for the person with IDD; and when the connection between the intervention and the person's goals or values is relatively easy for the person to make.

For other types of health decisions, many persons with IDD will be capable of directing decisions so long as there are close and trusted people who can reliably support them to communicate what matters most to them (i.e., their goals or values) and help them apply this knowledge to consider the relative benefits, burdens, and risks of proposed and available medical options. This was the case in Pat's story.

Still other patients are unable to participate very much or at all in the decision-making process regarding most health care decisions, even when supports are available. They might be unable to communicate their need or desire for such supports when accommodated to do so. Or they might be unable to express, verbally or through cues, what matters to them in ways that another person, even a trusted person, can reliably interpret.[48]

A tool has been developed for clinicians, *Decision Making in Health Care of Adults with Intellectual and Developmental Disabilities: Promoting*

Capabilities, that adapts typical cognitive assessments for decision-making capacity to adults with IDD using a solidarity model of health care relationships to distinguish among these various scenarios.[49]

This tool helps health care providers to think about, document, and implement adjustments to time, communication, and setting that people with IDD might need. It also facilitates communication with people with IDD, and their supporters as needed, about the patient's goals or values regarding a specific health care decision. It breaks the decision-making process down into several steps involving various tasks and assesses, for each step, the person's need and desire for one or more decision-making supporter to help them with each task.

The approach to assessing the appropriateness of supported decision-making offered by this tool goes beyond the typical cognitive or functional assessments used to determine legal capacity in health care settings. It is also conducted in consultation with other members of the health team and close and trusted supporters designated by the person with IDD.

The tool can also be used to enhance certain identified facilitators to using a supported decision-making approach with people with IDD, regardless of the legal regime. Facilitators include (a) developing the skills of health care providers to assess decision-making using a supported decision-making approach;[50] (b) coaching supporters regarding their role;[51] and (c) advocacy by health care providers for a supported decision-making approach in medical, legal, and other contexts that tend to exclude people with IDD with interdependent decision-making capabilities in favour of a substitute decision-making approach.

The tool also offers a systematic process for documenting and identifying support needs at each stage of the decision-making process. It is crucial to establish a systematic process for supported decision-making, even if this process might need to be adapted to the context of each person with IDD.[52] Douglas and Bigby[53] have proposed an evidence-based decision-making process for supporters that consists of seven steps:

1. knowing the person;
2. identifying and describing the situation;
3. understanding the person's will and preference;
4. refining the decision and taking account of constraints;
5. considering whether a self-generated, shared, or substitute decision is to be made;
6. reaching the decision and associated decisions; and
7. implementing a decision and seeking out advocates if necessary.

Sullivan and Heng[54] have also described a systematic process for supported decision-making of adults with IDD, with five steps analogous to those described by Douglas and Bigby but specifically relating to the context of a primary health care practice:

1. Enlist the help of caregivers and supporters to prepare the person with IDD for visits to the clinic.
2. Promote conditions in the clinic to optimize the person with IDD's communication (e.g., scheduling a time that is optimal for the patient and available for accompanying supporters, booking sufficient time, and accommodating noise or light sensitivities). As in the case of Pat, members of the health team should be aware that some persons with IDD might have difficulty expressing emotional distress relating to medical situations and procedures. The person with IDD might manifest this in the decision-making process by avoidance or resistance. The underlying causes of such reactions will need to be explored.
3. Discern (i.e., elucidate and clarify) the life goals or values of the person with IDD. As in the case of Pat, assess whether the person with IDD might need one or more close and trusted supporters to identify or communicate goals and values or to clearly distinguish between transient desires and more deeply rooted hopes (goals) and commitments (values). Adults with a severe to profound level of IDD might need people who know their life history to interpret goals (e.g., experiences or relationships that bring the person with IDD joy). Supporters can help to explain cultural or religious values that are important to the family or community to which the person with IDD belongs.
4. Deliberate on appropriate medical options to reach a shared decision. Assess whether the person with IDD might need support to weigh benefits, risks, and burdens of proposed available interventions in their life circumstances to approximate identified goals or values. It is important for the person with IDD and supporters, as needed, to feel that they have sufficient time. As in the case of Pat, this weighing of options might involve primary care providers and supporters in communicating benefits, risks, and burdens in ways that relate to what matters most in life to the person (i.e., not just medical facts). Complex decisions might need to be broken down into various steps for the person with IDD. When an intervention involves uncertainty or ambiguity regarding benefits, risks, or burdens to the person, a trial period for the intervention should be one of the proposed options. The primary care provider should also

propose as options alternative ways of administering interventions if they are likely to mitigate the burden of those interventions to the person with IDD.

5. Develop a care plan that outlines the role of the person with IDD, their various health care providers and caregivers, and the steps needed to implement the decision and identify a coordinator.

Mitigating Vulnerabilities of People with Intellectual and Developmental Disabilities Using a Supported Decision-Making Approach

The tool *Decision Making in Health Care of Adults with Intellectual and Developmental Disabilities: Promoting Capabilities* described earlier can be used in conjunction with assessing the vulnerabilities of people with IDD in a supported decision-making process in primary health care and addressing these vulnerabilities.

Primary care providers will always need to be attentive to, and address using available means, factors such as suggestibility, learned compliance, distorted thinking, and impulsive or compulsive behaviour that might undermine the voluntariness of a supported decision.[55]

Other vulnerabilities that primary care providers who adopt a supported decision-making approach should screen for include the potential risks of some members of the health team and supporters of the person with IDD inappropriately taking over decision-making, as discussed earlier.

There is need for a tool to assist health care providers in self-reflection and to assess risk factors that might undermine the quality or validity of a supported decision-making process involving people with IDD. In Table 13.1, we highlight some of these risk factors, give examples of screening questions, and propose some ways of mitigating decision-making vulnerabilities that these questions bring to light. The greater the implications of the decision to be made are for the overall well-being and personal integrity of the person with IDD, the greater the ethical responsibility for health care providers to screen for and address these risk factors. There are some types of decisions for which, in the opinion of the authors, neither a supported nor a substitute decision-making approach for a person with IDD is ethically appropriate (e.g., sterilization, medical assistance in dying).

Considerations regarding	Possible risk factors	Sample screening questions	Strategies for mitigating decision-making vulnerabilities
Adult with IDD	• Learned compliance or suggestibility • Cognitive distortions (emotional or conceptual) and fixations • Distress (e.g., trauma from past medical experiences) • Lack of experience and familiarity with the condition or medical intervention relevant to the decision • Impulsive or compulsive behaviours • Inability to communicate verbally	Would you like to know more about this [condition or intervention]? What do you like or not like about this [intervention]? What would happen if you didn't choose this [intervention]? Do you need more time to think about your decision?	• For learned compliance or suggestibility, promote reflective practices and coaching for members of the health team and supporters of the person with IDD regarding behaviours that overlook or dismiss the perspectives of the person with IDD. • Consider training for the person with IDD to build confidence in expressing, verbally or through other means, what matters to them. • Refer the person with IDD for mental health assessments and management by specialists who have clinical knowledge of and experience with people with IDD. • Consider adjustments to reduce stressors, relaxation and distraction techniques, and desensitization programs. • Communicate in terms of goals and values that the person with IDD can relate to. Increase decision-making supports as needed. • Seek collateral history from decision-making supporter(s). Consider therapies to address these patterns of thought and behaviour.
Health care provider proposing intervention(s)	• Proposing limited alternatives • Sharing information without discerning the goals or values of the person with IDD (informative model) • Ableism (paternalistic model regarding people with IDD) • Not considering relevant aspects of the person with IDD's life situation (e.g., life-phase transitions) in proposing options, such as palliative care	[For health care provider] Have I made my best efforts to facilitate a supported decision-making approach in solidarity with this person?	• Explore possible adjustments or alternatives to increase the range of available options. • Assess the need for supporter(s) to help to discern or interpret the goals, values, and preferences of the person with IDD. Communicate information regarding proposed options in relation to these goals, values, and preferences (e.g., using activity scripts). • Self-reflect and follow through with efforts to involve people with IDD in the decision-making process as much as possible. • Consider and discuss implications of intervention options in the context of life-phase transitions with the person with IDD and the person's supporters.

(Continued)

Table 13.1. (Continued)

Considerations regarding	Possible risk factors	Sample screening questions	Strategies for mitigating decision-making vulnerabilities
Decision-making supporters	• Unfamiliar with person with IDD • Not desired or trusted by person with IDD • Projection or imposition of supporters' goals, values, and preferences; inappropriate taking over of the decision-making process	Would you like this person/these people to help you with this [task]?	• Support the person with IDD to find an appropriate decision-making supporter. • Mentor and coach decision-making supporters regarding their appropriate role and the importance of self-awareness in that role; consider input from different supporters; mentor and coach the person with IDD to develop decision-making capabilities.
Life situation or environmental factors related to the social determinants of health	• Negative and traumatizing life experiences of the person with IDD that could be unduly affecting the decision • Environmental influences on the decision, such as policy and systemic pressures that negatively discriminate against or exclude people with IDD	Do you feel sad or upset by something that's happened? [For health care provider] Have I made my best efforts to maintain solidarity with this person and to practise and advocate for a supported decision-making approach?	• Seek collateral history. Enhance social supports and counselling (e.g., trauma-informed approaches, logo, narrative, dialectical, or solution-focussed therapies). • Increase advocacy (e.g., health care provider prepares a letter outlining the person's condition; what is required, current impact on accessibility, accommodation, or adaptation rights; and expected benefit when the person has better options and decides how their needs will be met. Show solidarity by making a commitment to review progress when needs are being addressed.)

IDD = intellectual and developmental disabilities.

Conclusion

Currently, 185 countries have ratified the UNCRPD, including Canada, which, as noted earlier, ratified it in 2010. The UNCRPD affirms the right of persons with disabilities, including those with IDD, to individual autonomy, including the freedom to make their own choices in health care and other areas of life (article 3). It also provides in article 12 that countries that are parties to the UNCRPD must recognize and take steps to operationalize the right of persons with disabilities to exercise legal capacity on an equal basis with others in all aspects of life. These principles are analogous to rights enshrined in Canada's *Charter of Rights and Freedoms*, specifically section 7's guarantee to life, liberty, and security of the person and section 15's equality rights.

Almost two decades after the publication of the UNCRPD, limited progress has been made in Canada to implement this right to autonomy for people with IDD in a fulsome fashion in primary care contexts. In our view, there are three reasons for this delay:

1. The lack of practical tools to facilitate implementing supported decision-making with people with IDD that are specifically adapted to primary care contexts. In this chapter, we have highlighted some tools that have recently been developed or can be developed.
2. Lack of reflection and framing work to articulate an ethical basis for supported decision-making that strives to integrate the right of people with IDD to exercise personal autonomy, with supports as needed, with the ethical responsibility of health care providers to promote the health and overall well-being of patients with IDD. The most prevalent concern raised in legal, medical, ethical, and other contexts is that supported decision-making may, in some instances, lead to harm suffered by the person with IDD. We have addressed such objections in our chapter by proposing a solidarity approach to supported decision-making. According to this model, a systematic process for assessing and addressing the need of people with IDD for decision-making supports while identifying and addressing decision-making vulnerabilities, using tools developed for these purposes, can promote the decision-making capabilities of people with IDD while avoiding or mitigating harm. In the solidarity model, the person with IDD, the health team, family, and other supporters are committed to a shared goal, namely, the health and overall well-being of the person concerned. This entails support for the person to discern life goals or values; to distinguish these goals or values from transient beliefs and desires; and to weigh benefits,

risks, and burdens of various options considering this knowledge. In this context, the attentive and iterative process by which health care providers and decision-making supporters interpret, educate, or coach the person should not be summarily dismissed as imposing undue influences on the person with IDD being supported.
3. Lack of acknowledgment that substitute decision-making models also carry risks. For example, the motives of substitute decision-makers might not always align with the best interests of the incapable person, and these motives may not be readily ascertainable by health care practitioners proposing a treatment. Substitute decision-makers themselves might be vulnerable to abuse, misrepresentation, or fraud by third parties, and these issues might also not be readily apparent to health care practitioners. Although Ontario's capacity and consent laws do create legal avenues to address these problems,[56] these legal mechanisms require being proactive and having emotional and economic resources that are not always available to the substitute decision-maker or the person determined to be incapable.

The solidarity model of supported decision-making entails expanding the range of options for people with IDD by adjusting typical ways of administering interventions according to preferences (e.g., acceptable types or levels of burden to the person concerned) to attain certain life goals or values of the person with IDD. At the same time, there should be a concomitant process to check for and address risk factors that might undermine the alignment of a particular decision with what matters most to the person with IDD in terms of their overall well-being and ability to flourish in life. If these factors cannot be addressed for certain decisions involving people with IDD, then, as a last resort, a substitute decision-making approach that considers best interpretations of the goals, values, and preferences of the person is, according to the solidarity model, ethically justified. For certain types of decisions in which the risk of harm to overall well-being and the integrity of the person concerned is significant and likely (such as sterilization or medical assistance in dying), we have argued that neither supported nor substituted decision-making with people with IDD is, according to the solidarity model, ethically justified.

NOTES

1 United Nations. Convention on the rights of persons with disabilities (Dec. 13, 2006). Treaty Series, vol. 2515, Article 3 [Internet]. Available from:

https://www.un.org/development/desa/disabilities/convention-on-the
-rights-of-persons-with-disabilities/convention-on-the-rights-of-persons
-with-disabilities-2.html.

2 United Nations. Convention on the rights of persons with disabilities
(Dec. 13, 2006). Treaty Series, vol. 2515, Article 12 [Internet]. https://
www.un.org/development/desa/disabilities/convention-on-the-rights
-of-persons-with-disabilities/convention-on-the-rights-of-persons-with
-disabilities-2.html.

3 *Canadian Charter of Rights and Freedoms*, s 7, Part 1 of the *Constitution Act*,
1982, being Schedule B to the *Canada Act* 1982 (UK), 1982, c 11 a; *Quebec
(Attorney General) v 9147-0732 Quebec Inc.*, 2020 SCC 32, paras. 31–34.

4 *R. v. Ewanchuk*, 1999 CanLII 711 (SCC), [1999] 1 SCR 330, para. 73.

5 Schalock RL, Luckasson R, Tassé MJ. Intellectual disability: definition,
classification, and systems of supports. 12th ed. Washington
(DC): American Association on Intellectual and Developmental
Disabilities; 2021.

6 Maulik PK, Lakhan R, Kishore MT, et al. Prevalence and aetiopathogenesis
of intellectual developmental disorders. In: Bertelli S, Munir DK,
Hassiotis A, et al. Textbook of psychiatry for intellectual disability and
autism spectrum disorder. Cham: Springer; 2022. p. 51–70. https://doi
.org/10.1007/978-3-319-95720-3_2.

7 Einfeld SL, Ellis LA, Emerson E. Comorbidity of intellectual disability and
mental disorder in children and adolescents: a systematic review. J Intellect
Dev Disability 2011;36(2):137–43. https://doi.org/10.1080/13668250.2011
.572548.

8 Emanuel EJ, Emanuel LL. Four models of the physician-patient relationship.
JAMA. 1992;26(16): 2221–6.

9 Emanuel EJ, Emanuel LL. Four models of the physician-patient relationship.
JAMA. 1992;26(16): 2221–6.

10 Emanuel EJ, Emanuel LL. Four models of the physician-patient relationship.
JAMA. 1992;26(16): 2221–6.

11 *Health Care Consent Act, 1996*, SO 1996, c 2, Sched A.

12 *Health Care Consent Act, 1996*, SO 1996, c 2, Sched A, s 4(2).

13 *Health Care Consent Act, 1996*, SO 1996, c 2, Sched A, s 4(1).

14 *Starson v. Swayze* 2003, SCC 32 (CanLII), para 76.

15 *Charter of Rights and Freedoms*, Part 1 of the *Constitution Act, 1982*, being
Schedule B to the *Canada Act 1982* (UK), 1982, c. 11; *Gligorevic v. McMaster*,
2012 ONCA 115, para. 58 to 60.

16 *Health Care Consent Act, 1996*, SO 1996, c 2, Sched A, s 32; *Substitute
Decisions Act, 1992*, SO 1992, c 30, s 3.

17 *Health Care Consent Act, 1996*, SO 1996, c 2, Sched A, s 11(1).

18 *Health Care Consent Act, 1996*, SO 1996, c 2, Sched A, ss 11(2) and (3).

19 *Health Care Consent Act, 1996,* SO 1996, c 2, Sched A, s 20 and *Substitute Decisions Act 1992,* SO 1992, c 30, Part II.

20 Enck GG. Healthcare decisions are always supported decisions. Am J Bioethics. 2021;21(11):32–35. https://doi.org/10.1080/15265161.2021.1980137.

21 Sullivan WF, Heng J, Bach M. Supported decision making: a new approach to promoting decision-making capabilities in health care of adults with intellectual and developmental disabilities. In: Khemka L, Hickson L, editors. Decision making in individuals with intellectual and developmental disabilities: integrating research into practice. New York: Springer; 2021. p. 46–64.

22 *Health Care Consent Act, 1996,* SO 1996, c 2, Sched A, s 42.

23 *Health Care Consent Act, 1996,* SO 1996, c 2, Sched A, s 21 and *Substitute Decisions Act 1992,* SO 1992, c. 30, s. 66.

24 *Substitute Decisions Act 1992,* SO 1992, c 30, s 66(5).

25 *Health Care Consent Act, 1996,* SO 1996, c 2, Sched A, s 33(1); *Substitute Decisions Act 1992,* SO 1992, c 30, s 46.

26 *Alberta Guardianship and Trusteeship Act,* SA 2008, c A-4.2, s 2(c).

27 *Alberta Guardianship and Trusteeship Act,* SA 2008, c A-4.2, s 6.

28 *Alberta Guardianship and Trusteeship Act,* SA 2008, c A-4.2, s 6.

29 *Adult Protection and Decision Making Act, Schedule A,* SY 2003, c 21.

30 *Adult Protection and Decision Making Act,* Schedule A, SY 2003, c 21, ss 2(d), 4, 5 and 6.

31 *Adult Protection and Decision Making Act,* Schedule A, SY 2003, c 21, s 5.

32 *Adult Protection and Decision Making Act,* Schedule A, SY 2003, c 21, s 6 to 13, especially 11.

33 *The Vulnerable Persons Living with a Mental Disability Act,* CCSM, c V.90.

34 *The Vulnerable Persons Living with a Mental Disability Act,* CCSM, c V.90, ss 1(1), 6(1).

35 *The Vulnerable Persons Living with a Mental Disability Act,* CCSM, c V.90, Preamble, s 6(2).

36 *The Vulnerable Persons Living with a Mental Disability Act,* CCSM, c V.90, ss 49, 53(1).

37 United Nations. Convention on the rights of persons with disabilities (Dec. 13, 2006). Treaty Series, vol. 2515, Article 3 [Internet]. Available from: https://www.un.org/development/desa/disabilities/convention-on-the -rights-of-persons-with-disabilities/convention-on-the-rights-of-persons -with-disabilities-2.html.

38 Human Rights Code, RSO 1990, c H.19.

39 Law Commission of Ontario. Concepts of legal capacity and approaches to decision-making: promoting autonomy and allocating legal accountability [Internet]. In: Legal capacity, decision-making and guardianship: final report . Toronto: The Commission; 2017. https://www.lco-cdo.org/en /our-current-projects/legal-capacity-decision-making-and-guardianship/.

40 Scholten M, Braun E, Gather J, et al. Combining supported decision-making with competence assessment: a way to protect patients with impaired decision-making capacity against undue influence. Am J Bioethics. 2021;21(11):45–7.

41 Law Commission of Ontario. Legal capacity, decision-making and guardianship: final report [Internet]. Toronto: The Commission; 2017. https://www.lco-cdo.org/en/our-current-projects/legal-capacity-decision-making-and-guardianship/.

42 Peterson A, Karlawish J, Largent E. Supported decision making with people at the margins of autonomy. Am J Bioethics. 2021;21(11):4–18. https://doi.org/10.1080/15265161.2020.1863507.

43 Kohn NA. Realizing supported decision-making: what it does – and does not – require. Am J Bioethics. 2021;21(11):37–40. https://doi.org/10.1080/15265161.2021.1980149.

44 Blumenthal-Barby J, Ubel PA. Supported decision making: a concept at the margins vs. center of autonomy? Am J Bioethics. 2021;21(11):43–4. https://doi.org/10.1080/15265161.2021.1981033.

45 Douglas, J, . and C. Bigby C. Development of an evidence-based practice framework to guide decision making support for people with cognitive impairment due to acquired brain injury or intellectual disability. Disabil Rehabil. 2020; 42(3:434–41). https://doi.org/10.1080/09638288.2018.1498546.

46 Cook S, Hole R. Trauma, intellectual and/or developmental disability, and multiple, complex needs: a scoping review of the literature. Res Dev Disabil. 115:103939. https://doi.org/10.1016/j.ridd.2021.103939.

47 Friedman C, Rizzolo MC, Spassiani NA. Self-management of health by people with intellectual and developmental disabilities. J App Res Intellect Disabil. 2019;32(3):600–9. https://doi.org/10.1111/jar.12554.

48 Sullivan WF, Heng J, McNeil K, et al. Promoting health care decision-making capabilities of adults with intellectual and developmental disabilities. Can Fam Physician 2019;65(Supplement 1):S27–S29. https://www.cfp.ca/content/65/Suppl_1/S27.long.

49 Decision Making in Health Care of Adults with Intellectual and Developmental Disabilities: Promoting Capabilities. In: Tools for the primary care of adults with intellectual and developmental disabilities [Internet]. Toronto: Surrey Place Centre; 2018. Available from: https://ddprimarycare.surreyplace.ca/tools-2/.

50 Sullivan WF, Heng J. Supporting adults with intellectual and developmental disabilities to participate in health care decision making. Can Fam Physician. 2018;64(Suppl 2):S32–S36. https://www.cfp.ca/content/64/Suppl_2/S32.long.

51 Bigby C, Douglas J, Smith E, et al. "I used to call him a non-decision-maker – I never do that anymore": parental reflections about training to support decision-making of their adult offspring with intellectual

disabilities. Disabil Rehabil. 2022;44(21):6356–64. https://doi.org/10.1080/09638288.2021.1964623.

52 Browning M, Bigby C, Douglas J. A process of decision-making support: exploring supported decision-making practice in Canada. J Intellect Dev Disabil. 2021;46(2):138–49. https://doi.org/10.3109/13668250.2020.1789269.

53 Douglas J, Bigby C. Development of an evidence-based practice framework to guide decision making support for people with cognitive impairment due to acquired brain injury or intellectual disability. Disabil Rehabil. 2020;42(3):434–41. https://doi.org/10.1080/09638288.2018.1498546.

54 Sullivan WF, Heng J. Supporting adults with intellectual and developmental disabilities to participate in health care decision making. Can Fam Physician .2018;64(Suppl 2):S32–S36. https://www.cfp.ca/content/64/Suppl_2/S32.long.

55 Heng J, Sullivan WF. Ethics of decision making and consent in people with intellectual and developmental disabilities. In: Wehmeyer ML, Brown I, Percy M, et al., editors. A comprehensive guide to intellectual and developmental disabilities. 2nd ed. Baltimore: Paul H. Brookes; 2018. p. 655–64.

56 *Substitute Decisions Act 1992*, SO 1992, c 30, ss 47(3), 53, 55, 61; *Health Care Consent Act, 1996*, SO 1996, c 2, sched A, ss 21(2), 21(6), 33, 35, 36, 37.

Conclusion

JENNIFER STONE AND RAMI SHOUCRI

Intractable Social Problems Demand an Interdisciplinary Approach

The patient stories provided throughout this text reveal many intractable social problems that can confound primary care providers. After years of global austerity, with income inequality now exacerbated by the COVID-19 pandemic, there is little doubt that ameliorating the social determinants of health (SDOHs) demands an interdisciplinary approach.

We hope that this text has inspired primary care providers to

- take an interest in and be curious about your patient's SDOHs and what legal resources are available in your community, and build partnerships with those legal service providers;
- be responsive to patient requests but also confidently approach case findings, screening for poverty, social histories, and narrative approaches, for the most common health-harming social issues that may have legal remedies:
  - *I* – income
  - *H* – housing
  - *E* – employment/education
  - *L* – legal status
  - *P* – personal safety;
- engage in ongoing training about implicit bias; and
- be aware of key patient populations, including Black and other People of Colour, those living with HIV, paediatric patients, Indigenous patients, and patients who are gender and sexual minorities. As discussed in this book, racialized, Indigenous, newcomer, 2SLGBTQ+, unattached, and female individuals are more likely to live in poverty, face discrimination at work, and live in precarious housing. These should be high priority-patient populations for case finding.

Case Example of a Partnership: The Health Justice Program at the St. Michael's Hospital's Academic Family Health Team

We hope that this text has increased health care providers' confidence in identifying and addressing their patients' health-harming legal needs. Health and justice partnerships represent an opportunity for primary care providers to facilitate access to legal services for these issues, as well as to meet interprofessional educational needs and identify and address organizational and systemic contributors.

The model and the approach are flexible and adaptable to whatever care setting you work in. Here, we elaborate on our particular partnership for the purposes of illustration but would like to emphasize that simply learning about what resources are available in your community and starting conversations with legal service providers can be the first steps to building your own partnership.

We are a primary care physician and a legal aid lawyer, respectively. Along with many other colleagues, we have worked to implement, support, and grow the Health Justice Program, a health and justice partnership (HJP) between four community legal aid clinics (Neighbourhood Legal Services, taking the lead role, supported by Aboriginal Legal Services, ARCH Disability Law Centre, and the HIV and AIDS Legal Clinic of Ontario) and the St. Michael's Hospital's Academic Family Health Team (SMHAFHT) in Toronto. This program began as a pilot in 2014, funded by Legal Aid Ontario with in-kind support from the SMHAFHT. In 2019 the funding became permanent. It is presently managed by Neighbourhood Legal Services as the lead community legal aid clinic.

The Health Justice Program is guided by a memorandum of understanding and is funded for the equivalent of one full-time lawyer and an intake paralegal. A physician and a social work clinical champion from the SMHAFHT get protected time to support the ongoing partnership. Our work is guided by an advisory Partners Committee.

The goals of the Health Justice Program are threefold:

1. To improve SDOH where a legal remedy exists for low-income patients of the SMHAFHT and in turn improve the access to justice (legal health) of this population through preventive, stabilizing interventions before their social or legal issues become crises. The direct service offered is the cornerstone of the program, and it helps to inform education and systemic advocacy initiatives. Health care providers at the SMHAFHT can easily refer their low-income patients for a legal consult or seek a secondary consultation themselves. We also provide a weekly drop-in.

2. To support and cultivate clinicians' abilities to recognize and effectively refer patients with legal issues that affect their health. As such, the education program continues to strengthen the capacity of the SMHAFHT and the related primary health care community to provide services with a knowledge of their patients' rights within the health care system and how to navigate appropriate legal resources in the community. In turn, the Health Justice Program aims to improve legal partners' ability to deliver services in a trusted primary care setting.
3. To identify and take action on collaborative systemic law reform issues that affect low-income patients' SDOHs and to bring together legal aid and medical partners in advocating for positive change for the betterment of the populations they jointly serve.

Direct Services

The origin story of the Health Justice Program came from health and legal service providers working together in the service of common patient-clients. The SMHAFHT is a large urban family health team with approximately 57,000 patients rostered; about 80 physicians and 100 other allied health care providers on staff; and five brick-and-mortar clinics across Toronto's downtown east communities. Approximately 30 per cent of its patient population lives under the Low-Income Measure. The SMHAFHT's catchment area maps almost exactly onto Neighbourhood Legal Services' geographical catchment area: the downtown east neighbourhoods of Toronto.

Neighbourhood Legal Services has only 9 full-time staff. The clinic serves approximately 1,500 people per year, with more than 300 of those coming by way of the Health Justice Program, now an embedded referral pathway for patients rostered at the SMHAFHT. Its core areas of practice are housing, income security, immigration, and employment law.

The complex social problems of Toronto's low-income communities in the downtown east call for interprofessional collaboration. This community is highly dense and made up mostly of renters, with more than 9,000 social housing units. Despite this, most people in Toronto's downtown east spend well over 30 per cent of their income on rent; therefore, housing precarity is common. There is a sizeable urban Indigenous population and many Indigenous-led organizations in Toronto's downtown east. The population is growing – quickly – and there are many seniors living alone. It is also the epicentre of Ontario's opioid crisis, with toxic drug overdoses common and their number increasing.

The population includes a great number of newcomers and a higher-than-the-Toronto-average number of non-permanent residents, so immigration status precarity is also a reality for many. Toronto's downtown east includes the neighbourhood with the highest child poverty rate in Canada.

These statistics reveal significant intersecting and overlapping social problems that exacerbate poor health and vice versa. We are proud promoters of the health and justice partnership model because we have seen firsthand the many benefits that flow from an interdisciplinary approach in a community like ours. The Health Justice Program develops and delivers support to address the legal issues of vulnerable individuals around their SDOHs; stabilize patient-clients' situations; and, where possible, prevent cascading problems.

To be sure, an interprofessional partnership has challenges that require dedicated staff and attention to ensure communication channels are open and clear while also protecting patient-client privacy. We firmly believe the effort pays off in more robust and early interventions to stabilize low-income patients' situations before they cascade into crises. We have also found that the Health Justice Program allows under-resourced legal aid services to get clients connected to wraparound supports provided by the SMHAFHT, such as social work, addictions counselling, psychology, chiropractic care, physiotherapy, diabetes education, income security health promotion, and more.

Education Opportunities

This text grew out of a 2019 lunch-and-learn series called *Health Justice Tuesdays*. We coordinated 11 workshops for primary health care providers, from within both the SMHAFHT and the broader medical community. The goals included building providers' capacity and confidence in spotting potential health-harming legal needs in order to make timely referrals to the Health Justice Program.

A health care provider and a lawyer jointly developed and delivered the material for each workshop. After the introductory workshop, each subsequent workshop centred on a legal issue that was regularly referred to the Health Justice Program. These workshops were supplemented by a few additional workshops focusing on the expertise of our specialty legal aid clinic partners. That content subsequently developed into the chapters you have read here, while exploring a few new topics as well. This, we understand, is the first text of its kind exploring health and justice partnerships in the Canadian context.

Advocacy

As we have noted, a third key pillar of the Health Justice Program involves identifying systems-level issues and advocating for change. Practically speaking, the issues we have worked on have arisen from common issues arising from direct services work as well as the particular expertise of the partners. A recent article summarized the advocacy activities of the Health Justice Program as well as an analysis of how these activities were chosen and why.[1] In our experience, the most effective advocacy involves long-term and intentional partnership with community-based and other advocacy-engaged organizations to contribute the particular expertise of our program to their work.

As we set out in chapter 1, no one health and justice partnership model will fit all settings. In the United States, where there are more than 450 health and justice partnerships, they are seen in a variety of settings, including veterans' hospices, children's hospitals, general hospitals and health care settings, and more.

All of these health and justice partnerships embody common principles, however, of wholistic service provision: targeting vulnerable populations, using an interdisciplinary approach, working across sectors, and seeking early intervention whenever possible

Health and Justice Philosophy of Care, Supported by a Growing Body of Research

Giving attention to health-harming legal needs is both intuitive and supported by a growing body of research.[2] Three recent reviews by Beardon et al.,[3] Jomaa et al.,[4] and Tobin-Tyler et al.,[5] in particular, comprehensively and concisely summarize the evidence to date of the impact of this approach.

Health and Justice Programs Improve Stress, Anxiety, and the Ability to Focus on Health

Beardon et al. highlight many positive legal and social outcomes that have been documented through high-quality peer-reviewed research, linking specific objectives of HJPs to outcomes. Notably, the studies have demonstrated improvements in mental health, stress, and engagement with health advice. A theory of change proposed is, thus, "that legal assistance brings about improved circumstances (material, financial and practical) which leads to reduced stress and anxiety, improved ability to focus on health and participate in daily life, and ultimately better mental and physical wellbeing."[6(p. 6)]

One area that has not yet demonstrated a definitive impact of HJPs is improvement in physical health. Effectively, improving recognized SDOHs through HJPs has been established in the literature, but biological health is harder to demonstrate.

> The impacts of HJPs on individual health has been the subject of debate. The reviewed publications had examined different health outcomes (mostly self-reported), among different patient groups, for different legal interventions and over different time periods. Broad generalization is therefore not possible from the current evidence. Health impacts are likely to depend on the patient population (e.g. age, health status) and legal issues addressed. However, overall there was strong evidence among the studies (both quantitative and qualitative) for improvements in mental health, particularly stress, depression, anxiety and wellbeing, and that these improvements occurred as a direct result of the legal interventions.[7(p. 7)]

Tobin-Tyler et al. also point out the challenges in evaluating health outcomes across different jurisdictions, focusing on different patient populations, to extract general findings. It could also be that we need to think critically about our arguably narrow definition of health. We hope providers will reflect on what chapter 3 offers in terms of a perspective on Indigenous SDOHs, too often missing from the research calculus, and adopt a more wholistic evaluation of health.

Health and Justice Partnerships Are Most Effective When They Target Vulnerable Populations

The Jomaa et al. scoping review notes that medical–legal partnerships "operate in a myriad of ways, yet all are designed to improve vulnerable peoples' health through greater access to justice."[8(p. 7)] This is particularly true for people with disabilities; Black, Indigenous, and People of Colour; and other marginalized people, who are most likely to benefit from intentional pairing of health and legal services.

"The medical-legal approach is gaining increasing traction in the U.S., Canada, the U.K., and Australia as legal professionals seek to respond to a growing evidence base suggesting that legal assistance services should be: 1) targeted to those most in need, 2) combined with other services (legal and non-legal), 3) provided in a timely manner (including early intervention and prevention) to minimize the impact of problems, and 4) designed for the ease of helping people."[9(p. 7)]

The authors of chapter 10 of this text point out that where there is intersectionality, the burden of illness is greater, as are the barriers to care.

An excellent example of the interplay between health and housing, and why targeted HJPs can make a key difference, was shown in chapter 4 of this text in discussing an older tenant with a disability:

> Clearly identifying Mrs. VH's disability-related needs and limitations – and possible solutions, where available – helps trigger the landlord's duty to accommodate her disability under provincial human rights legislation ... Setting out her other housing options if evicted – or dispelling potential myths about the availability of state-provided or otherwise institutional care – helps underscore (for a decision-maker) the need to grant relief from eviction if possible, and to make every effort to support Mrs. VH in her current housing. Connecting Mrs. VH with legal representation helps give her the chance to have these facts and arguments clearly explained to her landlord and a legal decision-maker in the eviction process. Being ready to testify within that process makes it far more likely that the facts relating to Mrs. VH's health are taken seriously and understood within the legal process.

Indeed, the Jomaa et al. scoping review recognizes that "a legal rights-based framework presents appropriate remedies for many health-harming social determinants such as unsafe housing, food insecurity, unstable income, and discrimination."[10(p. 9)]

Inter-professional education through HJPs enriches the next generation of primary care (and legal aid) providers.

The Tobin-Tyler et al. scoping review includes a great discussion of inter-professional education for the next generation. It discusses how collapsing disciplinary silos in the educational context provides an early opportunity for skills development. This includes building relationships across sectors, engaging in systems thinking, identifying root causes of health disparities situated in laws and policies and how to advocate for change, and implementing trauma-informed practice in a HJP setting.

Excitingly, the Tobin-Tyler et al. scoping review looks to the development of HJPs in Australia, the United Kingdom, and the United States and highlights burgeoning international collaboration on best practices for the HJP service delivery model, including regarding inter-professional education. The review also correctly notes how government-funded legal services in every jurisdiction are chronically under-resourced. HJPs can reduce the justice gap by tackling unresolved and overlooked legal needs with the institutional support of health institutions.

Future Directions

We wish to end this text with some calls to action. We have explored
the limitations and overwhelming benefits of HJPs, and we encourage
health care and legal sector leaders to consider the following:

- a call to government action for greater access to primary care
  - We saw how often legal rights will go unenforced but for health
    care providers' support. This obviously does not happen for the
    approximately 6 million people in Canada who do not have a
    primary care provider.
  - We call for expansion of team-based primary care to allow
    for interdisciplinary approaches, including health and justice
    approaches, to increasingly complex patient issues.
- a call to government action to invest in legal aid
  - Recognize that funding cuts to the realization and enforcement of
    legal rights for poor people simply results in externalities pushed
    onto the health care system.
- a call to government and institutional support for the adaptation of
  HJP approaches across Canada
  - As in the United States and Australia, it would be great to see a
    national HJP movement in Canada and something akin to the
    United States' National Centre on Medical-Legal Partnerships.
- the integration of health and justice interprofessional education
  into law schools, medical schools, and family medicine residency
  programs.

NOTES

1 Shah N, Radford K, Durant S, et al. Advocating for policy change:
   Examples emerging from a medical-legal partnership in primary care.
   J Health Care Poor Underserved. 2024;35(1):8–17.
2 See, for example, Pascoe P, Coumarelos C, Forell S, et al. Reshaping
   legal assistance services: building on the evidence base – a discussion
   paper. Sydney (NSW): Law and Justice Foundation of New South
   Wales; 2014; Genn H. When law is good for your health: mitigating the
   social determinants of health through access to justice. Curr Leg Probl.
   2019;72(1):159–202. https://doi.org/10.1093/clp/cuz003.
3 Beardon S, Woodhead C, Cooper S, et al. International evidence on the
   impact of health-justice partnerships: a systematic scoping review. Public
   Health Rev. 2021;42:1603976. https://doi.org/10.3389/phrs.2021.1603976.

4 Jomaa D, Ranasingh C, Raymer N, et al. The impact of medical legal partnerships: a scoping review. Univ Tor J Pub Health. 2022;1(1). https://doi.org/10.33137/utjph.v3i2.38094.

5 Tobin-Tyler E, Boyd-Caine T, Genn H, et al. Health justice partnerships: an international comparison of approaches to employing law to promote prevention and health equity. J Law Med Ethics. 2023;51(2023):332–43.

6 Beardon S, Woodhead C, Cooper S, et al. International evidence on the impact of health-justice partnerships: a systematic scoping review. Public Health Rev. 2021;42:1603976. https://doi.org/10.3389/phrs.2021.1603976.

7 Beardon S, Woodhead C, Cooper S, et al. International evidence on the impact of health-justice partnerships: a systematic scoping review. Public Health Rev. 2021;42:1603976. https://doi.org/10.3389/phrs.2021.1603976.

8 Jomaa D, Ranasingh C, Raymer N, et al. The impact of medical legal partnerships: a scoping review. Univ Tor J Pub Health. 2022;1(1). https://doi.org/10.33137/utjph.v3i2.38094.

9 Jomaa D, Ranasingh C, Raymer N, et al. The impact of medical legal partnerships: a scoping review. Univ Tor J Pub Health. 2022;1(1). https://doi.org/10.33137/utjph.v3i2.38094.

10 Jomaa D, Ranasingh C, Raymer N, et al. The impact of medical legal partnerships: a scoping review. Univ Tor J Pub Health. 2022;1(1). https://doi.org/10.33137/utjph.v3i2.38094.

Appendix 1: Legal Aid and Other Legal Resources in Canada

Table A.1. Legal Aid and Other Free or Low-Cost Legal Resources in Canada, by Province (as of December 2020)

Provinces	Areas of covered by legal aid plan	Eligibility*	Other free or low-cost legal resources
Alberta https://www.legalaid.ab.ca/	• Serious criminal charges • Charges under the *Youth Criminal Justice Act* • Family law issues • Child welfare matters • Immigration or refugee claims • Civil law matters (such as guardianship or trusteeship) and income support • Siksika Nation members (criminal charges, family law and child welfare matters, and advice on civil law issues)	• Can be eligible for legal representation if income falls within the following amounts, listed by family size, for monthly income or annual income, respectively: 1, $1,668 or $20,021 2, $2,066 or $24,788 3, $2,940 or $35,275 4, $3,178 or $38,134 5, $3,416 or $38,134 $\geq$6, $3,416 or $40,995 There is no financial eligibility requirement for duty counsel assistance for matters in criminal (adult and youth) courts, drug treatment courts (Calgary and Edmonton), disciplinary hearings at correctional facilities, and Mental Health Review panel hearings, as well as for some family matters at Provincial and Court of Queens Bench	• Pro Bono Alberta: https://www.pbla.ca/

| https://iss.bc.ca/ | • Child protection matters
• Some immigration issues
• Criminal law
• Mental health
• Prison law issues
• Aboriginal Legal Aid BC (including Gladue rights; fishing, hunting, and gathering; and family rights) | ...the amount shown below by family size for standard cases and CFSA and Criminal Early Resolution, respectively:

1, $1,660 and $2,660
2, $2,320 and $3,320
3, $2,990 and $3,990
4, $3,650 and $4,650
5, $4,310 and $5,310
6, $4,980 and $5,980
$\geq$7, $5,640 and $6,640

If one does not qualify for representation by a legal aid lawyer under financial requirements, they still may be eligible for legal advice services such as duty counsel for criminal, family, and immigration law | https://www.accessprobono.ca/ |
| Manitoba
https://www.legalaid.mb.ca/ | • Public interest
• Family
• Immigration and refugee
• Residential tenancies
• Child protection
• Mental health
• Government benefits
• Criminal | • Low-income adults and youth who financially qualify or have a case with merit are eligible.
• If individuals have enough money or assets to pay for legal fees, they may be eligible to receive legal aid through the Agreement to Pay program.
The financial guidelines for free legal aid by family size and gross family income are as follows:

1, $26,000
2, $30,000
3, $34,000
4, $37,000
5, $40,000
6 $43,000
$\geq$7, $46,000

Duty counsel services are offered regardless of financial circumstances, primarily in the areas of criminal defence and child protection. | |

(Continued)

Table A.1. (Continued)

Provinces	Areas of covered by legal aid plan	Eligibility*	Other free or low-cost legal resources
New Brunswick http://www.legalaid-aidejuridique-nb.ca/	• Criminal Law Services (trials, court duty counsel, and consulting from police station) • Family Services (family duty counsel, child protection proceedings, child and spousal support, custody and access, family advice lawyers) • Public Trustee Services (generally charge a fee for services, however it can be reduced by the Public Trustee)	• Generally, people with low income or those on social assistance qualify for covered services. Eligibility contribution by household size and based on gross annual income is as follows for no contribution, $150 contribution, $250 contribution, and not financially eligible: 1, 0–$14,400, $14,401–$22,800; $22,801–$31,200; and $\geq$$31,201 2, 0–$21,600; $21,601–$33,600; $33,601–$45,600; and $\geq$$45,601 3, 0–$22,800; $22,801–$34,800; $34,801–$46,800; and $\geq$$46,801+ 4, 0–$24,000; $24,001–$37,200; $37,201–$50,400; and $\geq$$50,401 5, 0–$25,200; $25,201–$39,600; $39,601–$54,000; and $\geq$$54,001 $\geq$6, 0–$27,600; $27,601–$42,000; $42,001–$56,400; and $\geq$$56,401 There are no financial eligibility requirements for duty counsel service for criminal matters, matters before mental health review boards, and family law matters.	

| Newfoundland and Labrador
https://www.legalaid.nl.ca/ | • Family law (including divorce, custody, access, child protection, and wardship)
• Criminal law (adult and young offenders) | • The *Legal Aid Act* does not provide specific income cut-offs for determining eligibility for legal aid in Newfoundland and Labrador.
• Applicants can receive legal aid coverage if they cannot afford to pay for a private lawyer without adversely affecting their ability to support themselves and their family.
• Individuals receiving social assistance are automatically eligible for legal aid coverage.
• Services are also available with respect to an individual's contribution for legal aid coverage; however, the level of contribution is also determined by several factors. Income guidelines are based on family size and net yearly income:

1 adult, $4,716
1 dependent, $5,808
2 dependents, $6,324
3 dependents, $6,804
4 dependents, $7,296
5 dependents, $7,836
6 dependents, $8,364
2 adults, $6,492
1 dependent, $6,960
2 dependents, $7,416
3 dependents, $7,920
4 dependents, $8,364
5 dependents, $9,012
6 dependents, $9,684 |

(Continued)

Table A.1. (Continued)

Provinces	Areas of covered by legal aid plan	Eligibility*	Other free or low-cost legal resources
Northwest Territories https://www.justice.gov.nt.ca/en/legal-aid/	• Criminal and *Youth Criminal Justice Act* charges • Serious offences under the Criminal Code and other federal laws • Less serious offences that may result in going to jail or losing way of making a living • Some appeals of court decisions • Child support, child custody, or access cases • Spousal support • Child welfare • Division of property and divorce related to child matters	• To qualify for legal aid, individuals must meet financial eligibility requirements. • Applicants may be required to pay some or all of the costs, depending on total household income and number of dependents. • The annual net income required depends on in which zone an individual resides: Zone 1, Yellowknife, Detah, N'dilo Zone 2, Behchokǫ Enterprise, Fort Smith, Hay River, Hay River Reserve, Fort Providence, Kakisa, Fort Liard, Fort Simpson, Jean Marie River, Fort Resolution, Nahanni Butte, Inuvik, Wrigley, Gamètì, Wekweètì, Whatì Zone 3: Sambaa K'e, Norman Wells, Aklavik, Fort McPherson, Tuktoyaktuk, Tsiigehtchic, Łutselk'e, Fort Good Hope, Tulita, Délįne, Paulatuk, Sachs Harbour, Ulukhaktok, Colville Lake The financial eligibility threshold is based on household size, zone (1–3), and annual net income, respectively; there is no contribution level: 1, $29,500, $34,033, or $41,025 2, $41,719, $48,130, or $58,018 3, $51,095, $58,947, or $71,057 4, $59,000, $68,066, or $82,050 5, $65,964, $76,100, or $91,734 6, $72,260, $83,364, or $100,490	

| Nova Scotia
https://www.nslegalaid.ca/ | • Criminal matters (youth court cases, any cases under Criminal Code, *Controlled Drugs and Substances Act*, or other federal Legislation)
• Family law (domestic violence, child protection, child custody, some divorces, and division of property)
• Social justice and civil law (such as Canada Pension Plan, Employment Insurance, or income assistance)
• Prison law | • To obtain full legal representation by a lawyer, individuals must meet financial, area-of-law, and merit-based qualifications. Financial eligibility is based on family size and gross annual income:

  1 adult, $12,804
  2 adults, $17,088
  1 adult, 1 child, $16,992
  2 adults, 1 child, $20,496
  1 adult, 2 children, $20,400
  2 adults, 2 children, $23,184
  1 adult, 3 children, $23,088
  2 adults, 3 children, $25,872

• Duty counsel lawyers are available to all Nova Scotians facing criminal or drug charges. |
| Nunavut
http://nulas.ca/en/ | • Family matters (including child custody, child support, DNA testing, division of property, spousal assault, etc.)
• Criminal
• Youth
• Poverty and civil law (landlord–tenant issues, employment law, and human rights complaints)
• Legal services are provided through three regional clinics | • An applicant is eligible for free legal aid if they receive most of their income from social assistance.
• Where the legal fees for services would reduce the individual's income to make them eligible for social assistance, the individual may be required to contribute towards the payment of costs. |

(Continued)

Table A.1. (Continued)

Provinces	Areas of covered by legal aid plan	Eligibility*	Other free or low-cost legal resources
	• The Legal Services Board's regional legal aid clinics are located in Cambridge Bay (Kitikmeot Law Centre), Rankin Inlet (Kivalliq Legal Services), and Iqaluit (Maliiganik Tukisiiniakvik)	Financial guidelines are based on household size and annual gross income: 1 person, $50,400.00 2 persons, $62,400.00 3 persons, $88,800.00 4 persons, $96,000.00 5 persons, $103,200.00 6 persons, $110,400.00 7 persons, $117,600.00 8 persons, $124,800.00 9 persons, $132,000.00 ≥10+ persons, $139,200.00 (http://nulas.ca/wp-content/uploads/2015/02/Family-Law-Coverage-and-Eligibility-Policy-September-2014.pdf) • All persons in criminal matters are automatically financially eligible for duty counsel services	
Ontario https://www.legalaid.on.ca/	• Family law • Refugee and immigration law • Criminal law • Mental health law • Clinic law (social assistance matters, housing, income, immigration, and some employment) • Other services include 20 min of free legal advice for family law matters; same-day court services, including duty counsel and representation by	• Legal aid services are only provided if the individual meets the financial eligibility test. To receive free legal aid, their gross income must be lower than the amounts provided below by family size, as of April 2020 (contribution options are also available depending on income and assets): 1, $16,239 2, $28,094 3, $32,026 4, $36,188 ≥5, $40,168	• Pro Bono Law Ontario's free legal advice hotline for non-unionized workers (www.probonoontario.org/work/; toll free: 1-855-255-7256) • Human Rights Legal Support Centre (https://hrlsc.on.ca/)

	- There is also a financial eligibility test for legal aid duty counsel services. An individual's annual gross income must be less than the amount specified below, by family size, as of April 2020: 1, $22,720 2, $32,131 3, $39,352 4, $45,440 $\geq$5, $50,803		- Workers' Action Centre (Toronto, Ontario; https://workersactioncentre.org/; does not provide legal advice but can provide information and referrals) - Law Society of Ontario's "Lawyer Referral Service" – up to 30 min of free legal advice regardless of income (https://lsrs.lso.ca/lsrs/welcome) - Some private bar lawyers offer contingency fees, lower rates, and deferred fee plans. Legal aid clinics should be able to provide some referrals.
Prince Edward Island https://www.princeedwardisland.ca/en/information/justice-and-public-safety/legal-aid	- Criminal law (youth and adults); PEI Legal Aid does not offer a duty counsel program at criminal courts - Family law - Some civil law matters closely related to family law (including domestic violence, child protection law, and involuntary hospitalization under mental health law)	- Family size is used to determine eligibility, and financial eligibility is based on before-tax income: 1, $17,632 2, $24,554 3, $30,072 4, $34,725 5, $38,823 6, $42,529 These are just two of the several factors considered; other factors can relate to urgency and seriousness of legal needs.	

(Continued)

Table A.1. (Continued)

Provinces	Areas of covered by legal aid plan	Eligibility*	Other free or low-cost legal resources
Quebec http://www.csj.qc.ca/	• Family matters • Youth protection • Representing youth in criminal matters • Prosecution of a criminal act • Claims regarding benefits • Some criminal matters if the case involves a probable prison sentence or loss of livelihood or when it is in the best interests of justice • Some administrative, civil, and immigration matters if there is a threat to physical or psychological safety or a threat to livelihood or if freedom is likely to be restricted	• Legal aid is provided free of charge if the individual's situation fits the eligibility criteria, listed by family size and gross annual income: Single person, $22,750 Family of 1 adult and 1 child, $27,834 Family of 1 adult and ³2 children, $29,714 Family of spouses with no children, $31,661 Family of spouses with 1 child, $35,424 Family of spouses with ³2 children, $37,306 • Contributory legal aid is also available, depending on financial circumstances	• Justice Pro Bono / Services juridique benevole: https://justiceprobono.ca/en/
Saskatchewan http://www.legalaid.sk.ca/	• Criminal matters • Family matters (divorce, custody, access, child protection, and adoption) • Full legal representation will be provided to individuals who meet the financial requirement. Youth are automatically eligible.	• Individuals are financially eligible for legal aid if they meet at least one of these requirements: If the individual is a youth; the individual receives social assistance; the individual receives band assistance; or net income is at or below social assistance levels. Income and asset guidelines by family size and by net annual income and maximum assets, respectively, are as follows: Single, $9,420 and <$1,500 Couple without children, $11,400 and $3,000 Family with 1 child, $12,300 and $3,500	• Pro Bono Law Saskatchewan: https://pblsask.ca/

| Yukon
https://www.yukonlegalaid.ca/ | • Criminal matters (likelihood of jail; mental disorder; *Youth Criminal Justice Act, Extradition Act, Fugitive Offenders Act* matters)
• Civil matters (child protection proceedings; proceedings under *Mental Health Act*, family matters in which children are involved in issues of custody, access, and child support) | Family with 2 children, $15,000 and $3,500
Family with 3 children, $17,700 and $3,500
Family with 4 children, $20,400 and $3,500
Family with 5 children, $23,100 and $3,500
Family with 6 children, $25,800 and $3,500
Family with 7 children, $27,900 and $3,500
Family with 8 children, $30,420 and $3,500
• *General*: Legal Aid SK provides general summary advice to anyone (up to discretion of each office as to whether they offer these services).
• *Custody*: Three types of in-custody service are offered to any client regardless of financial situation: phone service, duty counsel advice, and duty counsel service.
• Legal aid is free to individuals who fall within the eligibility guidelines.
• In general clients are eligible if they have no income, receive social assistance benefits, or their net income is comparable with social assistance benefits.
• If an individual's financial circumstances are slightly over the guidelines, they may be required to contribute to the costs for legal aid assistance.
Financial eligibility is based on the number of adults and youth and annual net household income:
1 adult, $21,600
2 adults, $26,400
For every additional adult, add $5,400
1 adult, 1 youth, $25,200
1 adult, 2 youth, $28,800
1 adult, 3 youth, $32,400 |

(Continued)

Table A.1. (Continued)

Provinces	Areas of covered by legal aid plan	Eligibility*	Other free or low-cost legal resources
		For every additional youth, add $3,600 2 adults, 1 youth, $30,000 2 adults, 2 youth, $33,600 2 adults, 3 youth, $37,200 For every additional youth add $3,600	

* For further information about eligibility in each province and territory, see the Government of Canada's resource "Legal Aid Eligibility and Coverage in Canada," available at https://www.justice.gc.ca/eng/rp-pr/csj-sjc/jsp-sjp/rr03_la5-rr03_aj5/index.html.

Appendix 2: HELPS Brain Injury Screening Tool

Consumer Information: _______________________________________

____

____

Agency/Screener's Information: ________________________________

____

____

H Have you ever **Hit** your **Head** or been **Hit** on the **Head**? ☐ Yes ☐ No

Note: Prompt client to think about all incidents that may have occurred at any age, even those that did not seem serious: vehicle accidents, falls, assault, abuse, sports, etc. Screen for domestic violence and child abuse, and also for service related injuries. A TBI can also occur from violent shaking of the head, such as being shaken as a baby or child.

E Were you ever seen in the **Emergency** room, hospital, or by a doctor because of an injury to your head?   ☐ Yes ☐ No

Note: Many people are seen for treatment. However, there are those who cannot afford treatment, or who do not think they require medical attention.

L Did you ever **Lose** consciousness or experience a period of being dazed and confused because of an injury to your head?   ☐ Yes ☐ No

Note: People with TBI may not lose consciousness but experience an "alteration of consciousness." This may include feeling dazed, confused, or disoriented at the time of the injury, or being unable to remember the events surrounding the injury.

P Do you experience any of these **P**roblems in your daily life since you hit your head?   ☐ Yes   ☐ No

Note: Ask your client if s/he experiences any of the following problems, and ask when the problem presented. You are looking for a combination of two or more problems that were not present prior to the injury.

☐ headaches	☐ difficulty reading, writing, calculating
☐ dizziness	☐ poor problem solving
☐ anxiety	☐ difficulty performing your job/school work
☐ depression	☐ change in relationships with others
☐ difficulty concentrating	☐ poor judgment (being fired from job,
☐ difficulty remembering	arrests, fights)

S Any significant **S**icknesses?   ☐ Yes   ☐ No

Note: Traumatic brain injury implies a physical blow to the head, but acquired brain injury may also be caused by medical conditions, such as: brain tumour, meningitis, West Nile virus, stroke, seizures. Also screen for instances of oxygen deprivation such as following a heart attack, carbon monoxide poisoning, near drowning, or near suffocation.

Scoring the HELPS Screening Tool

A HELPS screening is considered positive for a *possible* TBI when the following 3 items are identified:

1) An event that could have caused a brain injury (yes to H, E **or** S), **and**
2) A period of loss of consciousness or altered consciousness after the injury or another indication that the injury was severe (yes to L or E), **and**
3) The presence of two or more chronic problems listed under P that were not present before the injury.

Note:
- A positive screening is **not sufficient to diagnose TBI** as the reason for current symptoms and difficulties – other possible causes may need to be ruled out
- **Some individuals could present exceptions** to the screening results, such as people who do have TBI-related problems but answered "no" to some questions
- Consider positive responses within the context of the person's self-report and documentation of altered behavioural and/or cognitive functioning

Appendix 3: Sample Advocacy Letter for Supported Decision-Making

---

To: Pat's family members, decision-making supporters, and Group Home Director

From: Dr. X, Pat's family physician (or other member of Pat's family health team)

Re: Pat's participation in decisions about receiving a vaccine to prevent COVID-19

I am writing to advocate for promoting Pat's involvement in the decision regarding his receiving a COVID-19 vaccine and to arrange to discuss the possibility of him visiting family and friends while he is not yet vaccinated.

Pat is a 33-year-old single male who has an intellectual and developmental disability in the moderate range (mental age equivalent to 5–7 years old). He is otherwise healthy.

Due to the risk to his health of being infected by the COVID-19 virus, and to the health of others in his group home, I understand that he is unable to visit in person with family or friends until after he is vaccinated against COVID-19. I am aware that Pat highly values such interactions.

I also appreciate that Pat is generally averse to receiving injections of any kind (possibly due to past trauma associated with such medical procedures). We hope, however, that with supports, he might be willing to accept a COVID-19 vaccine if it is provided in a way that he could tolerate and accept.

I would like to arrange a time for me, and possibly other members of Pat's family health team, to meet with Pat, involved family members, his decision-making supporter(s), and the director of his group home regarding a proposed approach to supporting his decision-making. This supported decision-making approach depends on a shared commitment to promoting Pat's involvement in this decision as much as possible while also identifying and reducing possible risks of this approach.[1]

I would also like to discuss the possibility that Pat does not, in the end, consent to receiving the COVID-19 vaccine or that, despite best efforts, he resists receiving the vaccine at the time of the procedure, in which case it would not be given. Given the significant burden on Pat of the group home's policy regarding being vaccinated against COVID-19 as a condition of visiting family and friends, could we explore other ways of minimizing the health risks to Pat and others of being infected by the COVID-19 virus so that such visits, which are important to his well-being, could occur even while he has not yet been vaccinated?

Sincerely, Dr. X

---

1 See chapter 13 for details regarding this approach.

Glossary

Note that this glossary relates to terms found throughout this text.

adverse childhood events (ACEs) – traumatic childhood events, such
as abuse, negligence, or household dysfunction, that can affect the
child's current health as well as future adult health

health and justice partnerships – the more internationally accepted
term to describe partnerships that "train and partner health, social
and legal service providers to explicitly identify, prevent and
respond to violations of legal rights that harm health and well-
being."[1(pp. 332–3)] *Medical–legal partnerships* was the term used in the
United States to describe similar partnerships, and it continues to
be widely in used in that context. In this text, we have tried to use
the term *health and justice partnerships* when not discussing U.S.
partnerships specifically.

Jordan's Principle – Jordan's Principle was named in response to
the death of five-year-old Jordan River Anderson, a child from
Norway Cree Nation who had a diagnosis of Carey-Fineman-
Ziter syndrome. Jordan died in 2005 after spending all five years
of his life in hospital as a result of a dispute between federal and
provincial authorities over responsibility for funding resources at
home. Jordan's Principle holds that First Nations children should
not be denied access to public services while governments fight
over who should pay. To ensure substantive equality, this can also
include services that are not ordinarily available to other children.

legal professional – Note from the editors: we have left this term
intentionally broad throughout the text. We chose a term that would
include, but go beyond, lawyers. We also chose this term for its
general application across Canada, given the practical reality that

bigger cities will of course have more legal professional options than smaller centres. The following notes supplement the chapters:

- Generally, low-income patients who cannot afford to pay a lawyer privately, unless a private law firm agrees to assist pro bono, might seek help from a non-profit community-based legal aid or advocacy organization. In the case of Ontario, there are 72 such clinics. Legal aid staff offices or university law student clinics are also a place to find support.

- For certain issues such as refugee and immigration matters, an authorized representative should be found. Lawyers or immigration consultants can be authorized representatives, as can paralegals in Ontario and notaires in Quebec.

- New rules brought in by the College of Immigration and Citizenship Consultants also require those who practice at the Immigration and Refugee Board to complete additional training through the college. Less ideal but practical, unpaid family members, friends, and community workers can act as representatives in certain situations.

Non-Insured Health Benefits (NIHB) – a federal health insurance program available to residents of Canada and one of the following: a registered Indian according to the *Indian Act*, an Inuk recognized by one of the Inuit Land Claim organizations, or an infant younger than age 18 months whose parent is an eligible client. In most provincial jurisdictions, NIHB navigators are located in various organizations, such as the Chiefs of Ontario, that can provide assistance in navigating benefits through NIHB

primary care – Primary care is the first point of consultation for all patients in the health care system. For the purposes of this text, *primary care* is used interchangeably with *primary health care*. Primary care often refers to check-ups, preventive care, and the treatment of common ailments, and it is usually provided at a clinic but can also include care provided in emergency departments. In contrast, secondary care often involves the referral of a patient to a specialist at a hospital for a closer assessment or treatment. Tertiary and quaternary care represent the most advanced form of health care and may include complex surgery, such as neurosurgery, cardiac surgery, plastic surgery, and transplantation, as well as neonatology, psychiatry, cancer care, intensive care, palliative care, and many other complex medical and surgical interventions.

primary health care provider – anybody who provides primary care, including physicians, nurses, nurse practitioners, social workers, pharmacists, dieticians, physiotherapists, income security health promoters, system navigators, and so forth. Team-based primary care has expanded the types of professionals involved in primary care. Primary health care providers can also be referred to as *clinicians*.

NOTE

1 Tobin-Tyler E, Boyd-Caine T, Genn H, et al. Health justice partnerships: an international comparison of approaches to employing law to promote prevention and health equity. J Law Med Ethics. 2023;51(2):332–43.

Contributors

Jamie Ahn is an associate at J K Hannaford Barristers. She earned her Juris Doctor from the University of Toronto, Faculty of Law, in 2022 and was called to the Ontario Bar in 2023. During her legal studies, Jamie was actively involved with the Health Justice Program at St. Michael's Hospital through Pro Bono Students Canada.

Gordon Arbess is a staff family physician in the St. Michael's Hospital Family Health Team (SMH FHT) and is on faculty in the Department of Family and Community Medicine at the University of Toronto. He is the clinical director of the HIV Program at the SMH FHT and is on staff at Casey House Hospital.

Anu Bakshi is a staff lawyer at the Income Security Advocacy Centre. She is one of the founders of the South Asian Legal Clinic of Ontario. Her focus is health justice and income benefits for vulnerable populations.

Michaela Beder is a psychiatrist at St. Michael's Hospital, the director of mental health and substance use care with Inner City Health Associates, and an assistant professor at the University of Toronto. Michaela is also a community organizer working together with allies at Health Providers Against Poverty and the Healthcare for All Coalition.

Christa Big Canoe is a First Nations woman, mother, and lawyer. She comes from Georgina Island First Nation, an Anishinabek community. Christa was policy counsel for Legal Aid Ontario and the lead on the organization's province-wide Aboriginal Justice Strategy before becoming Aboriginal Legal Services's (ALS's) legal director in 2011. In 2017 Christa took a two-and-a-half-year leave of absence so that she could be senior and then lead counsel for the National Inquiry into Missing and Murdered Indigenous Women and Girls before returning to ALS. She has been before all levels of court in Canada and provides inquest representation for Indigenous families.

Beth Bilson is Professor Emerita in Law and Legal Counsel at the University of Saskatchewan. She has served as dean in the Colleges of Law and Education and as university secretary. She has chaired the Saskatchewan Labour Relations Board, served as chair of the federal government Pay Equity Task Force, and chaired equity committees of the Canadian Bar Association at the provincial and national levels.

Gary Bloch is a family physician with St. Michael's Hospital Academic Family Health Team and Inner City Health Associates and an associate professor with the University of Toronto. His innovative program development, education, research, and advocacy focus on the role of primary care in addressing social determinants of health and health inequities.

Andrew Bond is the senior vice president and medical director at Green-Shield, Canada's only national non-profit health and benefits provider. Before his work at GreenShield, he was the executive medical officer at Inner City Health Associates in Toronto, one of the largest community medical organizations in Canada. Dr. Bond continues to practice as a primary care physician and is a faculty member of the Department of Family and Community Medicine at the Temerty Faculty of Medicine, University of Toronto. Originally from Winnipeg, Dr. Bond completed his undergraduate training at Queen's University, his MD at the University of Ottawa, postgraduate specialty training in Family Medicine at the University of Toronto, and a Master of Health Administration from the Johnson Shoyama Graduate School of Public Policy at the Universities of Saskatchewan and Regina. He is currently completing a Master of Business Administration at the Massachusetts Institute of Technology.

Dilan Brar is a graduate of the University of Toronto Faculty of Law. His passion for health care and the law led him to complete his Articling Term at the Centre for Addiction and Mental Health, Canada's largest mental health teaching hospital.

Christine Carthew is a Juris Doctor candidate at Osgoode Hall Law School at York University in Toronto, Ontario, Canada. She is deeply committed to public health and health equity and interested in exploring the role of law in advancing these aims. She earned her Master of Public Health at the University of Toronto in 2017.

Lee Ann Chapman was the pro bono Ontario lawyer at SickKids until her retirement in 2023. She is the originating lawyer at SickKids Family Legal Health Program, established in 2009, Canada's first medical–legal partnership, a free legal service to patients and families at Sick-Kids, addressing legal impediments to child health and recognized by Accreditation Canada as an innovative Leading Practice in health care. She is a member, and former vice chair, of the Canadian Coalition on the Rights of the Child, where she made submissions to the UN Committee on the Rights of the Child on shortfalls pertaining to child health in Canada. Before coming to SickKids, she was a lawyer at Justice for Children and Youth, where she represented young people on legal matters at all levels of courts and tribunals.

Naheed Dosani is a palliative care physician and health justice advocate dedicated to advancing equitable access to health care for structurally vulnerable populations, including those experiencing homelessness. He is the founder and lead of the Palliative Education and Care for the Homeless Program at Inner City Health Associates, serves as the medical director of Kensington Hospice (at Kensington Health), and works as a palliative care physician at St. Michael's Hospital (at Unity Health Toronto). In addition to his clinical work, he is a health equity expert advisor at the Canadian Partnership Against Cancer and Health Equity Lead at Kensington Health. Naheed is an assistant professor in the Department of Family and Community Medicine at the University of Toronto and contributes to research as an investigator with the MAP Centre for Urban Health Solutions at St. Michael's Hospital's Li Ka Shing Knowledge Institute. His leadership extends to serving on the Board of Directors for the Canadian Medical Association.

Kathleen Doukas is a family physician at St Michael's Hospital in Toronto. She completed medical school at McMaster University and went on to do residency at the University of Toronto, after which she pursued a fellowship in low-risk obstetrics and women's health. She holds a MScCH in health practitioner teacher education and has served as education lead at Inner City Health Associates. She is currently the undergraduate program director at St Michael's Hospital. She is a facilitator for EPOCH (Effective Prescribing of Opioids for Chronic Pain). Her clinical interests include adolescent medicine, mental health, and women's health.

Kate Forget is a member of Matachewan First Nation and grew up in New Liskeard, Ontario. She joined the Indigenous Justice Division (IJD) in 2016 to be on the MMIWG Team and represent Ontario at the National Inquiry into Missing and Murdered Indigenous Women and Girls. During this period, Kate was also seconded to the Office of the Independent Police Review Director's systemic review of the Thunder Bay Police Service. Kate has acted as inquest counsel on multiple inquests involving the deaths of Indigenous people. In 2021, she was seconded to the Office of the Chief Coroner (OCC) to act as inquest counsel and is on the OCC's Law Enforcement Team that is working on policing-related inquests. Before joining IJD, she worked as duty counsel in London, Ontario. Kate was a Gladue caseworker at Aboriginal Legal Services before and throughout law school. She is a proud Auntie.

Diana Gallego is a Colombian-trained lawyer with experience in advocacy, human rights, and social justice. In 2002, Diana was forced to flee Colombia with her husband and son. This experience shaped a new commitment and led her to work with immigrants and refugees. Diana obtained a diploma in community work from George Brown College in Toronto. She is a part-time professor in the Centre for Community Services at George Brown College. Diana Joined the FCJ Refugee Centre in 2015 and is now its senior director. Diana was elected in fall 2023 as the president of the Canadian Council for Refugees (CCR). She also serves on the Inland Protection steering committee of the CCR, where the social and economic integration of refugees and family reunification are two of the main focuses of her advocacy.

Sarah Gander is a social paediatrician in Saint John, New Brunswick, and founder of New Brunswick Social Pediatrics, a clinical, research, and advocacy not-for-profit aimed at mitigating and preventing adverse childhood experiences in New Brunswick. Dr Gander is an associate professor at Dalhousie University and an assistant professor at Memorial University of Newfoundland.

Ritika Goel completed medical school at McMaster University and a family medicine residency at St. Michael's Hospital and has a Master of Public Health from Johns Hopkins University's School of Public Health. She has served as both the lead physician at the Inner City Family Health Team and the population health lead for Inner City Health Associates (ICHA). Her clinical work with ICHA is based at Sistering, a women's drop-in centre, and FCJ Refugee Centre, working with uninsured migrants. She is a board member of the Scarborough Community Volunteer Clinic for the Uninsured and Canadian Doctors for Medicare and co-chair of the Ontario College of Family Physicians' Poverty and

Health Committee. Ritika has been involved in health-related activism since medical school. She is currently part of the steering committee for the OHIP for All campaign, as well as the Decent Work and Health Network.

John Heng serves as chair of the Department of Philosophy at King's University College, Western University, London, Ontario, and also teaches ethics in the Department of Thanatology and the Department of Disability Studies. He partakes in the Ethics Special Interest Research Group of the International Association for the Scientific Study of Intellectual and Developmental Disabilities.

Promise Holmes Skinner is a criminal lawyer and adjunct professor in the University of Toronto's Faculty of Law and Centre for Criminology and Sociolegal Studies. Having overcome personal experiences of traumatic brain injury, Promise has argued at the Supreme Court of Canada and the Ontario Court of Appeal, contributing to major changes to Canadian law.

Paula Hutchinson, PhD, is a credentialed evaluator and researcher working in Kjipuktuk, Mi'kma'ki territory (Halifax, Nova Scotia), with Horizons Community Development Associates and Dalhousie University. She has been involved in several rights-based projects in Canada; a public review of Nova Scotia's *Adult Capacity and Decision-Making Act*; Exploring Experiences of COVID-19 Restrictions with People First Nova Scotia; My Home, My Rights with self-advocate researchers; and All about Inclusion: Expanding Capacity with Visual Aids for Supported Decision-Making. She also brings to her work practical insights and lived experience as a parent of a young man with autism spectrum disorder.

Caitlyn E. Kasper (deceased 2024) was originally from Chippewas of Georgina Island First Nation in the land now known as Ontario and worked as an Indigenous senior staff lawyer with Aboriginal Legal Services in Toronto. Her contributions to this work and many other health justice initiatives leave a powerful legacy. She is deeply missed.

Melanie Laking (she/her) is Ojibwe with European ancestry and a member of Shawanaga First Nation. Melanie holds a Master of Social Work degree from the University of Toronto and an Honours Bachelor of Arts degree, specializing in Indigenous studies. She is a registered social worker with the Ontario College of Social Workers and Social Service Workers and a member of the Ontario Association of Social Workers.

Sara Mainville is a partner at JFK Law and is a member of the Ontario bar (2005) and the British Columbia bar (2022) with specific matter approvals to practice in Nunavut and Quebec. Sara has a management and public administration degree (Lethbridge) and a Bachelor of Laws from Queen's University. She has a LLM from the University of Toronto, an advanced negotiations certificate from Harvard University, and a certificate in entertainment law from Osgoode Professional Development.

Edgar-Andre Montigny completed his doctorate in Canadian history in 1993 and spent several years teaching history and Canadian studies before he decided to study law at the University of Toronto Faculty of Law, graduating in 2003. He was a staff lawyer at ARCH Disability Law Centre. He served on the Advisory Board that helped produce the Law Commission of Ontario's report on legal capacity, decision-making and guardianship in Ontario. In 2017 Ed established his own practice to focus on issues of consent, capacity, and substitute decision-making and estate issues. Recently, he merged his practice to become Montigny Munk Law. He volunteers with St. Michael's Hospital's Academic Family Health Team's Health Justice Program, helping to prepare wills and power-of-attorney documents for low-income persons. Ed has been an adjudicator with the Toronto Licensing Tribunal since 2019. In 2022 he was appointed as a part-time member of the Ontario Animal Care Review Board.

Luis Alberto Mata is immigration specialist head of AMIGRAR Immigration Consulting. He has been a settlement worker and coordinator of an anti-human-trafficking program for migrant workers and a member of the Migrant Rights Network and the Collaborative Network to End Exploitation. He was co-chair of the Immigration Settlement Working Group of the Canadian Council for Refugees and is former chair of the Toronto Counter Human Trafficking Network. Luis has a MA in human rights and multiculturalism. He is committed to social justice and has lectured and written on human rights and the origins of the Colombian conflict.

Flora I. Matheson is the Endowed Chair in Homelessness, Housing, and Health at St. Michael's Hospital. She leads the Justice and Equity Lab at MAP Centre for Urban Health Solutions and as a sociologist builds community-embedded solutions to reduce social and health inequities for people experiencing problem gambling and imprisonment.

Devan Nambiar, MSc, is an education and training specialist on 2SLG-BTQ+ health and HIV prevention, testing, and care for organizations, clinicians, and allied health professionals. He also has a consultancy, GHIS.CA. He draws from more than 30 years of HIV activism, advocacy, and service. His expertise includes developing and leading education and training initiatives to improve queer and trans health, directed to social service agencies and health care providers. Devan serves on various committees, including as community co-lead on cures and immunotherapies at the Canadian Institutes of Health Research Canadian HIV/AIDS & STBBI Clinical Trials Network, Community Liaison Subcommittee of the Scientific Program Committee at Conference on Retrovirus and Opportunistic Infections, Patient Advisory Committee at the Canadian Drug Agency, and Community Advisory at Ontario Caregiver Organization. He is involved in six research studies on people living with HIV, anal cancer, and human papilloma virus; 2SLG-BTQ Health Hub; mpox; and prophylactic doxycycline use among gay, bisexual, and other men who have sex with men.

Robin Nobleman is a staff lawyer at the Income Security Advocacy Centre (ISAC). Before joining ISAC, Robin was a staff lawyer at the HIV & AIDS Legal Clinic Ontario, where she represented individual clients living with HIV at courts and tribunals and argued interventions at all levels of court. Robin holds a master's degree in health, community, and development from the London School of Economics and teaches public health law as an adjunct professor at the University of Toronto.

Ryan Peck has been the executive director of the HIV & AIDS Legal Clinic Ontario since 2007. He has worked as a staff lawyer at the Advocacy Centre for the Elderly and in the Tenant Duty Counsel Program at the Advocacy Centre for Tenants Ontario. Ryan also served as criminal duty counsel at Toronto's Old City Hall.

Mercedes Perez is a lawyer and managing partner at Perez Procope Leinveer LLP in Toronto, Ontario. She was called to the bar in 2003 after receiving her law degree from McGill University. She also completed a Bachelor of Arts at the University of Toronto and a Master of Arts at the University of Chicago. Mercedes has represented clients before a range of administrative tribunals and at all levels of court in Ontario, the Federal Court, and the Supreme Court of Canada. Her practice is varied but with a heavy focus on mental health, capacity, *Charter* and disability rights, and victim representation in criminal matters. She is an adjunct professor at Osgoode Hall Law School, where she co-instructs the law and psychiatry course.

Andrew Pinto is the founder and director of the Upstream Lab, a research team focused on tackling social determinants of health, population health management, and using data science to enable proactive care. He holds the Canadian Institutes of Health Research (CIHR) Applied Public Health Chair in Upstream Prevention. He is a public health and preventive medicine specialist and family physician at St. Michael's Hospital in Toronto and an associate professor at the University of Toronto. He is the associate director for clinical research at the University of Toronto Practice-Based Research Network, the lead for clinical research of Ontario's POPLAR network, and the founder of the Canadian Primary Care Trials Network. He serves on the Institute Advisory Board of CIHR's Institute for Population and Public Health, is an adjunct scientist at the Institute for Work and Health, and an honorary senior lecturer at St. Andrews University in Scotland.

Nabila F. Qureshi is a staff lawyer at the Income Security Advocacy Centre, a specialty legal clinic in Toronto funded by Legal Aid Ontario. She works on test cases and appeals relating to low-wage and precarious workers' rights, poverty and human rights law, and various income security benefit programs. Nabila is passionate about improving the lives of vulnerable workers and has argued before various courts, including the Ontario Court of Appeal and the Supreme Court of Canada.

Debbie Rachlis is an immigration and refugee lawyer at Debbie Rachlis Law. She graduated from Osgoode Hall Law School in 2015 and was called to the bar in Ontario in 2015. Debbie represents clients in applications to Immigration, Refugees and Citizenship Canada and Canada Border Services Agency, before all divisions of the Immigration and Refugee Board, and before the Federal Court of Canada. She has also represented interveners at the Federal Court and the Supreme Court of Canada. Debbie is a former staff lawyer at the HIV & AIDS Legal Clinic Ontario.

Vanessa Redditt is a staff family physician at the Crossroads Clinic. Vanessa is interested in enhancing the health of marginalized individuals and communities through clinical care, health system improvement, and tackling social inequities. She is a lecturer at the University of Toronto's Department of Family and Community

Medicine (DFCM) and Dalla Lana School of Public Health. Her current research focuses on better understanding the health of newly arrived refugees and their experiences in the health care system, with a goal of improving clinical practices, care delivery models, and social services to better support this population. She also serves on the board of directors of Sojourn House refugee shelter, on the steering committee of the Together Project refugee social integration program, and on the Social Accountability Committee at the DFCM. Vanessa has also previously worked in Rwanda with Partners in Health and the Ministry of Health in primary care system strengthening and health worker training.

Benjamin Ries, BA, JD, LLM, is executive director of South Etobicoke Community Legal Services, a non-profit community legal clinic serving low-income residents of Toronto's far west end. He leads a small team of legal professionals, staff, and students providing advice and representation in the areas of housing, social assistance, employment, and immigration. Formerly the supervising lawyer for housing law at Downtown Legal Services from 2014 through 2022, Ben recently served as president of the Association for Canadian Clinical Legal Education and is almost as passionate about teaching and mentoring students as he is about poverty lawyering.

Rami Shoucri, MD, LLM, JD, is a family physician at the St. Michael's Academic Family Health Team in Toronto and was the Clinical Champion for the Health Justice Program between 2016 and 2024, a physician member for the Consent and Capacity Board of Ontario since 2019, and a board member for Community Legal Education of Ontario since 2021, elected chair in 2023.

Suzanne Shoush is a First Nations/Black physician, mother, and advocate who lives and works in Toronto's downtown core where she has spent more than a decade working in the city's shelter systems. She is the inaugural director of the Indigenous Health Program for Inner City Health Associates, where she is the lead physician for community and culture-based, trauma-informed, culturally safe, and low-barrier comprehensive primary care clinics, including Nameres, Auduzhe Mino Nesewinong, Ode'I min, the Call Auntie Clinic, and the Indigenous Health Organization Outreach Program. She is also the Indigenous health faculty lead for the Department of Family and Community Medicine with the University of Toronto Faculty of Medicine.

Louise Simbandumwe is co-director at SEED Winnipeg and played a lead role in working with partner organizations to develop SEED's financial empowerment programs. A former refugee, Louise is passionate about human rights and social justice. Her volunteer commitments include the Immigration Winnipeg Partnership Council and the Immigration Matters in Canada Coalition. She also served on the advisory committee for Manitoba's poverty reduction strategy and the Ministerial advisory committee for Canada's first poverty reduction strategy. Louise holds a Bachelor' of Commerce from the University of Saskatchewan and a Master of Comparative Social Research from Oxford University, where she studied as a Rhodes Scholar.

Jennifer Stone is the executive director of Neighbourhood Legal Services (NLS) and manager of the Health Justice Program. She was NLS's staff immigration lawyer from 2011 to 2018. Before joining NLS she co-founded the Hong Kong Refugee Advice Centre (now Justice Centre HK), which advocates for the rights of refugee claimants and other migrants in the Hong Kong Special Administrative Region. Until November 2018 she had spent four years on the Executive Committee of the Canadian Council for Refugees (CCR), and from 2018 to 2024 she co-chaired the CCR's Legal Affairs Committee. Jennifer is an adjunct professor at the University of Toronto's Faculty of Law, supervising health law externs and co-teaching public health law.

William F. Sullivan, MD, PhD, CCFP, FCFP, serves as the Joseph P. Kennedy Senior Chair in Bioethics, Kennedy Institute of Ethics, Georgetown University. He brings to this position qualifications and experience in family medicine and a doctorate in philosophy (bioethics). Before this appointment, he was professor in the Department of Family and Community Medicine at the University of Toronto. In his clinical and bioethical work, Dr. Sullivan focuses on promoting ethical primary health care and public health care of people with intellectual and developmental disabilities. He is also interested in developing methods for effective collaborative research on complex clinical and public health care ethical questions.

Douglas Varrette is an Algonquin Anishinaabe lawyer at Mississauga Community Legal Services (MCLS) and currently practices in housing and social assistance. He serves as the legal case coordinator for income maintenance at MCLS and, before joining MCLS in 2022, he worked at Aboriginal Legal Services as a staff lawyer. He recently became a member of the provincial inter-clinic Steering Committee on Social Assistance.

Anita Volikis is a partner at J K Hannaford Barristers. She graduated from the University of Toronto with her Bachelor of Laws in 1999 and was called to the bar of Ontario in 2001. Anita represents and advises clients on all aspects of separation and divorce and has extensive experience dealing with complex financial and parenting issues. She has appeared in all levels of court in Ontario. She was a long-standing co-author of *The Annotated Ontario Children's Law Reform Act* and served as associate editor of *Evidence in Family Law* for many years.

Index

accommodate, duty to, 42–50,
112–13, 125, 130, 485; children,
378, 380–2, 393; failure to
accommodate, 125–6, 395; health
care provider responsibilities,
49–50, 91–2, 125, 129–31, 217–
18, 315–17, 378–83, 399–400;
immigrants, 216–8; individuals
with disabilities, 45–50, 105, 112,
460, 466, 485; individuals living
with HIV/AIDS, 314–17, 321–2
adverse childhood experiences
(ACEs), 244, 372
affidavits, expert medical opinion, 95–6
Anishinaabe wheel, 59–60

barriers to income security, 147–50;
access to identification, 150–2;
failure to file taxes, 152–3; precarious
immigration status, 153–4
Beardon, S., 483
Benai, Elder Benson, 58
best interests of child, 219, 241, 247,
253–60, 263-4, 281, 374–6, 380, 393
Bigby, C., 462, 468–9
Blackstock, Cindy, 385
Blumenthal-Barby, J., 461
Borrows, John: *Revitalizing
Anishinaabe Inaakonigewin (Law)*, 59

Bryce, Peter: Bryce Report, 65
burial costs, 428, 431–2, 434, 441, 443

Canada Child Benefit (CCB) program,
119, 142–4, 148t, 149–50, 163t, 397
capacity, decision-making, 255, 373–7,
409–11, 414, 418–23, 432, 454, 457–61,
467–8; tools to promote, 467–70
Charter of Rights and Freedoms,
Canadian, 31–3, 35–44, 62, 196,
292, 374, 380, 454, 457, 473; and
housing, 93–5, 97–8
children's rights, 373–7; and
immigration status, 219, 392–4;
duty to accommodate, 378, 380–2,
393; to child support, 245–6; to
consent, 255, 373–7, 379; to
education, 380–3; to safety and
protection, 257–9, 377–9; under
Youth Criminal Justice Act, 383–4
citizenship status, 188–9, 196–8,
204t, 210t, 212t, 220; application
documentation, 220–1; pathways
to, 188–9
class action suits, housing, 96
common law vs. civil law, 34–5, 38,
82–4, 311, 318, 321, 324
consent, 22–5, 90, 183–4, 215, 262,
318, 322–7, 334, 373–6, 383, 411,

consent (*continued*)
414, 418–20, 457–61, 466; and
capacity, 411, 418–21, 457–9; and
OCL, 257; lock box, 323; to disclose
child's medical information, 254–6
Consent and Capacity Board, 376–7,
421, 457
Constitution, Canadian, 30–4, 36–8,
41, 44, 62, 290–1, 374, 387, 457
Cook, S., 464
criminal-legal system, 290–3, 296;
bail, 292–3; parole, 299–300;
probation, 300–1; health care
provider role, 291, 293–6, 298–9,
301; sentencing, 296–9; *Youth
Criminal Justice Act*, 383–4
cultural competency/safety, 70–2,
137, 183

Dauvergne, Catherine, 186, 196
*Decision Making in Health Care
of Adults with Intellectual and
Developmental Disabilities:
Promoting Capabilities*, 470
digital divide, 51, 157
disabilities, individuals with, 44,
90–1, 145–6, 182–3, 196, 313–14, 317,
349, 454. *See also* intellectual and
developmental disabilities (IDD),
individuals with; children, 380–3,
397–8, 400; criminal-legal system,
286; discrimination, 125–6, 287,
313–15, 472; duty to accommodate,
45–50, 105, 112, 314, 460, 466, 485;
Henson trust, 398; homelessness,
80; immigration issues, 349; income
support/benefits, 125, 143, 145–7,
148f, 156, 158, 160, 162–70, 172,
248, 342–4t, 415, 434–5, 437; legal
definition of disability, 165t; poverty,
149t, 150, 156–7; SDOHs, 466–7, 472t

disclosure of medical information,
21–4, 130, 190, 261, 323–4, 390,
482; child's medical information,
254–6, 374–5; HIV/AIDS status,
315, 318–35, 348–9; legislation,
254–6, 318–21, 323, 383; lock box,
323; remedies for breach, 326–8
discrimination, 32, 35–6, 42–5, 62,
106; definition, 43, 313; HIV/
AIDS status, 312–15, 317–18,
330–1, 350–1; Indigenous Peoples,
38–40, 56, 61–2, 64, 66t, 67–8, 71–2,
111–12, 182–4, 385–6; individuals
with disabilities, 125–6, 287, 313–
15, 472; migrants, 202, 208, 212t,
345, 350–1; race-based, 310–11;
workplace, 109–18, 122–4
divorce/separation, 238–45, 250, 252,
493t, 496t; child support, 240–2,
245–8, 250, 267t, 492–3t, 497t;
Divorce Act, 259–60; housing security,
251–2; parenting, 240–1, 253–9, 261,
264–5, 267t; health care provider role,
242–4; spousal support, 240–1, 245,
248–50, 267t, 490t, 492t
Douglas, J., 462, 468–9

Echaquan, Joyce, 68–9
Emanuel deliberative model, 455–7
Emanuel, Linda L., 456
Emanuel, Ezekiel J., 456
end-of-life planning, 406–9; health
care provider role, 407–9
exclusive possession orders, 263–4
executors/estate trustees, 406–7,
425–7, 432, 434–6, 438, 443–5; role
of, 439–42

family reunification, 189f, 193, 195,
215, 218
Friedman, C., 467

Gladue decision, 9–10, 297–8, 489t
government-assisted refugees (GARs),
    145, 191, 195, 198, 201t, 210t, 348
guardians, court-appointed, 414–19,
    458, 463

harassment, 41, 43, 87t, 89, 106, 243,
    260, 389; in workplace, 109–10,
    113, 115, 118t, 122–4, 126–7
health and justice partnerships (HJPs),
    6, 18–20, 22, 24–6, 78, 88–90, 92, 96–9,
    172, 372–3; benefits of, 480, 482–6
Health Justice Program, 480–3
HIV/AIDs, individuals living with,
    310–12; access to medication, 337–
    44, 352; criminal-legal system, 286,
    321, 328–34; disclosure of status,
    315, 318–35, 348–9; discrimination,
    312–15, 317–18, 330–1, 350–1; duty
    to accommodate, 314–17, 321–2;
    impact on immigration issues,
    345–53; health care provider role,
    322, 333–4; testing, reporting
    and contact tracing, 334–5; travel
    outside Canada, 351–2
Hole, R., 464
homelessness, 80–3, 88, 93f, 96–9,
    283, 286, 377, 389, 406–7
housing law, 82–9; homelessness,
    94–5; legal assistance, 86–9
housing, transitional, 83f, 93f
human rights commissions, 41–2, 93,
    317, 381, 395; Canadian (CHRC),
    41–2, 114t; provincial/territorial,
    42, 114–15t, 291, 380–1
human rights legislation, 39–45,
    52, 62, 196, 312–14, 327, 380,
    395, 460; housing related, 84,
    91, 94; immigration related, 217;
    influence of international law,
    35–7, 84, 93–4, 454; workplace

related, 105, 107, 109–15, 125–7,
    129, 353
humanitarian and compassionate
    applications, 188–90, 209, 345–7,
    350, 393; medical documentation,
    218–19, 400

identification of issues, 14–17, 128–9
iHELP (Income, Housing,
    Employment and education,
    Legal status, Personal and family
    stability), 16, 479
immigration and refugee law, 35, 51,
    188, 191, 196, 345–53, 488–9t, 494t,
    496t; family sponsorship, 349;
    health care provider role, 347–9;
    medical examination, 348–9;
    medical inadmissibility, 345–8
immigration categories, 122, 188–97.
    See also individual categories
immigration detention, 190, 203,
    209–12, 221, 223–4
immigration status, 35, 153–4,
    189f, 194–6, 220, 392–3; access to
    education, 203–7; access to health
    care, 197–201, 204f, 213–15, 220,
    223–4, 338, 348–9, 352–3, 392–3;
    access to identification documents,
    150–1; criminal-legal system,
    189t, 190, 209–12; discrimination,
    202, 208, 212t, 345, 350–1;
    duty to accommodate, 216–8;
    employment, 105–6, 153–4, 208–10;
    income/poverty, 145, 153–4, 157t,
    159, 208–10; personal safety, 202–4,
    214, 260; program availability, 145,
    148t, 154, 186, 210t; SDOHs, 186,
    188, 196–8, 209, 214
Inaakonigewin (Anishinaabe law), 58–9
income security, 18, 139, 142–5,
    172–4; barriers to, 147–50, 154–5;

income security (*continued*)
  health care provider role, 161–71,
    174; screening for, 140–2
income supports/benefits, 15–16, 98,
  127, 138–9, 142–50, 341–3t, 488t;
  barriers to, 157–60, 174; Canada
  Child Benefit (CCB) program,
  119, 142–4, 148t, 149–50, 163t, 397;
  Canada Pension Plan (CPP), 125,
  127, 144, 146, 148–9, 154, 160, 163–5,
  441, 493t; community organizations,
  172–4; disability benefits, 125, 143,
  145–7, 148f, 156, 158, 160, 162–70,
  172, 248, 342–4t, 415, 434–5, 437;
  Employment Insurance (EI), 107, 115,
  119–20, 127–8, 146, 148f, 159, 165t,
  208, 210t, 395–6; for life transitions,
  147–8, 160; health care provider role,
  161–72, 174; Indigenous support
  programs, 144, 148t, 156; refugee/
  new immigrant support programs,
  145, 148t, 154, 186, 208, 210t; seniors'
  benefits, 144, 147–9, 154, 163t, 340–3t;
  social assistance supplements, 145,
  148t; student benefits, 146–8
Indigenous Peoples, 9–10, 144, 148t,
  155–7, 450–2; child welfare, 39, 66t,
  144–5, 148f, 150–1, 279–81, 375–6,
  384–6, 388; criminal-legal system,
  209, 283, 285, 287–8, 295, 297–8,
  330; cultural safety in health
  care, 71–2, 183–4, 386–8, 450–1;
  discrimination, 38–40, 56, 61–2,
  64, 66t, 67–8, 71–2, 82–4, 111–112,
  385–6; divorce/separation issues,
  280–1; employment, 108, 136–7;
  health care inequity, 56, 66t, 155,
  182–5, 287, 384–6; intimate
  partner/family violence, 260;
  poverty, 150, 154–7, 280; SDOHs,
  61–2, 65–7, 136, 182–3, 385, 484;
  self-identification, 279; support

programs/benefits, 144, 148t, 156,
  184–5, 268t, 341t, 386; traditional
  beliefs and health care, 56–8,
  182–3, 450–1; wills and estates,
  428, 451–2
Indigenous rights legal framework/
  law, 32, 34, 37–40, 44, 83–4, 279–82
information sharing, issues, 22–5,
  258, 320t, 322–3, 383, 471t
informed consent, 22, 334, 457–8,
  460, 466
intellectual and developmental
  disabilities (IDD), individuals
  with, 454–67, 473–4; health care
  provider role, 467–70; SDMs,
  456–62, 465, 468, 470, 474;
  SDOHs, 466–7, 472t; supported
  decision-making, 455–62, 465–74
Interim Federal Health Program
  (IFHP), 145, 187, 197–9, 201t, 213,
  221–2, 224, 339t, 392, 394

Jomaa, D., 483–5
Jordan's Principle, 39, 66t, 144,
  148f, 385–6, 388; Jordan River
  Anderson, 144, 182, 385

Karlawish, J., 461
key life events/transitions, 15–17,
  147, 148t, 244
Kohn, N. A., 461

Largent, E., 461
legal aid clinics, community, 18, 20,
  41, 50–1, 86–8, 91, 170, 173, 208–9,
  211, 215, 373, 378, 384, 395–6, 414,
  480–2, 488–98t
legal information vs. legal advice,
  20–2
legal services (Canada), 17–19, 50–1,
  82, 86, 90, 172–3, 208–9, 310, 372–3,
  395, 480–1, 493–4t

letter/report writing, 25–6, 162,
166–8, 174, 472t; advocating
for patients, 91, 97, 218–19,
224, 293–5, 388, 391, 399–400,
501–2; criminal-legal system,
293–6, 298–301, 384; employment
related, 395–7, 400; to support
accommodation, 129–30, 158,
316–17, 378, 380–4, 399; to support
disability application, 158; to
support immigration application,
216–21, 347, 351, 393, 400
LGBTQ2S+ individuals/youth,
390–1; access to health care, 69–70,
136–7, 388–91; poverty, 150, 479

maanadamon, bibikadamon, 57, 60–2
marriage, cohabitation and
separation law, 239–40
medical colonialism, 37, 57, 60–2, 65–8,
72–3, 137, 155–6, 183, 385, 387, 450
migrant workers. *See* temporary
foreign workers
Mills, Aaron: *Revitalizing Anishinaabe
Inaakonigewin (Law)*, 59
mino bimaadiziwin (the good life), 57–8

National Inquiry into MMIWG,
63, 68–9
No One Is Illegal (NOII) report, 202,
205, 223

Office of the Children's Lawyer
(OCL), 254, 256–7
Ontario Disability Support Program
(ODSP), 162, 165t, 169–70, 248,
250, 342t, 349, 415, 434–5, 437

permanent residence status, 151t,
153–4, 188–91, 194–6, 345–7, 393;
access to education, 203–7; access to
health care, 201t; access to income
support and housing, 208–10;
criminal-legal system, 195–6, 204t,
212t; personal safety, 204t
Peterson, A., 461
poverty, 138–9; criminal-legal system,
283, 286, 293; debt load, 145, 147–48,
158–9, 173, 427; homelessness,
81, 93f, 98; immigration status,
145, 153–4, 157t, 159, 208–10,
213; income supports, 138–40,
142–50, 159–61; individuals with
disabilities, 149t, 150, 156–7; legal
issues, 6–7, 18, 51, 84–5, 87–8, 90;
racialized individuals, 81, 108–9,
150, 154–5, 479; screening for, 15,
140–2, 171, 401, 479
power of attorney, 374–5, 408, 411–19,
421–2, 439–40; for personal care
(POAPC), 411, 414, 418, 420–2,
432, 442; for property (POAP), 411,
413–14, 416, 419, 421–3, 426–7, 442
Prairie Sky (Levi Foy), 136–7
privately sponsored refugees (PSRs),
145, 189f, 191, 195, 198, 201t, 210t,
348
probate, 425–9, 431–2, 436–9
public guardian and trustee (PGT),
377, 414–16, 419, 423, 427, 438–9,
444–6
public health orders, 335–7, 353

racialized individuals, 5f, 63, 186,
202, 260, 285–7, 372; clinician bias,
166; criminal-legal system, 209,
285–6, 291; poverty, 81, 108–9, 150,
154–5, 479
racism, anti-Indigenous, 37, 56–7,
68–9, 156, 313–14, 385–7, 451;
health care, 60–2, 65, 68–9, 71–3,
155–6; laws, 62–5
referral, patient, 15–16, 22–6, 87,
90–1, 132, 171–3, 214, 280, 310, 388,

referral, patient (*continued*)
394, 481–2; referral letters, 25–6;
self-referral option, 24
refugee claimants, 145, 148f, 150, 153,
159, 188–9, 191–2, 195–6, 349–50;
access to education, 203–7; access
to health care, 197–9, 201t, 224,
338–9, 345, 392–4; access to income
support and housing, 208–10;
criminal-legal system, 212t; living
with HIV/AIDS, 345, 350–2;
medical documentation to support,
216–19; personal safety, 204t, 214
rent geared to income (RGI), 84, 87t,
89–90, 94
residential school system, Indian,
61–2, 64–5, 151, 452
Rizzolo, M. C., 467

Scholten, M., 461
Seven Sacred Laws, 58–9
Sinclair, Brian, 68, 182
Sixties and Millennial Scoop(s), 61, 64,
151, 280
social determinants of health
(SDOHs), 4–6, 20, 26, 398, 479–82,
484; children, 372–4; criminal-legal
system involved individuals,
283, 286; definitions, 4, 104;
housing/homelessness, 80–2,
97; IDD individuals, 466–7, 472t;
immigration status, 186, 188, 196–
8, 209, 214; Indigenous Peoples/
Indigenous people, 61–2, 65–7, 136,
182–3, 385, 484; individuals living
with HIV/AIDS, 310–12; work/
employment status, 104–6, 209
social housing, 17, 83f, 84t, 87f,
89–90, 94, 481
solidarity model of health care
relationships, 455–8, 461–2, 467–8,
473–4

Spassiani, N. A., 467
Stark, Kekkek Jason: *Anishinabe
Inaakonigewin*, 58
structural determinants of health,
214, 283, 286
substitute decision-makers (SDMs),
255, 374–7, 409–11, 415–16, 418,
420–1, 439; IDD individuals,
456–62, 468, 474
supported decision-making, 455–62,
465–74

tax credits, 142–5, 148t 159;
Disability Tax Credit, 143, 146,
148t, 150, 152, 163t, 165t, 397
tax-related benefits, child, 397–8
temporary foreign workers,
122–3, 153, 188–9, 191–4; access
to education, 206–7t; access
to health care, 201t; access to
income support, 210t; criminal-
legal system, 212t; health care
provider role, 131–2; Home
Child Care program, 192; Home
Support Worker program, 192;
personal safety, 204t, 214; Seasonal
Agricultural Worker Program
(SAWP), 191–3
Tobin-Tyler, E., 483–5
*Tools for the Primary Care of Adults
with Intellectual and Developmental
Disabilities*, 467–70
trauma-informed care, 72, 202–3,
213, 452, 464, 472t, 485
traumatic brain injury (TBI),
283–5; criminal-legal system,
283, 285–6, 288–90, 292, 297, 300,
302; definition, 285; SDOHs, 283;
symptoms of, 283, 286
Truth and Reconciliation
Commission report, 68,
280–1, 288

Ubel, P.A., 461
undocumented immigrants, 122,
    187–90, 192, 203–5, 208, 212t
undue hardship, 45–8, 113, 125,
    314–15, 380
uninsured patients, 197, 199–201

violence-informed care. *See* trauma-
    informed care
violence, intimate partner/family,
    90, 142, 174, 202–3, 221, 243–4, 252,
    254, 259–68; duty to warn/report,
    243, 261–2; health care provider
    role, 266; relocation, 264–5;
    resources, 267–8t; restraining
    orders, 263; safety plans, 243, 252,
    262, 266, 268t, 337

Walia, Harsha: *Border and Rule*, 186, 191
Welfare in Canada report, 147–9
wills, 414, 423–7, 429–38. *See also*
    executors/estate trustees; probate;
    alternatives to, 428–9; formal,
    423–6, 432, 439, 443; holographic,
    424–5, 431–2, 435–6, 438–9, 443;
    intestacy, 423, 427, 429–35, 437–9

work/employment status, 105–6;
    constructive dismissal, 124–5;
    precarious work, 105–6, 108,
    119–20, 122, 129, 155, 166, 394;
    SDOHs, 104–6, 209; termination,
    123–4
worker (mis)classification, 107,
    119–20, 127–8
workplace law, 107; Employment
    Insurance (EI), 107, 115,
    119–20, 127–8, 148, 165t, 395–6;
    employment standards legislation,
    107–11, 123–4, 127, 192, 395;
    human rights legislation, 105, 107,
    109–15, 125–7, 129, 352–3; migrant
    workers, 122–3; occupational
    health and safety legislation,
    107, 113–120, 126; worker's
    compensation, 107, 117t, 120–2,
    126–8
World Health Organization, 81,
    372; Commission on the Social
    Determinants of Health, 5;
    Housing and Health Guidelines, 81t

Zuckerman, Barry, 19